KT-500-047

# Becoming a Nurse in the 21st Century

LIBRARY & INFORMATION SERVICE
HARROGATE DISTRICT HOSPITAL
Tel: 01423 553104

This book is due for return on or before the last date shown below.

19 FEB 2008
CANCELLED
CANCELLED
25 JUN 2008
26 AUG 2008
CANCELLED
CANCELLED
- 6 MAY 2009
CANCELLED
13 APR 2010
17 AUG 2010
CANCELLED
CANCELLED
- 4 JAN 2012
- 8 JUN 2023

610.73 PEA

# Becoming a Nurse in the 21st Century

**IAN PEATE**

*With a Contribution by Dr Maxine Offredy*

John Wiley & Sons, Ltd

Copyright © 2006 John Wiley & Sons Ltd
The Atrium, Southern Gate, Chichester,
West Sussex PO19 8SQ, England
Telephone (+44) 1243 779777

Email (for orders and customer service enquiries): cs-books@wiley.co.uk
Visit our Home Page on www.wiley.com

Reprinted February 2007

All Rights Reserved. No part of this publication may be reproduced, stored in a retrieval system or transmitted in any form or by any means, electronic, mechanical, photocopying, recording, scanning or otherwise, except under the terms of the Copyright, Designs and Patents Act 1988 or under the terms of a licence issued by the Copyright Licensing Agency Ltd, 90 Tottenham Court Road, London W1T 4LP, UK, without the permission in writing of the Publisher. Requests to the Publisher should be addressed to the Permissions Department, John Wiley & Sons Ltd, The Atrium, Southern Gate, Chichester, West Sussex PO19 8SQ, England, or emailed to permreq@wiley.co.uk, or faxed to (+44) 1243 770620.

Designations used by companies to distinguish their products are often claimed as trademarks. All brand names and product names used in this book are trade names, service marks, trademarks or registered trademarks of their respective owners. The Publisher is not associated with any product or vendor mentioned in this book.

This publication is designed to provide accurate and authoritative information in regard to the subject matter covered. It is sold on the understanding that the Publisher is not engaged in rendering professional services. If professional advice or other expert assistance is required, the services of a competent professional should be sought.

***Other Wiley Editorial Offices***
John Wiley & Sons Inc., 111 River Street, Hoboken, NJ 07030, USA
Jossey-Bass, 989 Market Street, San Francisco, CA 94103-1741, USA
Wiley-VCH Verlag GmbH, Boschstr. 12, D-69469 Weinheim, Germany
John Wiley & Sons Australia Ltd, 42 McDougall Street, Milton, Queensland 4064, Australia
John Wiley & Sons (Asia) Pte Ltd, 2 Clementi Loop #02-01, Jin Xing Distripark, Singapore 129809
John Wiley & Sons Canada Ltd, 6045 Freemont Blvd, Mississauga, ONT L5R

Wiley also publishes its books in a variety of electronic formats. Some content that appears in print may not be available in electronic books.

***Library of Congress Cataloging-in-Publication Data***

Peate, Ian.
Becoming a nurse in the 21st century / Ian Peate ; with a contribution by Maxine Offredy.
p. ; cm.
Includes index.
ISBN-13: 978-0-470-02729-5 (alk. paper)
ISBN-10: 0-470-02729-0 (alk. paper)
1. Nursing. 2. Nurses. I. Title.
[DNLM: 1. Nursing Care. 2. Nurse's Role. 3. Nursing. WY 100 P363b 2006]
RT41.P43 2006
610.73–dc22

2006001919

***A catalogue record for this book is available from the British Library***

ISBN -13 978-0-470-02729-5 (PB)

Typeset by SNP Best-set Typesetters Ltd, Hong Kong
Printed and bound in Great Britain by TJ International Ltd, Padstow, Cornwall

This book is printed on acid-free paper responsibly manufactured from sustainable forestry in which at least two trees are planted for each one used for paper production.

I would like to dedicate this text to all student nurses past, present and future – go for it and make a difference.

# Contents

# Author

**Ian Peate EN(G) RGN DipN (Lond) RNT BEd (Hons) MA (Lond) LLM**
Associate Head of School
School of Nursing and Midwifery
Faculty of Health and Human Sciences
University of Hertfordshire

With a contribution from:
**Maxine Offredy PhD RN**
Senior Lecturer
School of Nursing and Midwifery
Faculty of Health and Human Sciences
University of Hertfordshire

# Acknowledgements

I would like to thank and acknowledge the help and support offered to me by Jussi Lahtinen. Without his support and understanding all of my endeavours would never have come to fruition. To Frances Cohen, who has been a constant source of motivation to me for many years, as well as an excellent proofreader and cake maker. To Lyn Cochrane and her outstanding ability to create graphs and figures.

# Introduction

This text is primarily intended for nursing students, health-care assistants, those undertaking SNVQ/NVQ level of study, or anyone who intends to undertake a programme of study leading to registration as a nurse. Throughout the text the terms 'nurse', 'student' and 'nursing' are used. These terms and the principles applied to this book can be transferred to a number of health-care workers at various levels and in various settings, in order to develop their skills for caring.

## A NOTE ON TERMINOLOGY

The term 'patient' has been used throughout this text and refers to all groups and individuals who have direct or indirect contact with all health-care workers and, in particular, registered nurses, midwives or health visitors. 'Patient' is the expression that is used commonly within the NHS. While it is acknowledged that not everyone approves of the passive concept associated with this term, it is used in this text in the knowledge that the term is widely understood. Other terms could have been used, for example service user, client or consumer, but for the sake of brevity patient will be used.

The term 'carer' is also used in this text. The term can be used to describe those who look after family, partners or friends in need of help because they are ill, frail or have a disability. Carer can mean health-care provider; that is, care workers or those who provide care that is unpaid. It is estimated that there are over six million unpaid carers in the UK (Carers UK, 2005). It must be noted and acknowledged that unpaid carers can also be young people aged under 18.

The phrase 'specialist community public health nurse' will also be used in the text. The NMC decided to establish a part of the register for specialist community public health nurses, as it felt the practice undertaken by these nurses has distinct characteristics that require public protection (NMC, 2004c).

## THE NURSING AND MIDWIFERY COUNCIL (NMC) AND QUALITY ASSURANCE (EDUCATION)

The programme of study you have embarked on, or are going to embark on, must meet certain standards. There are internal standards within your educational institution, for example your own university's policies and procedures relating to quality assurance and external influences. The NMC and the Quality Assurance Agency (QAA) standards must be satisfied before a programme of study can be validated and deemed fit for purpose (Quality Assurance Agency for Higher Education, 2000). Other external factors that must be given due consideration are the orders provided in the guise of European Directives. Two European Directives, 77/453/EEC and 89/595/EEC, and their implications are discussed.

It is the responsibility of the NMC to set and monitor standards in training (Nursing and Midwifery Order 2001). The NMC has produced a framework for quality assurance of education programmes (NMC, 2005). The framework relates to all programmes that lead to registration or to the recording of a qualification on the professional register.

The Nursing and Midwifery Order 2001 provides the NMC with powers in relation to quality assurance and, as a result of this, the production of a framework by which those education providers (for example universities) who offer, or intend to offer, NMC-approved programmes leading to registration or recording on the register have to abide. There are many provisions in place in the UK that ensure the quality of education programmes. In Northern Ireland, Scotland and Wales, agents are appointed by the NMC. They carry out quality assurance services on behalf of the NMC. In England, visitors are the preferred option. They are registrants from practice and education who undertake the approval and annual monitoring activities on behalf of the NMC.

The NMC has to be satisfied that its standards for granting a person with a licence to practice are being met as required and in association with the law. It does this by setting standards to be achieved in order to maintain public confidence, as well as protecting them. By appointing agents and visitors it can be satisfied that it is represented during the quality assurance process in relation to the approval, reapproval and annual monitoring activities associated with programmes of study.

Each programme of study (for pre-registration nursing) must demonstrate in an explicit and robust manner that it has included the extant rules and standards of the NMC so that those who complete a recognised programme of study are eligible for registration. The Standards of Proficiency for Pre-registration Nursing Education (NMC, 2004a) are examples of some standards that must be achieved prior to registration. See Table 1 for a summary of the standards for pre-registration nursing.

## BECOMING A PROFICIENT NURSE

Those who wish to study to become a nurse, register with the NMC and afterwards practise as a nurse must undertake a three-year (or equivalent) pro-

**Table 1** Summary of some of the standards for pre-registration nursing (NMC, 2004a)

| | |
|---|---|
| Standard 1 | Age of entry |
| Standard 2 | General entry requirements |
| Standard 3 | Accreditation of prior (experiential) learning |
| Standard 4 | Admission with advanced standing |
| Standard 5 | Transfer with accreditation of prior (experiential) learning |
| Standard 6 | Structure and nature of educational programmes |
| Standard 7 | First-level nurses – nursing standards of education to achieve NMC standards of proficiency |
| Standard 8 | Second-level nurses – nursing standards of proficiency |

*Source*: NMC, 2004a.

gramme of study. The programme of study must by law comprise 2300 hours of practice and another 2300 hours of theory.

The title 'registered nurse' is a protected title in law. This means it can only be used by a person who is registered with the NMC and their name must appear on the national register. There are three parts to the professional register:

- nurses
- midwives
- specialist community public health

Four distinct disciplines, each specialising in its own field of practice, are associated with nursing:

- learning disabilities nursing
- adult nursing
- children's nursing
- mental health nursing

Regardless of the branch the student has chosen, all students undertake a 12-month common foundation programme (CFP). When the student has successfully completed the CFP, having met all of the proficiencies dictated by the NMC, this allows the student to undertake the branch programme. The branch programme is two years in duration – this then becomes a branch-specific programme.

The student who wishes to undertake nurse education must meet the NMC's requirements for age of entry. Those entering a programme of pre-registration nursing education must be no less than 17 years and six months of age on the first day of the commencement of the programme. However, in certain exceptional circumstances and related to specific programmes, the NMC may agree to an earlier age, but this will never be less than 17 years.

As well as having to satisfy the NMC's age requirements, general entry requirements must also be satisfied. Educational requirements are set by each educational institution, and there must also be evidence of literacy and numeracy. How these requirements are set is the prerogative of the educational institution; however, the NMC must agree and permit these requirements. Those wishing to practise in Wales must be able to demonstrate proficiency in the use of the Welsh language where this is required. On entry all applicants must demonstrate, on an ongoing basis and on completion of their programme, that they have good health and good character sufficient for safe and effective practice. It is the responsibility of educational institutions to have processes in place to ensure assessment of good health and good character. Any convictions or cautions related to criminal offences that the applicant may hold must be declared. There are several ways in which this can be achieved, for example self-disclosure and/or criminal record checks conducted by accredited organisations.

Completion of the programme and successful achievement of the proficiencies means that the student will graduate with both a professional qualification – Registered Nurse (RN) – and an academic one. The academic qualification may be at diploma or degree level. The NMC requires a self-declaration of good health and good character from all those entering the register. The good character and good health declaration is made on an approved form provided by the NMC. This must also be supported by the registered nurse whose name has been notified to the NMC as being responsible for directing the educational programme at the university, or his/her designated registered nurse substitute.

Once registered with the NMC the nurse becomes accountable for his/her actions or omissions. He/she is subject to the tenets enshrined in the Code of Professional Conduct (NMC, 2004b). Important issues that must be legally undertaken, such as participating in continuing professional development and the maintenance of a personal professional portfolio, are addressed. This text provides you with insight into how to become a proficient nurse. All of the NMC proficiencies cited in standard seven (NMC, 2004a) are considered.

## THE PROFICIENCIES

Standard seven of the NMC's Standards of Proficiency for Pre-registration Nursing Education (NMC, 2004a) contains the nursing standards required to be achieved to demonstrate proficiency to the NMC. There are four domains:

- professional and ethical practice
- care delivery
- care management
- professional development

**Table 2** The four domains and the subsequent sub-sections

| *Domain I* Professional and Ethical Practice | *Domain II* Care Delivery |
|---|---|
| 1. Professional Practice<br>2. Ethical and legal issues<br>3. Diversity and culture | 1. Therapeutic relationships<br>2. Health promotion<br>3. Assessment of needs<br>4. Partnerships<br>5. Evidence-based practice<br>6. Sociocultural issues<br>7. Evaluating care<br>8. Clinical decision making |
| *Domain III* Care Management | *Domain IV* Personal and Professional Development |
| 1. Quality care<br>2. Inter-professional working`<br>3. Competence, accountability and delegation<br>4. Key skills | 1. Continuing professional development<br>2. Teaching, learning and supervising |

*Source*: Adapted from NMC, 2004a.

## THE CHAPTERS

Each chapter of this text addresses the content of each of the domains as prescribed by the NMC (NMC, 2004a). The domains and the subsections provide a framework for this text. See Table 2 for an outline of the domains and the subsequent subsections.

## THINK POINTS

Each chapter provides the reader with think points. These are included to help encourage and motivate you, as well as for you to assess your learning and progress. They are recognised by this symbol:

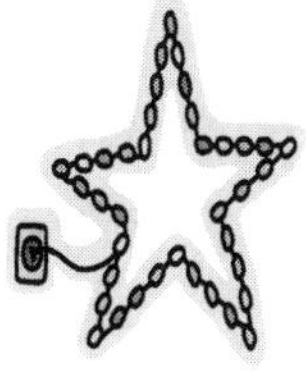

Most of the think points provide you with answers or suggestion for responses. You are encouraged to delve deeper and to seek other sources, human and material, to help with your responses.

The aim of this text is to encourage and motivate you and to instil in you the desire, confidence and competence to become a registered nurse. To become a member of the nursing profession bestows on you many demands, and the key demand is the desire to care with compassion and understanding.

## REFERENCES

Carers UK (2005) *A Manifesto for Carers.* Carers UK. London.

Nursing and Midwifery Council (2004a) *The Standards of Proficiency for Pre-registration Nursing Education*. NMC. London.

Nursing and Midwifery Council (2004b) *The NMC Code of Professional Conduct: Standards for Conduct, Performance and Ethics*. NMC. London.

Nursing and Midwifery Council (2004c) *Standards of Proficiency for Specialist Community Public Health Nurses*. NMC. London.

Nursing and Midwifery Council (2005) *QA Factsheet A/2005UK*. NMC. London.

Quality Assurance Agency for Higher Education (2000) *Code of Practice for the Assurance of Academic Quality and Standards in Higher Education*. QAA. Gloucester.

# I Professional and Ethical Practice

# 1 Professional Practice

Nursing is both an art and a science. It is associated with caring and helping. One aspect of the nurse's role is to help the patient achieve or carry out those activities of living they are incapable of doing for themselves. There are many facets associated with the role and function of the nurse. It is a fluid and dynamic entity and this makes it difficult to define.

There are several definitions of nursing. One is that of Henderson, which has been used since the 1960s:

> *The unique function of the nurse is to assist the individual, sick or well, in performance of those activities contributing to health or its recovery (or to a peaceful death) that he would perform unaided if he had the necessary strength, will or knowledge and to do this in such a way as to help him gain independence as rapidly as possible.* (Henderson, 1966)

This definition is succinct and to the point. It attempts to encompass and encapsulate many of the roles the nurse performs, such as carer and health educator. Such a definition, although not exclusively, could be seen as the nature of nursing. A more recent definition provided by the Royal College of Nursing (RCN) is:

> *The use of clinical judgment in the provision of care to enable people to improve, maintain, or recover health, to cope with health problems, and to achieve the best possible quality of life, whatever their disease or disability until death.* (RCN, 2003)

This chapter is concerned with professional nursing practice. An overview is provided of the development of nursing from what was an unstructured, *ad hoc* approach to caring to what has become a regulated profession. The student nurse and unqualified practitioners are not subjected to the rigours of professional regulation. However, when you successfully complete your programme of study leading to registration, you will be subject to professional accountability and all that it entails. It is expected that the student nurse commits him/herself to the values of the profession and that he/she accepts and internalises the code of conduct as part of the process leading to registration. The code of professional conduct, performance and ethics will be discussed in detail, with emphasis on commitment to the principle that the primary purpose of the registered nurse is to protect and serve society.

## A BRIEF OVERVIEW OF THE HISTORY OF NURSING IN THE UNITED KINGDOM

This brief overview of how the practice of nursing has evolved over the years outlines some key stages in the development of the nursing profession from a British perspective. It must be remembered, however, that the evolution of nursing in the UK did not occur in a vacuum. There are several other international factors that have also helped to focus and shape where we are today and where we may be going tomorrow.

In order to understand contemporary nursing it is important to have an understanding of where nursing has come from, how nursing has emerged and how it continues to evolve (Craig and Daniels, 2004). Having an understanding of the way nursing has evolved and developed over the years may help you to appreciate:

- Why nursing is regarded as a profession in its own right.
- How by becoming empowered nurses are in a position to enable others to do things for themselves.
- That nurses have become autonomous practitioners.
- How nurses are called to account for their actions and omissions.

This aspect of the chapter makes use of a 'time line' in order to frame the discussion regarding the historical overview. A time line provides you with important dates and events that have occurred over the years and that have had an influence on the evolution of the nursing profession. The discussion centres on the significant events and key characters that have influenced the development of nursing over the ages.

### THE PREHISTORIC ERA

The practice of nursing predates history, according to Craig and Daniels (2004). Bullough and Bullough (1979) note that those who lived in the prehistoric period suffered similar conditions to those experienced by society today. Tribes in those early years took part in caring for their sick and wounded. Archaeologists have retrieved human remains that demonstrate that fractured limbs have been healed, suggesting therefore that some form of care provision occurred. Healers or shamans used various potions and magical concoctions to heal the sick. Those responsible for feeding and cleaning the sick were predominantly females.

The Bible makes reference to nurses and midwives, for example *Genesis* 35 and *Exodus* 1. In *Exodus* 2 there is evidence to suggest that nurses were paid for their services. *Numbers* 11 refers to males who undertook the caring role.

## THE ANCIENT GREEKS

In ancient Greece temples were erected to honour the goddess Hygeia, the goddess of health. Care at the temples was related to bathing and this activity was overseen by priestesses, who were not nurses. The foundation of modern medicine was laid down by Hippocrates during this period. Navel cutters – known as *omphalotomai* – were also practising at this time.

## THE ROMAN EMPIRE

The first hospitals were established in the Byzantine Empire, which was the first part of the Roman Empire. As the Roman Empire expanded hospitals were erected. It was Fabiola, a wealthy Roman, who was responsible for the introduction of hospitals in the West; she devoted her life to the sick and made nursing the sick and poor fashionable in Roman society. The primary carers in these hospitals were men, who were called *contubernails*. After the Roman invasion in approximately 2AD slave girls were known to assist Roman physicians. *Valetudinariums* – civilian hospitals – were kept clean and aired by bailiffs' wives, who would also watch over the sick.

## THE MIDDLE AGES

Throughout the middle ages military, religious and lay orders of men provided most of the health care. Kalisch and Kalisch (2003) note that some of these orders of men included the Knights Hospitalers, the Order of the Holy Sprit and Teutonic Knights. While these men provided care, charlatans and quacks provided treatment for money. The standard of care provided by the latter people often did more harm than good.

Several hospitals were opened during this period, for example St Thomas's, St Bartholomew's and Bethlem. Care provision that had been provided by nuns was now provided by local women, whose efforts were overseen by matrons. Their duties centred on domestic chores.

## THE ENLIGHTENMENT

The core period of the Enlightenment was the second half of the eighteenth century. Scientific endeavour flourished during the Enlightenment and philanthropists provided the means to open charity hospitals around the UK. In London for example, the London, Middlesex and Guy's hospitals provided care to the poor who were ill. These hospitals employed nurses who may have been paid or unpaid. These nurses again predominantly carried out domestic duties. Pay was low and it was not unusual for nurses to drink alcohol and take money from patients in order to pay for their alcohol. Nurses at this time were slovenly and lazy and reflected characters such as Sairey Gamp and Betsy Prig, caricatures devised by Charles Dickens. Alms houses depended on women to clean floors, make beds and bathe the poor. There were no standards for nurses to work towards.

Medical schools began to emerge as medical knowledge grew. The Royal College of Surgeons was formed in 1800 and at this time doctors were required to carry out some aspects of their training in hospitals.

## FLORENCE NIGHTINGALE

The founder of modern nursing was born in Italy in 1820 and died aged 90 in 1910. When she was 25 years old she told her parents she wanted to become a nurse. Her parents were totally opposed to the idea, as nursing was associated with working-class women and had historical links to domestic service and vocational work.

In March 1853, Russia invaded Turkey and Britain, concerned about the growing power of Russia, went to Turkey's aid. This conflict occurred in and around Scutari and became known as the Crimean War. Soon after British soldiers arrived in Turkey, they began to fall ill with malaria and cholera. Florence Nightingale volunteered her services to the war effort and was given permission to take a group of nurses to a hospital in Scutari based several miles from the front.

Mary Seacole, a Jamaican woman with much expertise in dealing with and caring for those with cholera, arrived in Scutari to offer her services to Nightingale, but these were refused. Undeterred, Seacole set up her own services and provided these to the British and Russian soldiers, often at the battle front.

In 1856 Florence Nightingale returned to England as a national heroine. She set about reforming conditions in British hospitals (in the first instance this was confined to military hospitals). She published two books, *Notes on Hospital* (1859) and *Notes on Nursing* (1859). Nightingale was able to raise funds to improve the quality of nursing. In 1860, she used these funds to found the Nightingale School and Home for Nurses at St Thomas's Hospital. She also became involved in the training of nurses for employment in the workhouses.

Nightingale acknowledged the influence of the environment on health. She suggested the environment should be one that promotes health and she campaigned for wards to be clean, well ventilated and well lit. She believed:

- There should be a theoretical basis for nursing practice.
- Nurses should be formally educated.
- A systematic approach to the assessment of patients should be developed.
- An individual approach to care provision based on individual patient needs was required.
- Patient confidentiality needed to be maintained.

Nightingale, together with the philanthropist William Rathbone, set up the first district nursing service in 1861. Queen Victoria gave her support to this venture and district nurses became Queen's Nurses. Caring for the well person was a concept Nightingale wanted to see developed, and in the late 1800s her thoughts came to fruition when courses were provided to teach women to develop an insight into sanitation in homes. These women, who had a duty to care for the health of adults, children and pregnant women (pre- and antenatal), could be seen as the first health visitors. In 1873 Nightingale wrote, 'Nursing is most truly said to be a high calling, an honourable calling.' She died in London in 1910.

## TOWARDS REGISTRATION

Throughout the 1890s pressure grew for the registration of nurses. In 1887, Ethel Bedford-Fenwick formed the British Nurses' Association, which sought to provide for the registration of British nurses based on the same terms as physicians and surgeons, as evidence of their having received systematic training. Bedford-Fenwick was a staunch supporter of professional regulation. Up until this time nurses remained relatively free from external regulation. In 1902, the Midwives Registration Act established the state regulation of midwives; this Act came about as a response to the concerns about the rising numbers of deaths of women in childbirth (Davies and Beach, 2000). A House of Commons Select Committee was established in 1904 to consider the registration of nurses.

The First World War (1914–18) provided the final stimulus to the creation of nursing regulation, partly because of the contributions made by nurses to the war effort. The College of Nursing (this later became the Royal College of Nursing in 1928) was established in 1916.

Eventually in 1919 the Nurses Registration Acts were passed for England, Wales, Scotland and Ireland. The General Nursing Council (GNC) for England, Wales, Scotland and Ireland and other bodies were established as a result of these Acts. The Councils were established in 1921 with clearly agreed duties and responsibilities for the training, examination and registration of nurses and the approval of training schools for the purpose of maintaining a Register of Nurses for England and Wales, Scotland and Ireland. The GNC had powers to undertake disciplinary procedures and remove the name of a nurse from the register if they were deemed to have committed an act of misconduct or 'otherwise' – conduct unbecoming of a nurse. The Register of Nurses was first published in 1922. The GNC and the other bodies survived intact until changes were made in 1979. These resulted in the creation of the United Kingdom Central Council (UKCC) and the four National Boards.

## THE ESTABLISHMENT OF A NATIONAL HEALTH SERVICE

The National Health Service was established on 5 July 1948. The 1949 Nurses Act allowed that the constitution of the GNC be amended; the general and male nurse parts of the Register were amalgamated.

## THE BRIGGS COMMITTEE

The Briggs Committee, a working group, was set up in 1976 to review the training of nurses and midwives. The work of this committee led to the Nurses, Midwives and Health Visitors Act 1979, which dissolved the GNC. The GNC was replaced by the UKCC for Nursing, Midwifery and Health Visiting, with four National Boards for England, Wales, Scotland and Northern Ireland.

## PROJECT 2000

Much of the work of Briggs in the 1970s paved the way for reform in relation to nurse education. In 1984 the UKCC set up a project to consider reforming nurse education, which became known as Project 2000. The UKCC's report, published in 1986 (UKCC, 1986), provided the Council's strategy. The strategy was implemented by the mid-1990s.

## THE PEACH REPORT

The Peach Report was published in response to the UKCC's desire to conduct a detailed examination of the effectiveness of pre-registration nurse education and determine if students were 'fit for practice' and 'fit for purpose' (UKCC, 1999). The report outlined several recommendations, for example:

- A reduction in the common foundation programme from 18 months to one year.
- An increase in the branch programme from 18 months to two years.
- To ensure that students experienced at least three months' supervised clinical practice towards the end of the programme.
- Longer student placements.
- The introduction of practice skills and clinical placements early on in the common foundation programme.
- Greater flexibility in entry to nursing programmes.

## CONTEMPORARY NURSING PRACTICE

Contemporary nursing practice is based on a sound, up-to-date knowledge base, with nurses applying the appropriate skills and attitudes when delivering nursing care. It was Nightingale who suggested that nursing was subordinate to medicine (Holton, 1984). However, this notion of the nurse as handmaiden to the doctor is changing and the various roles and functions undertaken by the nurse are testimony to this.

After the number of nurses became substantial and the essential nature of nursing was established in the UK, the need to regulate the practice of nursing under law grew evident. These laws are aimed at the protection of the public.

## NURSING AS A PROFESSION

### PROFESSIONALISM

The term 'professional' is used in many aspects of our society, and often its meaning is taken for granted. When the term professional is used it refers to a process that contains some gravitas, in which a group or individual works in a knowledgeable manner and with understanding. The word professional has other meanings in other contexts. A profession is defined and measured by using several sets of criteria and characteristics.

Etzioni (1969) considered occupations such as nursing, teaching and social work as semi-professional. Nursing, he suggested, was a semi-professional occupation due to the inadequate length of time for training and because of the lack of autonomy and responsibility for decision making. The ultimate justification of a professional act, according to Etzioni (1969), is that to the professional's knowledge, it is the best act. Burnard and Chapman (2003) state that there must be a high level of accountability and autonomy in order for an act to be professionally justified.

Salvage (2003) states that the nursing profession has often held an uncomfortable social space, as it tends to lie between being a 'true' and 'semi'-profession. She described the 'true' professions as male dominated, elitist and powerful, for example medicine and law, in contrast to proletarian occupations such as domestic work, health-care assistance and unpaid women's work in the home. However, new professions are emerging and they fit the changing circumstances in which society operates today (Salvage, 2002).

What makes a profession? Many people claim to belong to professions or they say they are professional. Can you make a list of professionals?

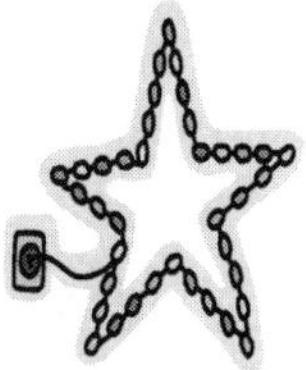

In your list you might have included some of the more obvious professions:

- clergy
- doctors
- solicitors
- barristers
- physiotherapists

But what about others who also profess to be professionals:

- footballers
- plumbers

**Table 1.1** Pyne's characteristics associated with a profession

| |
|---|
| • Its practice is based on a recognised body of learning. |
| • It establishes an independent body for the collective pursuit of aims and objectives related to these criteria. |
| • Admission to corporate membership is based on strict standards of competence attested by examination and assessed experience. |
| • It recognises that its practice must be for the benefit of the public, as well as that of the practitioners. |
| • It recognises its responsibility to advance and extend the body of learning on which it is based. |
| • It recognises its responsibility to concern itself with facilities, methods and provision for educating and training future entrants and for enhancing the knowledge of present practitioners. |
| • It recognises the need for members to conform to high standards of ethics and professional conduct set out in a published code with appropriate disciplinary procedures. |

*Source*: Pyne, 1998.

- teachers
- engineers
- architects
- diamond cutters
- carpenters

The terms professions and professional are dynamic and fluid, changing as time passes and as technology changes. Burnard and Chapman (2003) state that these days to be professional the occupation requires a degree of skill and/or specialist knowledge. Basford (2003) adds that that knowledge is gained through education.

The characteristics of a profession have changed over time. Pyne (1998) compiled a list of characteristics and these are presented in Table 1.1.

## NEW NURSING – NEW WAYS OF WORKING

The role and function of the nurse have changed and developed over the years. The first part of this chapter has demonstrated some of the transformations and the influences causing them. In order to meet the health-care needs of the nation, political and professional pressures have transformed the role of the nurse and other health-care professionals involved in the provision of health care, with the aim of developing their full potential. As a result of this, nursing has seen the creation of a number of new clinical roles, for example:

- family health nurses
- nurse endoscopists
- consultant nurses

- nutritional support nurses
- nurse prescribers

Cameron and Masterson (2003) and the NHS Modernisation Agency (2005) consider the role of the nurse at night and how the traditional role of night sister has changed considerably to become night nurse practitioner. The Hospital at Night Project (NHS Modernisation Agency, 2005) aims to redefine how medical cover is provided in hospitals during the night. The project requires a move from cover requirements defined by professional demarcation, to cover defined by competency; the night nurse practitioner is a competent practitioner. The project advocates that other staff, for example nurses, are taking on some of the work traditionally carried out by junior doctors.

Many of the new nursing roles listed above may not exist today if the nursing profession had not over the years sought to advance its professional practice and status. The key issues of clinical competence, clinical decision making and being aware of boundaries and limitations are central to the safety of the patient and the success of such roles.

Hood and Leddy (2003) suggest that the professional nurse has three intellectual properties:

1. A body of knowledge on which professional practice is based.
2. A specialised education to transmit this body of knowledge to others.
3. The ability to use the knowledge in critical and creative thinking.

## BODY OF KNOWLEDGE

Much of the work nurses carry out on a daily basis has a theoretical underpinning. However, nurses do not always articulate this theoretical basis from which they practise (Burnard and Chapman, 2003). Often the theories cited in Table 1.2, emerging from various disciplines and scientific perspectives, allow nurses to practise effectively and, above all, safely.

The examples cited in the table are theoretical examples reflecting a scientific perspective. Limiting caring to the scientific approach and neglecting experience could be detrimental to your patient's care. Professional nursing practice is also based on a body of knowledge that is derived from experience – expertise. The combination of knowledge related to science and experience has the potential to enable the nurse to make reliable clinical decisions (clinical decision making is discussed further in Chapter 11).

The use of expertise should never be undervalued however; having experience may not always be enough to help provide safe care. Nurses derive knowledge through:

- intuition
- tradition
- experience

**Table 1.2** Theoretical perspectives gained from other disciplines that are used when caring for the patient

| Theory basis | Example |
|---|---|
| Microbiology | Practices associated with aseptic nursing and infection control |
| Thermodynamics | Performance of duties associated with temperature taking and the care of the patient with a pyrexia or those who may have hypothermia |
| Psychology | The application of psychological theories when caring for a bereaved relative, or the importance of play in hospitalised children |
| Pharmacokinetics | Understanding drug therapies and how drugs are metabolised in the body |
| Physiology | Applying physiological theories to interpretation of nursing observations, for example physiological changes that occur if the patient has diabetes mellitus or a head injury |
| Sociology | Helping you to understand the patient's needs from a sociological perspective, for example understanding and addressing health inequalities |

*Source*: Adapted from Burnard and Chapman, 2003 and Hood and Leddy, 2003.

Benner (1984) discusses the subject of intuition as a form of expertise. Intuition can be described as just knowing and the just knowing comes from the individual. It is internal and can occur independently of experience or reason. It can become validated by experience and interaction with other nurses.

Consider the patient scenario below and then list the knowledge bases needed to care effectively for this patient.

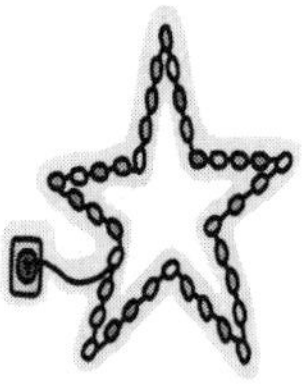

Mary Samonds, 86 years of age, is unconscious as a result of a head injury. She is totally dependent on the nursing staff for all her care. You are working with a registered nurse and you are going to provide care for Mary. She is incontinent of urine and faeces, so both you and the staff nurse are going to attend to her hygiene needs. Mary's husband is outside waiting for you to finish.

**Table 1.3** The various bodies of knowledge drawn on to care for a patient

| Bodies of knowledge drawn on |
|---|
| Expertise |
| Psychology |
| Sociology |
| Microbiology |
| Thermodynamics |
| Physiology |
| Pharmacokinetics |

In order for you to care effectively for Mary and to meet all of her needs, she will require much skilled care and you will need to draw on many bodies of knowledge to do this. There are many bodies of knowledge you could use and these will also include that important perspective – experience or expert practice. Table 1.3 lists some of the things you might have included.

## TRANSMITTING THE BODY OF KNOWLEDGE TO OTHERS

Transmitting the body of knowledge to others occurs at many levels. The educational programmes of study and the educational institutions where they take place are subject to statutory approval and scrutiny. This approval is through the NMC (see below). It is the members of the profession, therefore, who validate the programmes of study that will ultimately lead to registration. Registration conveys a message to the public that the nurse who is admitted to the register has reached and possesses a satisfactory level of competence (now called proficiency) along with a certain standard of behaviour – good character and good health.

## USING THAT BODY OF KNOWLEDGE IN CRITICAL AND CREATIVE THINKING

Nurses use their body of knowledge in order to provide the patient with care that has undergone critical scrutiny, or a systematic approach has been used to provide that care. Care becomes creative and innovative and provides nurses with new ways of thinking and addressing patient problems.

Advancing nursing practice ensures that nurses have the knowledge base and practical skills to provide specialist nursing care. Critical thinking allows nurses to see different approaches to clinical situations. Critical thinking occurs when nurses are faced with patients who have complex needs; the situation provides opportunities for nurses to develop and plan individual care.

PROFESSIONAL NURSING

The Hippocratic oath laid down the moral code of conduct for the practice of medicine and the underpinning principle of this code, as is the underpinning principle of any health-care code, is to treat the patient at all times as you would wish others to treat you.

Patients must be able to trust nurses with regards to their wellbeing. To justify that trust the nursing profession has a duty to maintain a good standard of practice and care, and to show respect for human life.

Professional nursing practice is not only judged by the recipient of care – the patient – but also by the profession itself. Professionals judge other professionals with regards to the quality and the appropriateness of care provided. There are many ways in which this judgement can occur, and one way is through the NMC. Deviation from the acceptable standards of practice may result in the nurse's name being removed from the professional register, ultimately resulting in the removal of the nurse's licence to practise.

## THE NURSING AND MIDWIFERY COUNCIL

In 1998 the government initiated a fundamental review of how the profession was regulated. The outcome of this review resulted in consultation with nurses and midwives regarding professional regulation and areas that needed to be addressed. Recommendations were suggested and acted on regarding self-professional regulation, regulatory mechanisms and procedural rules. The UKCC and the four boards were abolished; quality assurance elements were incorporated into the work of the NMC.

The Nursing and Midwifery Council (NMC) was set up by Parliament to ensure that nurses and midwives provide high standards of care to their patients. The Nursing and Midwifery Order 2001 (SI 2002/253) established the Council and it came into being on 1 April 2002.

Protection of the public is the key concern of the NMC. Its duties to society are to serve and protect, and this is done by:

- Maintaining a register listing all nurses and midwives.
- Setting standards and guidelines for nursing and midwifery education, practice and conduct.
- Providing advice for registrants on professional standards.
- Ensuring quality assurance related to nursing and midwifery education.
- Setting standards and providing guidance for local supervising authorities for midwives.
- Considering allegations of misconduct or unfitness to practise due to ill health.

**Table 1.4** The three parts of the professional register

| | |
|---|---|
| Sub-part 1 (for level 1 nurses) | Sub-part 2 (for level 2 nurses) |
| Midwives' part of the register | |
| Specialist community public health nurses' part of the register | |

## THE PROFESSIONAL REGISTER

The NMC maintains a register of around 650 000 qualified nurses, midwives and specialist community public health nurses (Dimond, 2005). The nurses', midwives' and specialist community public health nurses' names are held on a computer database. The information held includes personal details, educational qualifications and registration status. Personal details are never released by the NMC. All nurses, midwives and specialist community public health nurses who wish to practise in the UK must be on the NMC register.

The NMC's registration process enables nurses and midwives to be entered onto one or more parts of the register when they have completed an approved programme of study. The registration process begins from the day the student nurse commences a course, be it for initial registration or return to practice. The approved educational institute must ensure that accurate records of a student's progression throughout the course are maintained; this is often known as a transcript of training.

There are three parts of the professional register; see Table 1.4.

Admittance to the professional register provides the nurse with the privilege of performing certain activities with the public that might otherwise (outside of the professional relationship) be deemed unlawful. Members of the public have access to the professional register and can verify if a nurse is registered with the NMC.

## REGISTRATION – GOOD HEALTH AND GOOD CHARACTER

On completion of the approved programme of study, personal details of the applicant and the programme undertaken are transferred to the NMC. The approved educational institution is obliged to make a declaration of good health and good character in support of the applicant (see Appendix 1.1). All practitioners must demonstrate that their health and character are appropriate to allow them to register and stay on the register in order to practise. The good health and good character elements of getting onto and renewing an entry on the register are laid down in the legislation. The requirement of good character and good health was introduced by Parliament to enhance the protection of the public after a number of high-profile cases concerning the health and character of doctors and nurses (NMC, 2004b). The nurse must ensure that his/her good character and good health remain just that, 'good', throughout his/her period of time on the professional register. The applicant then pays a registration fee.

Having satisfied the criteria for admission to the professional register, for the nurse to remain on it (to remain on the 'live' register) he/she needs to abide by the tenets stated within the code of professional conduct. Furthermore, registration must be renewed on a three-yearly basis. Notification of practice must be made to the NMC and a declaration made that the nurse has met his/her post-registration education and practice (PREP) requirements for continuing professional development (NMC, 2004c). He/she must also provide the three-yearly fee. The issues of PREP and continuing professional development are considered in more detail in Chapter 16.

Each individual whose name is entered on the register is issued with a unique personal identification number (PIN) in card format and the date on which their registration expires. It must be noted that anyone who is newly qualified and who has not yet been registered is unable to practise as a registered nurse until their registration becomes effective. It is a criminal offence for anyone to falsely and deliberately represent themselves as a registered nurse. The newly qualified nurse should note that the entire registration process may take up to three weeks from the programme completion date (NMC, 2005).

## CONTEMPORARY NURSING

There are various aspects of care offered and provided by the National Health Service. These are often split between two areas of care:

- acute care
- chronic care

Care also occurs within the following health-care settings:

- primary
- secondary
- tertiary

### PRIMARY CARE SERVICES

Most care provision is carried out in the primary care sector; over 95 per cent of care is delivered in this sector. Care is delivered outside hospitals by a range of practitioners, for example:

- teams of nurses
- groups of doctors
- midwives
- health visitors

- dentists
- pharmacists
- optometrists
- occupational therapists
- physiotherapists
- speech therapists

For many patients, the professional health care they require will be provided in the community setting. In some situations, the care provided by and in the primary care sector may not be appropriate, or be able to meet the needs of the patient. Referral to other services may therefore be required – those services are offered by the secondary care sector.

## SECONDARY CARE SERVICES

This aspect of care provision occurs mainly through the acute hospital setting. The nursing and medical staff who work in this area have more readily available access to specialist and elaborate diagnostic aids and facilities, for example:

- X-ray department
- magnetic resonance imaging (MRI)
- computer axial tomography (CAT) scans
- operating theatres
- special care baby units (SCBU)
- microbiological laboratories

Those who provide care in the primary care setting, for example the community nurse and GP, could be seen as the 'gatekeepers' to care provision in the secondary care sector, as they may make the necessary referrals. The transition from primary care to secondary care should be a seamless move. The distinction between the two is becoming more blurred as the patient may visit the hospital for just a few hours before having follow-up care in the community.

## TERTIARY CARE SERVICES

In some larger hospitals there may be an opportunity to provide the patient with tertiary care. Tertiary care is provided by nurses, doctors and other health-care professionals with specialist expertise, equipment and facilities for caring for the patient with complex health-care needs, for example:

- intensive care units
- burns units
- oncology centres

Often staff working in these areas will have undertaken additional courses to enable them to further develop their skills and knowledge. It is important to remember that the majority of patients receive their care and have their needs met in the primary care setting. Only a few will require the services of those who work in the secondary care sector, and even fewer will need to access services provided in tertiary care.

Nurses can be found in all of these care settings. The biggest group of health-care professionals employed by the NHS are the 397 515 qualified nurses (Department of Health, 2005). *Making a Difference* (Department of Health, 1999) sets out the government's strategic intentions for nursing, midwifery and health visiting. These intentions include the establishment of a nursing career framework. The following descriptions of some nursing posts are provided only as a very brief explanation of the potential nursing career that may become available to you.

## CHIEF NURSING OFFICER

The Chief Nursing Officer (CNO) is the government's most senior nursing adviser and has the responsibility to ensure that the government's strategy for nursing, *Making a Difference* (Department of Health, 1999), is delivered. The CNO leads over 597 625 nurses, midwives and health visitors and other allied health professionals.

## NURSE CONSULTANT

Nurse consultants are very experienced practitioners. There is now a new range of these posts within all areas of nursing practice, both in the hospital and community setting. One of the key aims of the post is to strengthen professional leadership, with four main areas of responsibility (Department of Health, 1999):

- expert practice
- professional leadership and consultancy
- education and development
- practice and service development linked to research and evaluation

Most nurse consultants will spend approximately 50 per cent of their time in clinical practice, in direct contact with patients, and their remaining time may be spent undertaking research, teaching, leadership and evaluation activities.

## WARD SISTER/CHARGE NURSE

Ward sisters and their male counterparts, charge nurses, are experienced practitioners who have developed extensive skills and knowledge in their chosen area, for example:

- special care baby unit
- adolescent mental health unit
- oncology
- nursing within a general hospital, e.g. acute mental health admissions wards
- community practice, e.g. community team for learning disability
- intensive care unit

The ward sister/charge nurse has many responsibilities, including leadership; acting as a role model; and facilitating the learning of staff (such as registered nurses, student nurses and health-care assistants).

### STAFF NURSE

The staff nurse has completed a minimum of three years' education, usually at a higher education institution (HEI), and may be required as he/she gains more experience to act as deputy for the ward sister/charge nurse. Usually the staff nurse has his/her own group of patients to care for within the hospital or community setting. More experienced staff nurses can become facilitators/ mentors to other junior members of the team.

## THE CODE OF PROFESSIONAL CONDUCT

Groups recognised as professionals, according to Burnard and Chapman (2003), adopt codes of conduct that guide the members of that professional group with regards to their professional behaviour. Nurses are guided regarding standards for conduct, performance and ethics by way of *The NMC Code of Professional Conduct: Standards for Conduct, Performance and Ethics* (NMC, 2004a). The code has been reproduced as Appendix 1.2.

Professional codes for nurses aim to ensure that nurses work within ethical and moral frameworks. Codes of conduct are the collective and prevailing views shared by the profession, hence the NMC's code of conduct is the ethical standard that all nurses should be working towards (Kirby and Slevin, 2003; Fryer, 2004). The International Council for Nurses has produced its own code. *The ICN Code of Ethics for Nurses* was used to help devise the first *Code of Professional Practice* in 1983 (UKCC, 1983) and is based on ethical principles (ICN, 2000).

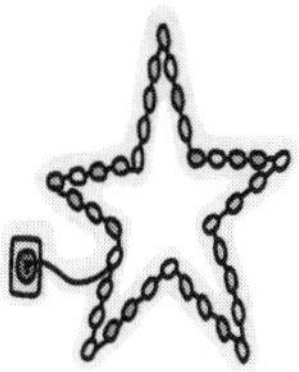

Take some time to devise what you think should be contained within a code of professional conduct for nurses. What do you think are the most important standards that nurses ought to aim to adhere to?

You can check your code of conduct against the NMC's code of conduct in Appendix 1.2.

Burnard and Chapman (2003) emphasise the fact that the code of conduct is not law, that there is no legal imperative, it is a guide. Codes of conduct do not solve problems, they reflect professional morality (Singleton and McLaren, 1995). They operate in such a way as to remind the practitioner of the standards required by the profession. However, breaching the code of conduct is in effect a breach of registration and may lead to removal of the nurse's name from the register, and consequently of the right to practise.

The purpose of the code of professional conduct is to:

- Inform the profession of the standard of professional conduct required of them in the exercise of their professional accountability and practice.
- Inform the public, other professions and employers of the standard of professional conduct that they can expect of a registered practitioner.

There are nine key facets incorporated within the NMC's code of conduct and they are arranged, broadly, under the following headings:

- An introduction – scope of the code.
- Respecting the patient and others.
- Information giving and consent.
- Team working and cooperating with others.
- Maintaining confidentiality.
- Maintaining competence and knowledge.
- Being trustworthy.
- Minimising risk.
- Indemnity insurance.

The principles enshrined within the code of conduct provide the professional framework from which practice is judged. Practice is judged with regards to professional standards – ethical and behavioural standards – when ensuring that public protection occurs and when the nurse is called to account for his/her actions or omissions. The code of conduct provides the nurse and the public with a clear message outlining personal accountability and a sense of moral responsibility.

## PROFESSIONAL ACCOUNTABILITY

To be accountable the nurse needs to be in possession of up-to-date knowledge and to possess the appropriate nursing skills. For this reason student nurses cannot be expected to be accountable as they may not have acquired the appropriate knowledge and skills.

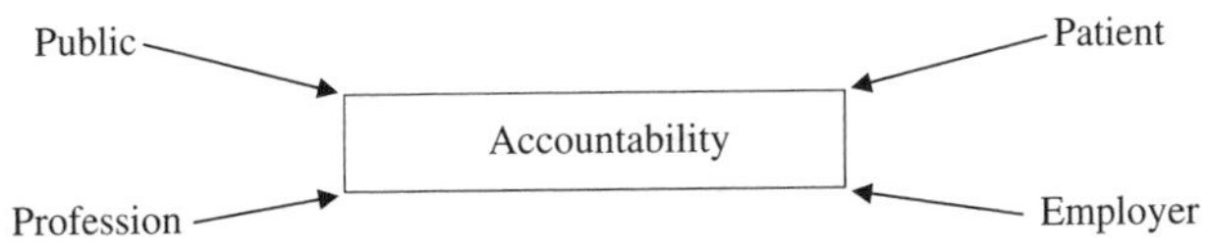


**Figure 1.1** The four areas associated with accountability
*Source*: Adapted from Dimond, 2005.

Professional accountability is unremitting. This means that a nurse is accountable at all times for his/her action or omissions, when on duty or off duty. The first section of the code of conduct makes it clear that as a registered nurse, midwife or specialist community public health nurse, you are personally accountable for your practice. This means that the nurse is answerable for his/her actions and omissions, regardless of advice or directions from another professional.

There are four arenas associated with accountability (Dimond, 2005) that nurses may be faced with (see Figure 1.1).

## PUBLIC ACCOUNTABILITY

Public accountability occurs through the criminal courts as defined by criminal law. In an instance where accountability is in question the police are likely to investigate and a decision may be made to prosecute the nurse for a criminal offence.

## ACCOUNTABILITY TO THE PATIENT

The injured party may seek a civil remedy via the criminal law in the criminal courts: the nurse may be sued for his/her actions or omissions – negligence. The complainant (the person making the complaint or bringing the action for negligence) can also, in certain circumstances, sue the NHS for the nurse's negligence (indirect liability). A sum in compensation may be paid to the injured party.

## EMPLOYER ACCOUNTABILITY

The employer expects the nurse to be accountable through the contract of employment. It is anticipated that every employee will obey the reasonable instructions of the employer and use due care and skill when carrying out his/her duties (Dimond, 2005). In some cases the employee may be in breach of contract if they have not acted with due care and skill and disciplinary action may ensue.

ACCOUNTABILITY TO THE PROFESSION

The nurse is professionally accountable to the NMC through its Conduct and Competence Committee. The NMC through the Conduct and Competence Committee will determine if a nurse is deemed incompetent through his/her actions or omissions.

## AUTONOMY

Parker and Dickenson (2001) define autonomy as self-determination, self-rule and being your own person. Dworkin (1988) adds a moral element to the term and suggests it is about choosing a moral position and accepting responsibility for the kind of person that you are. Hendrick (2004) equates autonomy with:

- integrity
- dignity
- independence
- self-assertion
- critical reflection

There are two perspectives associated with autonomy – a descriptive aspect and a prescriptive aspect. MacDonald (2002) suggests that descriptive autonomy is the capacity for self-governance and prescriptive autonomy is respect for autonomy, for example not interfering with a person's control over their own lives. According to Wade (1999), a professional nurse's autonomy is an essential attribute of a discipline striving for full professional status.

Professional self-regulation – the ability of a profession to self-regulate or 'control' itself – will only become a reality if the members of that profession have autonomy to practise. Self-regulation can be seen as an unwritten contract between society and the nurse (Hendrick, 2004). Accountability is the primary consequence of professional nurse autonomy (Wade, 1999). Becoming an autonomous and independent professional is dependent on what the nurse knows and what he/she realises she does not know. The nurse needs to be aware of his/her limitations as well as his/her clinical competence. It is important that the nurse understands that if there are any areas in which he/she is not clinically competent or he/she feels it is unethical to undertake, then it is his/her duty to decline to undertake them. This is true autonomy – being aware of one's limitations.

There are many new opportunities for nurses to develop advanced roles and skills to improve the quality of patient care. Finn (2001) has demonstrated that there is a direct correlation between job satisfaction among registered nurses and their degree of autonomy. It remains, however, the overriding responsibility of the nurse to ensure he/she is adequately prepared for any new role and ensure patient safety as the role expands.

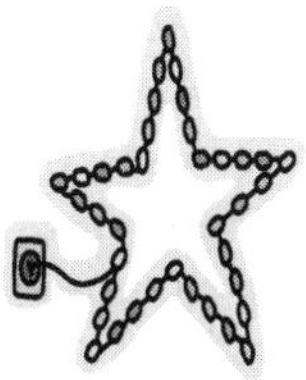

Thinking of the role of the nurse (in as many situations as you can), list the skills and the issues he/she needs to possess in order to perform his/her duties with due care and attention with the ultimate aim of protecting the patient. By being aware of these issues the nurse is better placed to act as an autonomous practitioner.

You must by now have a very long list. Just one nursing action, for example feeding a patient, would require the nurse to consider many issues in order to act in the patient's best interests (see Table 1.5). These are some of the skills that underpin safe nursing practice with respect to this one activity of living.

## PROFESSIONAL MISCONDUCT

Anyone can make a complaint about a nurse to the NMC. Complaints come to the NMC via various routes, for example the general public, fellow nurses, colleagues in other health-care professions and employees.

**Table 1.5** Some of the issues the nurse would need to take into account in order to perform safely and to act in the patient's best interests when feeding a patient

- The patient's likes and dislikes.
- Have the patient's nutritional needs been assessed?
- Does the nurse need to consult other health-care professionals such as:
  - nutritional nurse specialists
  - doctors
  - occupational therapists
  - speech and language therapists
  - dieticians?
- The patient's cultural beliefs (e.g. does he/she require a Halal-prepared meal).
- The patient's psychological/emotional status, e.g. does the patient have an appetite disturbance: anorexia nervosa, bulimia nervosa, obesity.
- The patient's ability to swallow – his/her physiological status.
- The patient's calorific needs – these vary with age.
- Does the patient require any aids to eating?
- The nutritional value of the meal being served – your understanding of a balanced diet.
- What is the patient's understanding of a balanced diet?
- Does the patient have the financial means to pay for a balanced diet – the patient may be living on a minimum income, if at all.
- The level of independence/dependence.
- The age of the patient, e.g. is the patient a neonate or an adolescent.
- Where the patient is being fed – eating is a part of social interaction, there may be customary influences.
- Is the patient being fed orally or by tube?
- Is a prescription needed for the nutrients the patient requires?

Professional misconduct can occur when the nurse has not abided by the rules set by the NMC, often in the form of the code of conduct, bearing in mind that nurses are also subjected to any of the elements of the general law that affect every citizen. The NMC has a legal duty to protect the public and in so doing has the power to exercise disciplinary procedures.

Bringing about disciplinary procedures cannot, and must not, be driven by professional self-interest – the patient first and foremost is the maxim. The key aim is to determine if that unwritten contract referred to earlier has been honoured, by ensuring that any nurse who is deemed to have failed to meet the trust that society places in him/her is not permitted to continue to practise if the allegation is proven.

The NMC will take action whenever a nurse's fitness to practise is impaired because of misconduct, illness, incompetence, criminal conviction or cautions. Fitness to practise is the nurse's suitability to be on the register without restrictions (NMC, 2004d) and Hendrick (2004) explains what the NMC might mean by this:

- Failing always to put the patient's interests first.
- Not being properly trained, qualified and up to date.
- Failing to treat patients with respect and dignity.
- Not speaking up for patients who cannot speak for themselves.

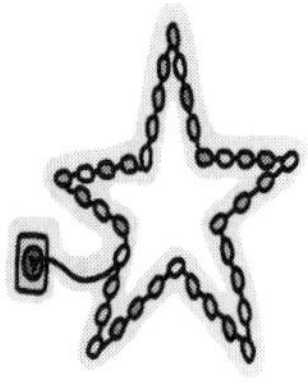

Make a list of what you think might be the most common examples of professional misconduct.

You may have some of the items below on your list. It is not possible to provide a definitive list of complaints the NMC investigates. However, the NMC (NMC, 2004d; NMC, 2004e) considers these to be the most common examples of allegations of unfitness to practise (this is not an exhaustive list):

- Physical, sexual or verbal abuse.
- Failure to provide adequate care.
- Failure to keep proper records.
- Failure to administer medicines safely.
- Deliberately concealing unsafe practice.
- Committing criminal offences.
- Continued lack of competence despite opportunities to improve.
- Health conditions.

### LACK OF COMPETENCE

A lack of competence relates to a lack of knowledge, skill or judgement of such a nature that the nurse is unfit to practise in a safe and effective manner. Some examples of lack of competence can include:

- A persistent lack of ability in correctly and/or appropriately calculating and recording the administration or disposal of medicines.
- A persistent lack of ability in properly identifying care needs and accordingly, planning and delivering appropriate care.

### CONVICTION OR CAUTION

The following may lead to a finding of unfitness to practise in relation to a conviction or caution:

- Theft.
- Fraud or other dishonest activities.
- Violence.
- Sexual offences.
- Accessing or downloading child pornography or other illegal material from the Internet.
- Illegally dealing or importing drugs.

### HEALTH CONDITIONS

There are certain health conditions that may lead the NMC to question a nurse's fitness to practise:

- Alcohol or drug dependence.
- Untreated serious mental illness.

## THE NMC COMMITTEES

Three committees handle and deal with all complaints of any allegation of unfitness to practise that are made against nurses. The three committees are:

- Investigating Committee.
- Conduct and Competence Committee.
- Health Committee.

The Investigating Committee deals with all allegations and the nurse is informed of the allegation(s) made against him/her. He/she is sent the allegation(s) and any other information that has been provided by the complainant. He/she is invited to respond in written form to the investigating panel. The panel then makes a decision to as to whether or not there is a case to answer.

If this panel determines that there is no case to answer then the case is closed. However, if it finds otherwise the case is then referred to either the Conduct and Competence Committee or the Health Committee (see Figure 1.2).

The panel convenes a hearing and the aim is to determine if the nurse's fitness to practise has been impaired and if this is the case then appropriate action is taken. Witnesses may be called to give their account of the situation; however, this is not always the case.

If a panel concludes that the nurse's fitness to practise has been impaired there are two options open to it. The panel can decide not to take any action or to make one of the following orders (see Figure 1.3):

- Striking off the register.
- A suspension order.
- A conditions of practice order.
- A caution order.

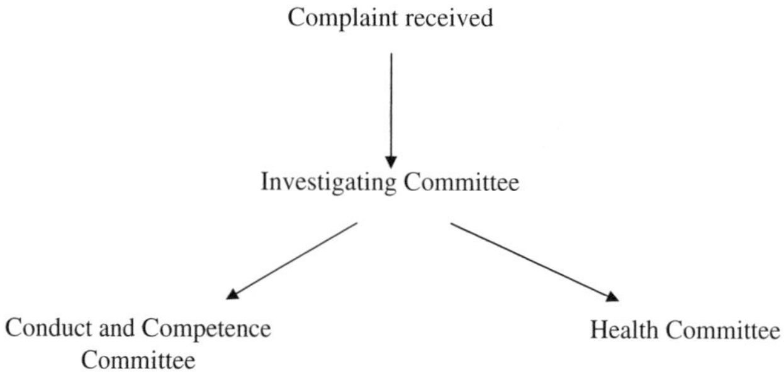


**Figure 1.2** The three committees handling allegations of unfitness to practise

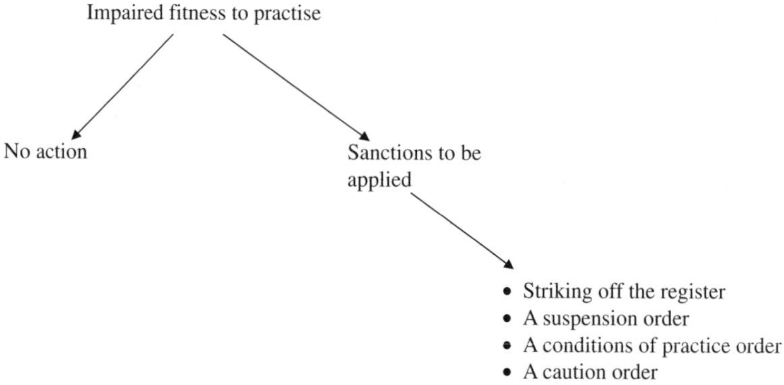


**Figure 1.3** Possible outcomes of the committee's findings

Interim suspension or interim conditions of practice orders can be made in exceptional circumstances. These orders can be made before either the Conduct and Competence Committee or the Health Committee has heard the case. Such orders usually mean the allegation is of a serious nature and there may be a risk to the public or to the nurse.

Restoration to the register can and does happen. Any nurse removed from the register has the right to apply to have his/her name restored. The Conduct and Competence Committee or the Health Committee considers cases of restoration. If restoration is to be granted the nurse must be able to demonstrate as a minimum that he/she:

- Understands and accepts the reason for his/her removal.
- Has undertaken appropriate action to address the problems that led to his/her removal.
- Has been working in a related field of care for a significant period of time and has demonstrated exemplary standards of conduct during that time.
- Supports his/her application for restoration with impeccable references from his/her current employer and, if deemed appropriate, from a medical practitioner.

Meeting the above conditions, however, does not provide an automatic restoration to the register. In some circumstances appeals to an appropriate court are possible against any of the sanctions stated earlier.

## CONCLUSIONS

Becoming a proficient registered nurse brings with it many privileges and one of those is the privilege of working with the public. From a historical perspective nurses and nursing have travelled a long way and nursing and nurses are now seen as being professionals.

The regulation of nurses has evolved since 1919 when the Nurses Registration Acts were passed. The regulatory framework enhances practice and serves to protect the public. Entry to the professional register also means that the nurse has the right to practise as an autonomous practitioner, but this has to be with the patients' best interests at the core of professional practice. Professional self-regulation – that is the ability of the nursing profession to self-regulate or 'control' itself – becomes a reality when nurses embrace the ability to practise in an autonomous manner. Self-regulation can be seen as an unwritten contract between society and the nurse.

Registered nurses are personally accountable for their practice. This means that they are answerable for their actions and omissions, regardless of advice or directions from another professional or any other party. No one else can answer for the actions or omissions and it is no defence for the nurse to say that he/she was acting on someone else's orders.

Students of nursing are never professionally accountable in the same way as they are when they become registered practitioners. It is the registered practitioner with whom the student nurse works who is professionally responsible for the consequences of the student's actions or omissions. Student nurses must always work under the direct supervision of a registered nurse or midwife (NMC, 2002).

A code of conduct is one hallmark of a profession. It must be remembered that the code of conduct is not law, there is no legal imperative, it is merely a guide. The code of conduct does not solve problems, it reflects professional morality and operates in such a way as to remind the nurse of the standards required by the profession. Furthermore, it guides nurses in the direction of their duties to patients. Breach of the tenets within the code of conduct is in effect a breach of registration and can lead to removal of the nurse from the register and the privileged right to practise.

Self-regulation serves to protect the public. To be seen to be effective those who fall short of upholding the good standing of the profession or bring the professional into disrepute may be found culpable of professional misconduct. Failure to put the patient's best interests first, failing to treat patients with respect and dignity and not being up-to-date with practice are examples of incompetence that can lead to sanctions being applied. There is a range of sanctions that may be imposed on a nurse whose fitness to practise has been impaired.

When complaints are received about a nurse's fitness to practise the case is referred to the Investigating Committee, which then decides if a case is to be answered. If no case is to be answered the complaint is dismissed. However, if the Investigating Committee considers that the complaint is to be investigated further, then the case is referred to either the Conduct and Competence Committee or the Health Committee. Interim suspension or interim conditions of practice orders can be made in exceptional circumstances, but this is rare. Such orders usually mean the allegation is of a serious nature and there may be a risk to the public or the nurse him/herself.

Restoration to the register can and does happen. Any nurse has the right to apply to have his/her name restored to the register. However, conditions must be met prior to restoration, as determined by either the Conduct and Competence Committee or the Health Committee. Appeals can be made to an appropriate court in respect to any sanctions applied.

## REVIEW

Attempt the following ten questions that are related to the code of professional conduct to test your knowledge. The answers can be found at the back of this book, in the section called 'Review Responses' (page 467).

1. What date was the current Code of Conduct published?
   a. 1994
   b. 2001
   c. 2004
   d. 2005

2. How many sections are there in the Code of Conduct?
   a. 10
   b. 9
   c. 14
   d. 16

3. The Code of Conduct is:
   a. A legal document
   b. A document produced to protect the nurse
   c. An advisory document
   d. A document used for disciplinary purposes for the student

4. Who does the document concern?
   a. Children and families
   b. Children's nurses
   c. All nurses, midwives and community public health nurses
   d. All health-care professionals

5. Where can copies be obtained?
   a. The university learning resource centre
   b. The NMC Web site
   c. The NMC
   d. All of the above

6. Which of the following are documents that the NMC does not produce?
   a. Administration of medicines
   b. Records and record keeping
   c. National service frameworks
   d. Manual removal of faeces

7. The key aim of the NMC is to:
   a. Protect and serve the public
   b. Protect the best interests of the nurse
   c. Provide an annual report to the ombudsman
   d. Generate income

8. How many parts are there to the professional register?
   a. 1
   b. 14
   c. 3
   d. 16

9. Which of the following statements is true?
   a. The NMC is a commercial enterprise
   b. All doctors must have live registration with NMC in order to practise
   c. The NMC is an organisation set up by Parliament to ensure nurses and midwives provide high standards of care to their patients and clients
   d. Membership to the NMC is open to all health-care professionals

10. When was the NMC created?
    a. December 2002
    b. April 2003
    c. April 2002
    d. December 2003

## REFERENCES

Basford, L. (2003) 'Professionalisation' in Basford, L. and Slevin, O. (eds) (3rd edn) *Theory and Practice of Nursing: An Integrated Approach to Caring Practice.* Nelson Thornes. Cheltenham. Ch 5 pp 85–96.

Benner, P. (1984) *From Novice to Expert.* Addison Wesley. Menlo Park.

Bullough, V. and Bullough, B. (1979) *The Care of the Sick: The Emergence of Modern Nursing.* Croom Helm. London.

Burnard, P. and Chapman, C. (2003) (3rd edn) *Professional and Ethical Issues in Nursing.* Balliere Tindall. London.

Cameron, A. and Masterson, A. (2003) 'Reconfiguring the clinical workforce' in Davies, C. (ed.) *The Future Health Workforce.* Palgrave. Basingstroke. Ch 4 pp 68–83.

Craig, C. and Daniels, R. (2004) 'Evolution of nursing practice' in Daniels, R. (ed.) *Nursing Fundamentals: Caring and Clinical Decision Making.* Thompson. New York. Ch 1 pp 2–23.

Davies, C. and Beach, A. (2000) *Interpreting Professional Regulation.* Routledge. London.

Department of Health (1999) *Making a Difference: Strengthening the Nursing, Midwifery and Health Visiting Contribution to Health and Health Care.* Department of Health. London.

Department of Health (2005) *Staff in the NHS 2004.* Department of Health. London.

Dimond, B. (2005) (4th edn) *Legal Aspects of Nursing.* Pearson. Harlow.

Dworkin, G. (1988) *The Theory and Practice of Autonomy.* Cambridge University Press. Cambridge.

Etzioni, A. (1969) *The Semi-Professions and Their Organization: Teachers, Nurses and Social Workers.* Free Press. New York.

Finn, C.P. (2001) 'Autonomy: An important component for nurses' job satisfaction'. *International Journal of Nursing Studies.* Vol 38, No 3, pp 349–357.

Fryer, N. (2004) 'Principles of professional practice' in Hinchliff, S., Norman, S. and Schober, J. (eds) (4th edn) *Nursing Practice and Health Care.* Arnold. London, Ch 2 pp 27–47.

Henderson, V. (1966) *The Nature of Nursing: A Definition and Its Implications for Practice, Research and Education.* Macmillan. New York.

Hendrick, J. (2004) *Law and Ethics.* Nelson Thornes. London.

Holton, S. (1984) 'Feminine authority in social order: Florence Nightingale's perception of nursing and health care'. *Social Analysis.* Vol 15, pp 59–72.

Hood, L.J. and Leddy, S.K. (2003) (5th edn) *Conceptual Bases of Professional Nursing.* Lippincott. Philadelphia.

International Council of Nurses (2000) *The ICN Code of Ethics for Nurses.* ICN. Geneva.

Kalisch, P.A. and Kalisch, B.J. (2003) (4th edn) *The Advance of American Nursing.* Lippincott. Philadelphia.

Kirby, C. and Slevin, O. (2003) 'Ethical knowing: The moral ground of nursing practice' in Basford, L. and Slevin, O. (eds) (3rd edn) *Theory and Practice of Nursing: An Integrated Approach to Caring Practice.* Nelson Thornes. Cheltenham. Ch 13 pp 209–254.

MacDonald, C. (2002) 'Nursing autonomy as relational'. *Nursing Ethics.* Vol 9, No 2, pp 194–201.

National Health Service Modernisation Agency (2005) *Hospital at Night: Patient Safety Risk Assessment Guide.* NHS Modernisation Agency. London.

Nursing and Midwifery Council (2002) *An NMC Guide for Students of Nursing and Midwifery.* NMC. London.

Nursing and Midwifery Council (2004a) *Code of Professional Conduct: Standards for Conduct, Performance and Ethics.* NMC. London.

Nursing and Midwifery Council (2004b) *Requirements for Evidence of Good Health and Good Character.* NMC. London.

Nursing and Midwifery Council (2004c) *The PREP Handbook.* NMC. London.

Nursing and Midwifery Council (2004d) *Reporting Unfitness to Practise: A Guide for Employers and Managers.* NMC. London.

Nursing and Midwifery Council (2004e) *Complaints About Unfitness to Practise: A Guide for Members of the Public.* NMC. London.

Nursing and Midwifery Council (2005) *Guidelines for Higher Education Institutions in England, Wales and Northern Ireland.* NMC. London.

Parker, M. and Dickenson, D. (2001) *The Cambridge Medical Ethics Workbook.* Cambridge University Press. Cambridge.

Pyne, R. (1998) (3rd edn) *Professional Disciplines in Nursing, Midwifery and Health Visiting.* Blackwell Scientific Publications. Oxford.

Royal College of Nursing (2003) *Defining Nursing:* def. *Nursing is. . . .* RCN. London.

Salvage, J. (2002) *Rethinking Professionalism: The First Step for Patient Focused Care.* Institute for Public Policy Research. London.

Salvage, J. (2003) 'Nursing today and tomorrow' in Hinchliff, S., Norman, S. and Schober, J. (eds) (4th edn) *Nursing Practice and Health Care.* Arnold. London. Ch 1 pp 1–24.

Singleton, J. and McLaren, S. (1995) *Ethical Foundations of Health Care Responsibilities in Decision Making.* Mosby. London.

United Kingdom Central Council (1983) *Code of Professional Practice.* UKCC. London.

United Kingdom Central Council (1986) *Project 2000 – A New Preparation for Practice.* UKCC. London.

United Kingdom Central Council (1999) *Fitness for Practice: The UKCC Commission for Nursing and Midwifery Education.* UKCC. London.

Wade, G.H. (1999) 'Professional nurse autonomy: Concept analysis and application to nursing education'. *Journal of Advanced Nursing.* Vol 30, No 2, pp 310–318.

# APPENDIX 1.1: THE SUPPORTING DECLARATION OF GOOD HEALTH AND GOOD CHARACTER FORM

**NURSING & MIDWIFERY COUNCIL**

Protecting the public through professional standards

**Declaration of Good Health and Good Character in Support of an Application for Admission to a Part of the NMC's Professional Register**

I ........................................................................................ NMC PIN ......................................

**to the best of my knowledge of:**

(full name of applicant) ..............................................................................................................

whose NMC PIN is ......................................................................................................................

believe the above named student's health and character are sufficiently good to enable safe and effective practice and that there is an intention to comply with the *Code of professional conduct: NMC Standards for conduct, performance and ethics.* I also support their application to be entered in the professional register for nurses and midwives.

Signature* ........................................................................... Date ................................................

Post held ......................................................................................................................................

Stamp of education/
Training institution

* The individual signing this form must be registered with the NMC and should be the nursing registrant responsible for directing the educational programme. For Midwifery programmes this should be the lead midwife for education. In signing this supporting declaration of good health and good character, the individual should take account of the personal responsibilities and accountability that professional registration confers upon those practitioners registered with the NMC.

Please fold back along perforated stub, detach & return appropriate copies

INVESTOR IN PEOPLE
23 Portland Place, London W1B 1PZ
Telephone 020 7333 9333 Fax 020 7636 6935 www.nmc-uk.org
INVESTOR IN PEOPLE

*Source*: The Nursing & Midwifery Council. This is Crown copyright material which is reproduced with the permission of the Controller of HMSO and the Queen's Printer for Scotland.

# APPENDIX 1.2: THE NMC CODE OF PROFESSIONAL CONDUCT: STANDARDS FOR CONDUCT, PERFORMANCE AND ETHICS

## PROTECTING THE PUBLIC THROUGH PROFESSIONAL STANDARDS

As a registered nurse, midwife or specialist community public health nurse, you are personally accountable for your practice. In caring for patients and clients, you must:

- Respect the patient or client as an individual.
- Obtain consent before you give any treatment or care.
- Protect confidential information.
- Co-operate with others in the team.
- Maintain your professional knowledge and competence.
- Be trustworthy.
- Act to identify and minimise risk to patients and clients.

These are the shared values of all the United Kingdom health care regulatory bodies.

The *Code of professional conduct* was published by the Nursing and Midwifery Council in April 2002 and came into effect on 1 June 2002. In August 2004 an addendum was published and the *Code of professional conduct* had its name changed to *The NMC code of professional conduct: standards for conduct, performance and ethics*. All references to 'nurses, midwives and health visitors' were replaced by 'nurses, midwives and specialist community public health nurses' and a new section on Indemnity Insurance was included. This updated version of the code was published in November 2004.

1 Introduction.

1.1 The purpose of *The NMC code of professional conduct: standards for conduct, performance and ethics* is to:

- Inform the professions of the standard of professional conduct required of them in the exercise of their professional accountability and practice.
- Inform the public, other professions and employers of the standard of professional conduct that they can expect of a registered practitioner.

1.2 As a registered nurse, midwife or specialist community public health nurse, you must:

- Protect and support the health of individual patients and clients.
- Protect and support the health of the wider community.

- Act in such a way that justifies the trust and confidence the public have in you.
- Uphold and enhance the good reputation of the professions.

1.3 You are personally accountable for your practice. This means that you are answerable for your actions and omissions, regardless of advice or directions from another professional.

1.4 You have a duty of care to your patients and clients, who are entitled to receive safe and competent care.

1.5 You must adhere to the laws of the country in which you are practising.

2 As a registered nurse, midwife or specialist community public health nurse, you must respect the patient or client as an individual.

2.1 You must recognise and respect the role of patients and clients as partners in their care and the contribution they can make to it. This involves identifying their preferences regarding care and respecting these within the limits of professional practice, existing legislation, resources and the goals of the therapeutic relationship.

2.2 You are personally accountable for ensuring that you promote and protect the interests and dignity of patients and clients, irrespective of gender, age, race, ability, sexuality, economic status, lifestyle, culture and religious or political beliefs.

2.3 You must, at all times, maintain appropriate professional boundaries in the relationships you have with patients and clients. You must ensure that all aspects of the relationship focus exclusively upon the needs of the patient or client.

2.4 You must promote the interests of patients and clients. This includes helping individuals and groups gain access to health and social care, information and support relevant to their needs.

2.5 You must report to a relevant person or authority, at the earliest possible time, any conscientious objection that may be relevant to your professional practice. You must continue to provide care to the best of your ability until alternative arrangements are implemented.

3 As a registered nurse, midwife or specialist community public health nurse, you must obtain consent before you give any treatment or care.

3.1 All patients and clients have a right to receive information about their condition. You must be sensitive to their needs and respect the wishes of those who refuse or are unable to receive information about their condition. Information should be accurate, truthful and presented in such a way as to make it easily understood. You may need to seek legal or professional advice or guidance from your employer, in relation to the giving or withholding of consent.

3.2 You must respect patients' and clients' autonomy – their right to decide whether or not to undergo any health-care intervention – even where a refusal may result in harm or death to themselves or a fetus, unless a court of law orders to the contrary. This right is protected in law, although in circumstances where the health of the fetus would be severely compromised by any refusal to give consent, it would be appropriate to discuss this matter fully within the team and with a supervisor of midwives, and possibly to seek external advice and guidance (see clause 4).

3.3 When obtaining valid consent, you must be sure that it is:
- Given by a legally competent person.
- Given voluntarily.
- Informed.

3.4 You should presume that every patient and client is legally competent unless otherwise assessed by a suitably qualified practitioner. A patient or client who is legally competent can understand and retain treatment information and can use it to make an informed choice.

3.5 Those who are legally competent may give consent in writing, orally or by co-operation. They may also refuse consent. You must ensure that all your discussions and associated decisions relating to obtaining consent are documented in the patient's or client's health-care records.

3.6 When patients or clients are no longer legally competent and have lost the capacity to consent to or refuse treatment and care, you should try to find out whether they have previously indicated preferences in an advance statement. You must respect any refusal of treatment or care given when they were legally competent, provided that the decision is clearly applicable to the present circumstances and that there is no reason to believe that they have changed their minds. When such a statement is not available, the patients' or clients' wishes, if known, should be taken into account. If these wishes are not known, the criteria for treatment must be that it is in their best interests.

3.7 The principles of obtaining consent apply equally to those people who have a mental illness. Whilst you should be involved in their assessment, it will also be necessary to involve relevant people close to them; this may include a psychiatrist. When patients and clients are detained under statutory powers (mental health acts), you must ensure that you know the circumstances and safeguards needed for providing treatment and care without consent.

3.8 In emergencies where treatment is necessary to preserve life, you may provide care without consent, if a patient or client is unable to give it, provided you can demonstrate that you are acting in their best interests.

3.9 No-one has the right to give consent on behalf of another competent adult. In relation to obtaining consent for a child, the involvement of those with parental responsibility in the consent procedure is usually necessary, but will depend on the age and understanding of the child. If the child is under the age of 16 in England and Wales, 12 in Scotland and 17 in Northern Ireland, you must be aware of legislation and local protocols relating to consent.

3.10 Usually the individual performing a procedure should be the person to obtain the patient's or client's consent. In certain circumstances, you may seek consent on behalf of colleagues if you have been specially trained for that specific area of practice.

3.11 You must ensure that the use of complementary or alternative therapies is safe and in the interests of patients and clients. This must be discussed with the team as part of the therapeutic process and the patient or client must consent to their use.

4 As a registered nurse, midwife or specialist community public health nurse, you must co-operate with others in the team.

4.1 The team includes the patient or client, the patient's or client's family, informal carers and health- and social-care professionals in the National Health Service, independent and voluntary sectors.

4.2 You are expected to work co-operatively within teams and to respect the skills, expertise and contributions of your colleagues. You must treat them fairly and without discrimination.

4.3 You must communicate effectively and share your knowledge, skill and expertise with other members of the team as required for the benefit of patients and clients.

4.4 Health care records are a tool of communication within the team. You must ensure that the health-care record for the patient or client is an accurate account of treatment, care planning and delivery. It should be consecutive, written with the involvement of the patient or client wherever practicable and completed as soon as possible after an event has occurred. It should provide clear evidence of the care planned, the decisions made, the care delivered and the information shared.

4.5 When working as a member of a team, you remain accountable for your professional conduct, any care you provide and any omission on your part.

4.6 You may be expected to delegate care delivery to others who are not registered nurses or midwives. Such delegation must not compromise existing care but must be directed to meeting the needs and serving the interests of patients and clients. You remain accountable for the appropriateness of the delegation, for ensuring that the person who does the work is able to do it and that adequate supervision or support is provided.

4.7 You have a duty to co-operate with internal and external investigations.

5 As a registered nurse, midwife or specialist community public health nurse, you must protect confidential information.

5.1 You must treat information about patients and clients as confidential and use it only for the purposes for which it was given. As it is impractical to obtain consent every time you need to share information with others, you should ensure that patients and clients understand that some information may be made available to other members of the team involved in the delivery of care. You must guard against breaches of confidentiality by protecting information from improper disclosure at all times.

5.2 You should seek patients' and clients' wishes regarding the sharing of information with their family and others. When a patient or client is considered incapable of giving permission, you should consult relevant colleagues.

5.3 If you are required to disclose information outside the team that will have personal consequences for patients or clients, you must obtain their consent. If the patient or client withholds consent, or if consent cannot be obtained for whatever reason, disclosures may be made only where:

- They can be justified in the public interest (usually where disclosure is essential to protect the patient or client or someone else from the risk of significant harm).
- They are required by law or by order of a court.

5.4 Where there is an issue of child protection, you must act at all times in accordance with national and local policies.

6 As a registered nurse, midwife or specialist community public health nurse, you must maintain your professional knowledge and competence.

6.1 You must keep your knowledge and skills up-to-date throughout your working life. In particular, you should take part regularly in learning activities that develop your competence and performance.

6.2 To practise competently, you must possess the knowledge, skills and abilities required for lawful, safe and effective practice without direct supervision. You must acknowledge the limits of your professional competence and only undertake practice and accept responsibilities for those activities in which you are competent.

6.3 If an aspect of practice is beyond your level of competence or outside your area of registration, you must obtain help and supervision from a competent practitioner until you and your employer consider that you have acquired the requisite knowledge and skill.

6.4 You have a duty to facilitate students of nursing, midwifery and specialist community public health nursing and others to develop their competence.

6.5 You have a responsibility to deliver care based on current evidence, best practice and, where applicable, validated research when it is available.

7 As a registered nurse, midwife or specialist community public health nurse, you must be trustworthy.

7.1 You must behave in a way that upholds the reputation of the professions. Behaviour that compromises this reputation may call your registration into question even if it is not directly connected to your professional practice.

7.2 You must ensure that your registration status is not used in the promotion of commercial products or services, declare any financial or other interests in relevant organisations providing such goods or services and ensure that your professional judgement is not influenced by any commercial considerations.

7.3 When providing advice regarding any product or service relating to your professional role or area of practice, you must be aware of the risk that, on account of your professional title or qualification, you could be perceived by the patient or client as endorsing the product. You should fully explain the advantages and disadvantages of alternative products so that the patient or client can make an informed choice. Where you recommend a specific product, you must ensure that your advice is based on evidence and is not for your own commercial gain.

7.4 You must refuse any gift, favour or hospitality that might be interpreted, now or in the future, as an attempt to obtain preferential consideration.

7.5 You must neither ask for nor accept loans from patients, clients or their relatives and friends.

8 As a registered nurse, midwife or specialist community public health nurse, you must act to identify and minimise the risk to patients and clients.

8.1 You must work with other members of the team to promote health-care environments that are conducive to safe, therapeutic and ethical practice.

8.2 You must act quickly to protect patients and clients from risk if you have good reason to believe that you or a colleague, from your own or another profession, may not be fit to practise for reasons of conduct, health or competence. You should be aware of the terms of legislation that offer protection for people who raise concerns about health and safety issues.

8.3 Where you cannot remedy circumstances in the environment of care that could jeopardise standards of practice, you must report them to a senior person with sufficient authority to manage them and also, in the case of midwifery, to the supervisor of midwives. This must be supported by a written record.

8.4 When working as a manager, you have a duty toward patients and clients, colleagues, the wider community and the organisation in which you and your colleagues work. When facing professional dilemmas, your first consideration in all activities must be the interests and safety of patients and clients.

8.5 In an emergency, in or outside the work setting, you have a professional duty to provide care. The care provided would be judged against what could reasonably be expected from someone with your knowledge, skills and abilities when placed in those particular circumstances.

9 Indemnity insurance.

9.1 The NMC recommends that a registered nurse, midwife or specialist community public health nurse, in advising, treating and caring for patients/clients, has professional indemnity insurance. This is in the interests of clients, patients and registrants in the event of claims of professional negligence.

9.2 Some employers accept vicarious liability for the negligent acts and/or omissions of their employees. Such cover does not normally extend to activities undertaken outside the registrant's employment. Independent practice would not normally be covered by vicarious liability, while agency work may not. It is the individual registrant's responsibility to establish their insurance status and take appropriate action.

9.3 In situations where employers do not accept vicarious liability, the NMC recommends that registrants obtain adequate professional indemnity insurance. If unable to secure professional indemnity insurance, a registrant will need to demonstrate that all their clients/patients are fully informed of this fact and the implications this might have in the event of a claim for professional negligence.

November 2004

## SUMMARY

As a registered nurse, midwife or specialist community public health nurse, you must:

- Respect the patient or client as an individual.
- Obtain consent before you give any treatment or care.
- Co-operate with others in the team.
- Protect confidential information.
- Maintain your professional knowledge and competence.
- Be trustworthy.
- Act to identify and minimise the risk to patients and clients.

*Source*: Nursing & Midwifery Council (2004). The Department of Health. This is Crown copyright material which is reproduced with the permission of the Controller of HMSO and the Queen's Printer for Scotland.

# 2 Ethical and Legal Issues

Ethical issues impinge on all aspects of care. An understanding of ethics will help the nurse when caring for patients and managing their care appropriately. Every aspect of nursing intervention has the potential to impinge on the patient's physical and psychological wellbeing and a constant awareness of this, regardless of how fleeting the interaction with the patient may be, is required. Nurses and nursing students are concerned with the ethical practice of nursing and are confronted with ethical issues, challenges and dilemmas nearly every day. This chapter provides knowledge of contemporary ethical issues and their potential impact on nursing and health care.

An overview of the various ethical principles will be considered. Much emphasis will be placed on confidentiality, for example regarding information the nurse acquires in a professional capacity. The expectation is that the student will be able to ensure the patient's best interests and wellbeing with respect to confidentiality.

There are few areas of health care that are untouched by the law and involvement with the legal process. The subsequent aspect of this chapter will briefly consider the legal process in order to develop an understanding of the law and its impact on nursing and health care. In this chapter the law as applied to England and Wales is the main thrust of the legal debate. The legal systems in Scotland and Northern Ireland have their own traditions and although different from the English and Welsh arrangements, there are a range of comparisons. The key issues associated with the relevant legislation and health and social policy related to nursing practice will be identified and discussed.

You may recall in Chapter 1 that nurses are accountable for their own practice regardless of the advice and directions given to the nurse by another health-care professional, for example a doctor. If a nurse acts on the directions of another health-care professional, this does not relieve him/her of personal responsibility, if the act he/she carried out was unethical or unlawful. It is important therefore that the nurse is aware of the legal and ethical issues surrounding patient care. Nurses need skills in ethical reasoning along with an understanding of the law and the demands made by the nursing profession.

The overall aim of the chapter is to ensure that the student practises in accordance with and within an ethical and legal framework.

## ETHICS IN NURSING PRACTICE

Several ethical perspectives need to be considered by the nurse when working with patients in any setting. Ethical dilemmas arise when there is or may be conflict between various interests and interested parties. Nurses often need to make decisions, prioritise care, manage resources (both human and material) and address conflict. Carrying out these tasks will inevitably involve ethical considerations, and increasingly these decisions transcend technical and professional concerns (Kennedy-Schwarz, 2000).

Every individual is important and deserves to be treated with respect. The Royal College of Nursing (RCN, 2004) suggests that this value – respect – is upheld in law and should underpin all aspects of nursing practice.

## DEFINING KEY TERMS

### ETHICS

Defining the term ethics is not easy, just as the definition of professional in the previous chapter proved challenging. Most definitions incorporate the term 'morals'. For example, Kirby and Slevin (2003) in their definition suggest that ethics is the study of moral thinking: it is about the values we hold and our actions. Dictionary definitions of ethics also incorporate morals – the *New Oxford Dictionary of English* defines ethics as 'Moral principles which govern a person's behaviour or the conduct of an activity' (*New Oxford Dictionary of English*, 2001). Philosophers provide differing explanations of ethics. Beauchamp and Childress (2001) suggest that ethics involve a systematic examination of moral life and allow us to look for and provide justification for our moral actions and the moral decisions we make.

According to Hope et al. (2003) most of us have gut reactions as to what we think is morally right or wrong in certain situations. Often these reactions are a result of our upbringing. When these rights or wrongs are related to dilemmas that occur during nursing practice the reasons are sometimes associated with what we have learnt during our professional apprenticeship – during our nursing education. These reactions, the reactions that help us decide what is right or wrong, must be examined further.

Ethics and morals applied to nursing practice are primarily concerned with the decisions made about whether something is right or wrong, good or bad. They affect matters associated with how decisions are made and how nurses carry them out in practice. All of this is conducted within the confines of the law and often the issues are complex (Cribb, 2002).

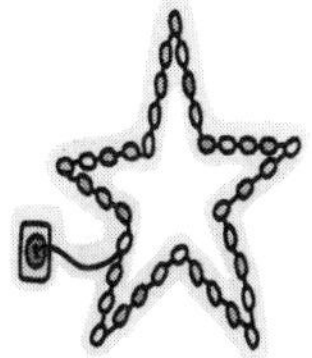

Think about the following:

- Are some things always wrong? What are they?
- Why should you be good?
- Is abortion right or wrong?

It may have taken you seconds to respond to the above statements, conversely you might have mulled over them for some time. For many centuries the answers (if there are any) to these questions have been fiercely deliberated and are still being debated today. In your response to the first question you may consider that sometimes some things are wrong depending on the situation. For example, you may think murder is wrong, however there are situations where it may be defensible. You might think that abortion is right or wrong and is related to an individual's particular perspective or point of view, for example their religious beliefs or values, cultural values and personal values.

## VALUES

Values are derived from many sources; see Figure 2.1. There are several ways of expressing individual or collective values, for example in nonverbal and verbal communication, and through codes of professional conduct.

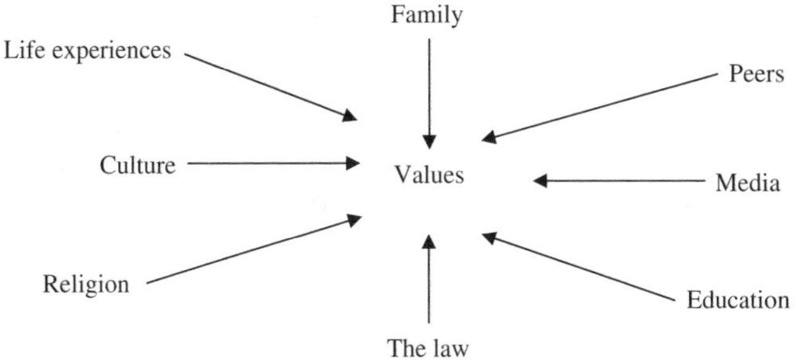


**Figure 2.1** Some factors that influence and shape the way we develop our values systems

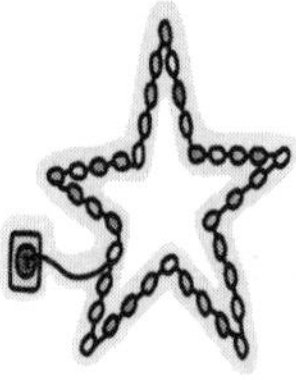

Consider a particular value that your parents or other people have taught you. What kind of an influence did that person or people have on your life and how did that individual (it may have been more than one person) persuade you to think?

Of course, there are many people who have influenced and persuaded you, for example your parents, your teachers and your friends. The person or people may have influenced you at an early age or at a period in your life when you were vulnerable or open to persuasion. It is possible to discover how the values that you hold dear today have been formed, shaped and moulded. As you develop and grow as an individual, these values may change – new ideas and influences can affect them and change them. Reflect on some values that you held dear to you: have they changed? Consider why they may have changed.

Every nurse will be influenced by his/her own value system, which has been shaped over time. Values are a part of who you are and what makes you worthwhile (Hendrick, 2004). Values have the potential to motivate and guide a person's choices and decision-making abilities – understanding your own value system may help when making an ethical decision regarding nursing practice.

Just as nurses have their own value systems so do patients, and often these are informed by the influencing factors outlined in Figure 2.1. Because of this, they may be similar or can differ significantly. There is therefore a potential for conflict. When this conflict does arise the nurse must respect the values of others, ensuring that a balance has been achieved in relation to the patient's rights and the nurse's professional duties (Fry and Johnstone, 2002).

Table 2.1 summarises the definitions of ethics, morals and values.

## ETHICAL THEORIES

Ethical theories are complex theories that philosophers use to reflect on moral beliefs and practices. Utilitarianism and deontology are two ethical theories that will be briefly discussed here.

### UTILITARIANISM – THE GREATEST GOOD FOR THE GREATEST NUMBER

Utilitarianism is one of the most widely used ethical theories today (Mason and Whitehead, 2003). One of the basic insights into utilitarianism is that the

**Table 2.1** An overview of morals, values and ethics

| Term | Definition | Example |
|---|---|---|
| **Ethics** | • Promotes ideal human behaviour<br>• Considers what ought to be done<br>• Aims to provide guidance or principles on which to direct human action | • Exploration of ethical principles and moral standards related to conduct<br>• Having high regard to the concept that humans are unique beings who have unique experiences |
| **Morals** | • Standards of conduct that reflect ideal human behaviour<br>• Norms of conduct identified by society<br>• Expected conduct regardless of the consequences of the individual | • An expectation that society will tell the truth and be honest in all situations despite the fact that there may be negative consequences<br>• Behaviours that are judged to be the 'right or correct' thing to do |
| **Values** | • Ideals and beliefs associated with patterns of behaviour that are held dear by individuals<br>• Behaviours that have been learned and acquired over a period of time from various influences, e.g. family and peers | • Personal values<br>• Professional values |

*Source*: Adapted from Harkreader and Hogan, 2004.

aim of morality is to make the world a better place. It is about producing good consequences, not having good intentions. The emphasis in utilitarianism is on consequences and not intentions: society should do whatever brings the most benefit to all humanity. The most often used maxim to sum up the utilitarian perspective is 'the greatest good for the greatest number' – always acting in such a way that will produce the greatest overall amount of good in the world. The focus or the moral position emanating from utilitarianism is to put aside our own self-interests for the sake of the whole.

Jeremy Bentham, a legal philosopher (1748–1832), believed that we should try to increase the overall amount of pleasure in the world. However, John Stuart Mill, another philosopher (1806–1873), disagreed with Bentham's philosophy. Despite pleasure being easy to quantify it was of short duration and was associated with the lower levels of our existence (sensual/physical pleasures). Mill felt that the term happiness should be used instead of pleasure. Happiness is associated with the higher levels of human existence (rational/mental pleasures). However, happiness as opposed to pleasure is not so easy to measure and quantify.

There are two types of utilitarianism: see Table 2.2 for an overview of these approaches.

**Table 2.2** An overview of act and rule utilitarianism

| Act utilitarianism | Rule utilitarianism |
|---|---|
| Each individual action a person takes should be assessed in relation to its rightness when the outcome (the utility) has been maximised. There are no moral rules apart from one, and that is that we should always strive to seek the happiness of the greatest number in all situations. | The right actions are those actions that are consistent with rules that would maximise the outcome. The rules formed are rules that use utilitarian principles, i.e. the greatest good for the greatest number. Deference to predefined rules and exceptions to these rules are acceptable. |

Utilitarianism can be considered as 'cost and benefit' and how alternative courses of action can produce the best overall outcomes. If a nurse uses a utilitarian approach in respect to truth telling for example, he/she would have to take into account, when making a decision, the consequence or the outcome of truth telling, and whether the act (telling the truth) would produce more happiness than unhappiness. In this circumstance, even if a decision is made to tell the truth in order to arrive at the greatest good for the greatest number, this may not necessarily be the morally correct theory to justify the action. A deontological approach may prove to be more appropriate.

### DEONTOLOGY

While utilitarianism is concerned with consequences, deontology contrasts with this theory and focuses on the individual's intentions. Immanuel Kant (1724–1804), a German philosopher, argued that an action is morally right only if the individual is motivated by 'good will'. If the proposed action is not motivated by good will then it is wrong, despite the consequences. There are key rules that have to be followed and hence deontologists are concerned with motive as opposed to consequence (Whaite, 2002).

Generally, deontologists are bound by constraints, for example the prerequisite not to kill, but they are also given options, for example the right not to donate money to a charity if they do not wish to. Strict utilitarians, in contrast, recognise neither constraints nor options, and the aim of the utilitarian is to maximise the good by any and all means necessary.

The above discussion deals with the subject in a superficial manner and the reader should note that the issues are complex. Problems and challenges associated with the philosophical theories were briefly described. Fry and Johnstone (2002) discuss in more detail the advantages and the disadvantages regarding both ethical approaches.

## PRINCIPLES OF HEALTH-CARE ETHICS

It is vital to be aware of the various ethical theories, but it is also important to understand that their application to nursing practice can be complicated

(McAthie, 1999). Principles of health-care ethics can help to guide and direct our behaviour when ethical issues arise. We choose what principles to apply to what situation depending on the context of care and the situation that has arisen. The following principles are discussed in the next aspect of the chapter:

- autonomy
- beneficence and nonmaleficence
- justice
- veracity
- fidelity

Two other issues relating ethical relationships with patients will also be discussed:

- confidentiality
- consent to treatment

## AUTONOMY

The term autonomy is derived from the Greek and is broadly defined as self-determination or self-rule (Parker and Dickenson, 2001). Dworkin (1988) suggests that the term is often used in a broad manner and is associated with the qualities of liberty, self-assertion, freedom from obligation and an absence of external causation. An autonomous patient, it could be suggested, is a patient who rules him/herself and no one rules him/her; an independent person.

You may recall that autonomy was discussed in Chapter 1, but this was primarily in relation to the autonomous practice of the nurse. Patient autonomy and the principle of respect for a patient's autonomy is central to the nurse–patient relationship. It can be seen as the opposite of paternalism, and allows the nurse to practise patient-centred nursing care.

Paternalism can be said to be acting for another person without their agreement or consent. The person acting paternalistically is assuming that he/she knows best and that his/her actions are in the patient's best interests. Autonomy can be overridden or not respected when a person acts paternalistically. Mason et al. (2002) believe that in the past paternalistic behaviour towards patients was the norm, however this situation is now changing and it is becoming far less acceptable.

Beauchamp and Childress (2001) suggest that respecting patients' autonomy means that they are treated as people, as individuals and not as mere objects. The nurse provides the patient with the opportunity to make his/her own decisions related to his/her health-care needs.

Husted and Husted (1995) suggest that being autonomous is about being yourself. Autonomy, they state, allows the nurse to relate to the person – by allowing the patient to experience what he/she wants. Their comments point to the fact that each individual deserves respect and is equal to every other person.

The importance of the freedom of an individual and the freedom to make a decision uncoerced has been discussed by Berlin (1969). He considers the ability to be free to choose and not to be chosen is what makes human beings human beings. This, he says, is an inalienable ingredient of humanness. His definition points to a need for liberty, liberty that is free from unwanted and unwelcome interference.

Seedhouse (2002) states that autonomy is not absolute, it can be found on a continuum ranging from absolute freedom (total control) to no freedom (no control); see Figure 2.2. The degree of freedom, Seedhouse contests, will depend on several circumstances and situations.

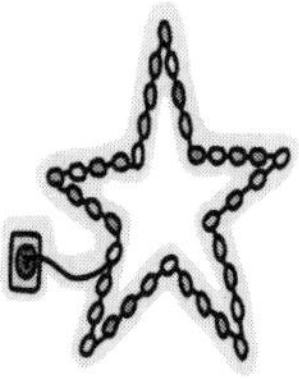

How free are you to make choices? To what extent are you an autonomous person? Think of the last time you made a choice – did you really have total autonomy or were there other things that stood in the way, 'unwanted interference'?

You may have thought you had total autonomy to make choices and to do what you wanted. However, this is not always the case as there are often constraints placed on us such as:

- Do we have enough money?
- Are we acting within the law?
- Do we know what other choices are out there?

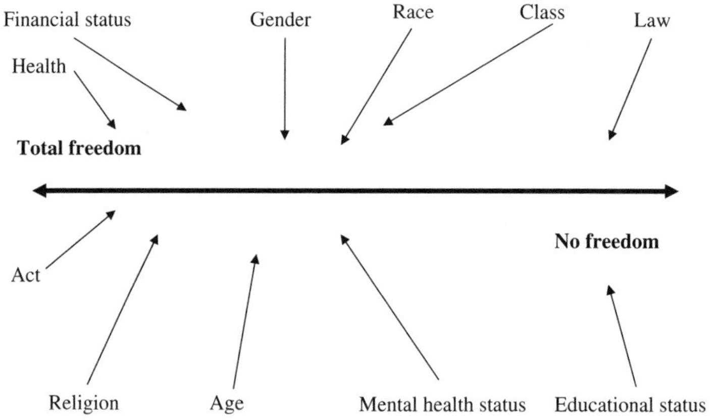


**Figure 2.2** The absolutes of freedom, with factors that will impinge on the degree of freedom experienced by a patient

- Do we have the understanding (the mental capacity) to grasp what the consequences of autonomous action are likely to be?
- Do we have the ability to act on the choices we have made or chosen?

Often it is not easy making choices and acting without unwanted interference if we do not fully understand the choices being offered (or sought) and the options or alternatives available to us. For certain reasons some choices are not available to us, for example a 17 year old may desire or want to act in an autonomous manner in order to purchase alcohol, but the law dictates that he/she is not legally able to do that.

When a patient is admitted to hospital some of his/her ability to make autonomous decisions may be taken away from him/her. Often hospital admission can result in a loss of a person's autonomy or some of the autonomous decision-making abilities that person possesses. He/she may no longer be able to decide when and what time to eat or drink or what clothes he/she wishes to wear, as ward routine may dictate this. Working with the patient and family to ensure that as much autonomous decision making as possible is retained by the patient is a key aspect of the nurse's role – acting as a patient's advocate.

Respecting a patient's autonomy can result in conflict, raise ethical dilemmas and may not be straightforward (Hope et al., 2003). Any competent adult patient can refuse treatment; note the word 'competent' – competency is dealt with later in this chapter when considering consent. If a patient is deemed incompetent then the overriding of his/her wishes may be permitted, however this is a serious action and must be fully justified both professionally and legally. Interfering in this manner (unwanted interference) is protected in some circumstances in the law relating to consent. In this instance there is conflict between the issue of autonomy and beneficence.

## BENEFICENCE AND NONMALEFICENCE

The term beneficence, according to Thompson et al. (2003), is associated with a duty to avoid doing no harm to others (both physically and psychologically), acting in a way so as not to cause harm; they compare beneficence with the saying 'Do unto others as you would have them do unto you'. On the face of it this seems like a reasonably straightforward statement (Hendrick, 2004); when summed up it is the duty of care (Hendrick, 2004; Thompson et al., 2003). The nurse owes a duty of care to the patient – section 1.2 of the code of conduct dictates this (NMC, 2004) – the nurse is obliged to help others (Edwards, 1996). Beneficence, therefore, is a duty to care or to do good.

Nonmaleficence, according to Rumbold (1999), places an obligation on nurses to do no harm to patients in their care (both physically and psychologically). This principle, suggest Hope et al. (2003), is the flip side of the coin of the beneficence principle.

Both beneficence and nonmaleficence, according to Thompson et al. (2003), complement respect for personal rights and justice; they also justify the minimum requirements for a coherent system of ethics. Beneficence and nonmaleficence, it could be suggested, are the foundations on which the code of conduct is built.

Employing the principles nonmaleficence and beneficence raises the questions:

- What harm is to be avoided?
- Who judges what is best for the patient?
- What and who deem the patient's best interests?

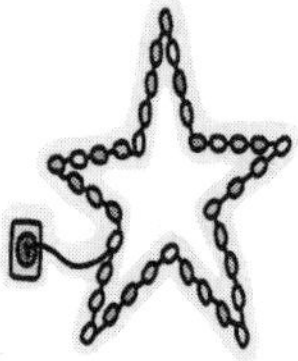

Think about giving a patient an intra-muscular injection, while also trying to bring into play the two principles of beneficence (to do good) and nonmaleficence (to do no harm).

With all the good will in the world, the administration of an intra-muscular injection is going to cause pain, if not hurt, to the patient. By attempting to carry out the principle of doing good (beneficence) you are invoking the principle of doing harm (maleficence) – are you therefore not acting in the patient's best interests?

There are other examples that could also have been used. For example, when you administer a prescribed drug to a patient, the key aim may be to do the patient good but there may also be side effects associated with that particular medication, which could result in harm to the patient. All nursing interventions have the potential to help and also harm the patient.

The example cited demonstrates how easy it is to harm the patient when attempting to do good. It is important therefore that during any nursing interaction or intervention you perform, you balance and weigh up the harm versus hurt equation, considering all options open to you. The aim should be to take the option that causes the least harm and promotes the most good, ensuring that the risks to be taken are never worse than the potential benefits to be gained.

Olson (2004) offers suggestions that may minimise harm that may be caused to a patient (see Table 2.3).

## JUSTICE

Being fair and right is something most people would aim for. However, when justice is discussed in a health-care arena there are many other factors that will influence whether we are being fair and right, for example inequalities in

**Table 2.3** Issues to be considered when attempting to minimise any harm to the patient

| |
|---|
| • The treatment must offer the patient a reasonable prospect of benefit.<br>• The treatment must not leave the patient in excessive pain or other inconvenience.<br>• The patient must be fully informed about any side effects, potential consequences of treatment and if appropriate the costs. |

*Source*: Adapted from Olson, 2004.

access to health care. Fletcher and Buka (1999) suggest that issues concerning justice tend to be related to the wider community as opposed to individuals and often centre on the allocation of resources. Other terms that you may come across that are also associated with justice are:

- fairness
- desert (what is deserved)
- entitlement

It may help to define the term justice. Beauchamp and Childress (2001) suggest that justice is the fair, equitable and appropriate treatment of all people in light of what is owed them. The underpinning principle associated with justice, therefore, is that everyone is valued equally and treated alike. Being fair and equitable will also depend on what we feel is owed to others – it is therefore subjective and can be loaded with values and judgements. Justice to individuals also means nondiscriminatory care based on sex, sexual orientation, gender, race or religion, age or illness (physical and psychological).

Seedhouse (2002) states that justice can be understood in more than one way and it can be interpreted in ways that contradict each other. There are three perspectives associated with justice:

- egalitarian
- libertarian
- rights

The egalitarian perspective is concerned with the distribution of health-care resources in association with individual need. In this perspective individual need should be met by equal access to services. The most important tenet of a libertarian perspective is liberty and choice. Justice is associated with how hard an individual has worked in order to earn heath care; they are judged on merit. Finally, the rights perspective implies that the state has an obligation to provide care and that the patient should suffer no harm as a result of that provision. People's rights have to be upheld in order to meet the criteria associated with a rights perspective.

The NHS is frequently cited in the media as being unjust in so far as it may not have sufficient resources to meet the needs of all of its patients. Often news stories centre on the number of people on waiting lists and the adverse effects the wait has on the patient.

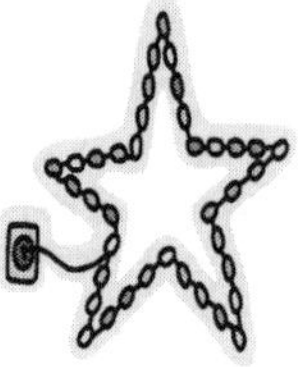

In the scenario outlined in Table 2.4, decide to whom you would allocate the resource.

Having made your decision you must now justify it.

Such a scenario is not unheard of. Table 2.5 provides other examples that may have implications for resource allocation, where patients may need to compete against each other for the use of limited resources.

## VERACITY

Veracity is the obligation to tell the truth and avoid deception. Thiroux (1995) includes veracity and honesty as part of the principles of ethics that can be applied to any situation. The key principle behind veracity is truth telling or information disclosure. Some health-care professionals often cite the main reason for not telling the patient the truth as being that disclosure of bad news may shatter the patient's hope. However, the disclosure of information and access to that information is the patient's right (see for example the Data Protection Act 1998). There are, however, some exceptions to the right to access information.

**Table 2.4** Making a decision with regards to the allocation of resources

- A 10-year-old boy needs to have a lung and heart transplant. He has been waiting for a donor for 18 months now.
- A 56-year-old man also requires a lung and heart transplant. He has suffered with chronic heart and lung disease for 20 years despite being advised to cut down on his smoking habits.
- A donor becomes available and the opportunity of transplantation is a possibility. However, only one of them will be able to have the transplant.

**Table 2.5** Examples of situations that could have consequences for the allocation of scarce resources

- A liver transplant in a patient who continues to drink alcohol to excess.
- A reversal of a sterilisation.
- A soft tissue injury as a result of engaging in extreme sporting activity.
- A spinal injury as a result of refusing to wear a protective helmet when horse riding.
- A patient wanting tattoos removed that she had had done when she was younger.

At first it may seem easy to uphold the principle of truth telling, as it seems right that the patient should be told the truth. It is, however, difficult in certain circumstances to achieve. Veracity underpins and is a key component of the concept of informed consent. Problems arise, nevertheless, when the nurse needs to decide on how much should be told, to whom and in what circumstances (Olsen, 2004).

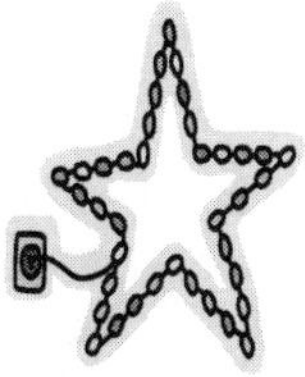

In the situation in Table 2.6, should the patient's mother be told the truth?

**Table 2.6** To tell the truth and to whom

| |
|---|
| Marie is 15 years of age and is pregnant. She visits her GP and decides she wants to have a termination of pregnancy. She refuses to tell her parents and asks the practice nurse to arrange the appointment at the clinic to have the termination. A week later Marie is brought to the GP surgery by her mother complaining of abdominal pain. |

You must remember that Marie is a minor. Does she have any rights? Do her parents have rights?

### FIDELITY

According to Fry and Veach (2000) the ethical principle of fidelity is concerned with the keeping of promises, the obligation to ensure a trusting relationship and the duty to maintain confidentiality. It is concerned with maintaining the duty of care even when the circumstances the patient finds him/herself in are difficult. Gastmans (2002) suggests that fidelity is the ethical framework on which the nurse–patient relationship is based, as it is concerned with faithfulness. Confidentiality is discussed in detail in the next section of this chapter.

To demonstrate that he/she is acting in a faithful manner towards the patient, the nurse has to function as the patient's advocate. Being the patient's advocate means that the nurse has to speak up for the patient or act in his/her best interests. Olsen (2004) outlines the acts that he considers would uphold the principle of fidelity (see Table 2.7).

## CONFIDENTIALITY

Many of the ethical theories discussed above come to the fore when the nurse attempts to deal with confidentiality. Ethical debates abound and often there

**Table 2.7** Nursing actions that may uphold the ethical principle of fidelity

| |
|---|
| • The nurse represents the patient's views to other members of the multidisciplinary team. |
| • The nurse avoids letting his/her own values and beliefs influence the ability to advocate for the patient. |
| • Regardless of what decision the patient makes, the nurse will support this even if it conflicts with his/her own preferences or choices. |

*Source*: Adapted from Olsen, 2004.

are no right or wrong answers to the questions surrounding this very complicated principle. Confidentiality is closely related to the ethical principle of fidelity (Hendrick, 2004). This confirms the often used saying that 'confidentiality is the cornerstone of nursing'.

Protecting confidentiality can be seen as respect for privacy (Stauch et al., 2002). The right to a private life is upheld in the Human Rights Act 1998. Patients have a legitimate expectation that the nurse will respect their right to privacy and that he/she will act in an appropriate way when addressing and dealing with privacy and confidentiality.

An element of trust is needed by both the patient and the nurse in order for confidentiality to exist. In some instances that element of trust may not be able to be agreed by the patient, as he/she may not be competent to enter into a bilateral trust agreement. When this is the case the duty owed should never be diminished. Mason and Whitehead (2003) point out that there must be an element of trust between both parties if there is to be an honest exchange of information and maintenance of secrecy. Without trust the therapeutic relationship between nurse and patient would be put in jeopardy: the patient may not be open and honest with the nurse. Patients place much trust in nurses and other health-care workers, for example doctors, so much so that patients permit nurses to perform intimate procedures on them and ask them personal questions in order to describe and reveal symptoms and problems they may be experiencing (Hope et al., 2003; Department of Health, 2003).

There have been many changes in the ways in which health care has been delivered over the years; this has resulted in devising new ways of protecting patient information. The Department of Health ordered NHS organisations to appoint a Caldicott Guardian who was to be charged with specific responsibility for ensuring that confidential information was protected within their organisation (Department of Health, 1997). The Caldicott Report (Department of Health, 1997) led to the production of an NHS code of practice concerned with the issue of confidentiality (Department of Health, 2003).

Section five of the NMC code of conduct (NMC, 2004) is solely dedicated to the issue of confidentiality and states clearly:

> *As a registered nurse, midwife or specialist community public health nurse, you must protect confidential information.*

While it is commendable for any nurse to seek to ensure that the important ethical principle of confidentiality is maintained, this is often a complex issue and there may be many situations where this will be challenged (Burnard and Chapman, 2003). Confidentiality is not an absolute principle, that is to say there are certain occasions when exemptions can be applied, and the confidence can be broken and the nurse overrides individual considerations, particularly when there may be implications for others – these instances are known as qualifications (Mason and Whitehead, 2003). Respect for a person's autonomy is an important component of confidentiality, however when the confidence is broken the nurse could be said to be acting in a paternalistic manner: 'nurse knows best'. When maintaining a confidence nurses are using the deontological ethical theory by keeping the patient's secret; conversely, they are acting in a utilitarian manner if they breach a confidence in order, for example, to safeguard the patient or others. In this instance nurses are operating in a maleficent manner (causing harm) as opposed to acting beneficently (the avoidance of doing harm).

If confidentiality is violated an individual has the right to sue through the civil courts. The individual can also make a complaint to the Information Commissioner if there has been a breach of the Data Protection Act 1998 (RCN, 2003). The patient has a right to confidentiality in law:

- common law
- Data Protection Act 1998
- Human Rights Act 1998

The patient can also complain about the nurse's alleged breach of confidentiality to the NMC and/or the employer (see Figure 2.3).

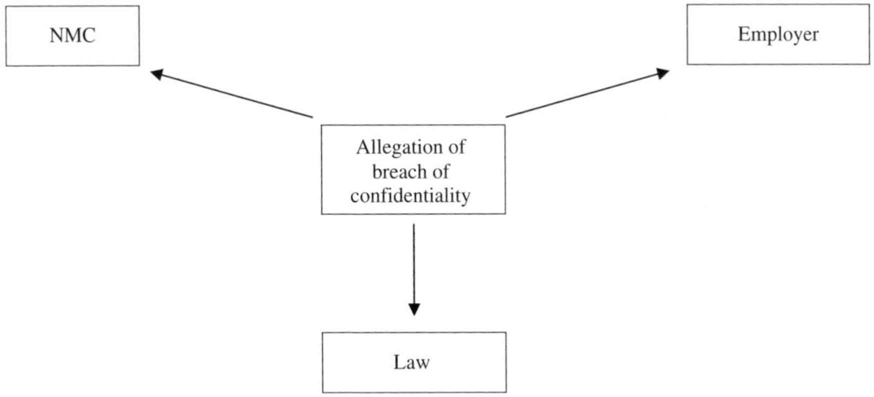


**Figure 2.3** Ways in which the patient may pursue a claim alleging a breach of confidentiality

## WHAT IS CONFIDENTIAL?

This question is not an easy one to answer. Information is provided to nurses in a variety of ways in a range of situations from many people. Beauchamp and Childress (2001) suggest that confidentiality is present when one person (the patient) discloses information to another (the nurse), and the nurse who has been given this information by the patient pledges not to disclose it to a third party without the patient's permission. The nurse has already agreed or pledged not to disclose the information by virtue of being on the professional register and adhering to the tenets of the code of conduct.

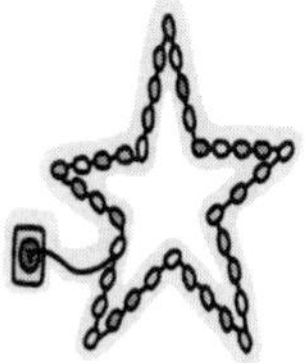

A nurse goes home after a busy day working on an oncology ward and tells her partner about the events of day. She happens to tell her partner that a patient she has been nursing that day has developed a urinary tract infection.

Clearly a breach of confidentiality has occurred: the nurse has disclosed confidential information to a third party without the patient's permission. How serious do you think this breach of confidentiality is?

Now consider this: A nurse goes home after a busy day working on an oncology ward and tells her partner about the events of the day. She happens to tell her partner that a patient she has been nursing that day has tested positive for HIV.

Again a breach of confidentiality has occurred. How serious do you think this breach of confidentiality is?

You may have felt that on both counts the confidence breached was serious. You may have thought that telling her partner about a patient developing a urinary tract infection was not as serious as telling her partner about a patient with HIV. Why? Was it because the implications of having HIV may be considered more serious than a urinary tract infection or that there is potential for stigma to arise because of being HIV positive? In both cases a confidence was violated.

Often nurses understand and are aware of the need to maintain confidentiality. Dimond (2005) suggests that challenges occur when issues concerning disclosure arise: what are the exceptions to maintaining confidentiality and the circumstances that would allow the duty to be violated? The NMC (2004) stipulates that improper disclosure should be avoided at all times. Permission needs to be granted by the patient for the nurse to disclose the information to a third party. In practical terms it is not always possible to seek permission to disclose information, but you must make the patient aware that there may be instances when the information obtained may be shared. There are many ways in which this can happen, for example by making explicit statements outlining the organisation's policy on the management of confidential information.

## THE CONFIDENTIALITY MODEL

The Department of Health has produced a model to help health-care professionals provide patients with a confidential service (Department of Health, 2003). The model informs staff that they must inform patients of the intended use of the information they provide, offer patients the choice to consent to or withhold their consent, as well as protecting the information that has been given (see Figure 2.4).

## DISCLOSURE OF CONFIDENTIAL INFORMATION

There are seven exceptions to the duty of confidentiality, according to Dimond (2005). These are detailed in Table 2.8.

### The Patient's Consent

The duty to maintain consent or to provide a confidence is owed to the patient, and as such the patient has the authority to allow disclosures to be made. When the patient provides the nurse with permission to disclose then there is no obligation to secrecy owed by the person receiving that consent (Mason and McCall Smith, 2005). The nurse should check with the patient to whom information may be disclosed, for example family members and employers.

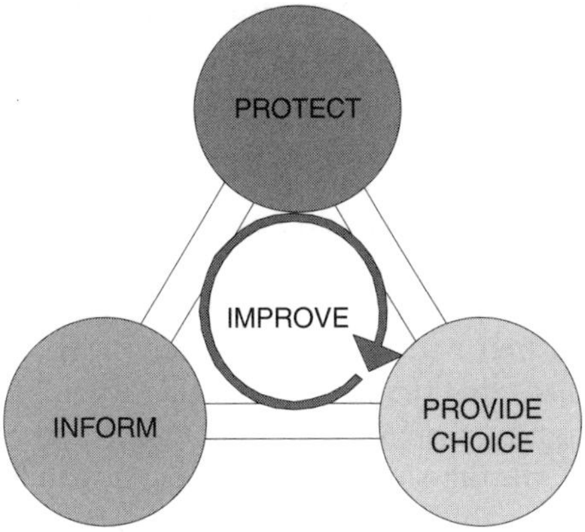


**Figure 2.4** The model of confidentiality
*Source*: Department of Health, 2003.

**Table 2.8** Seven exceptions that may allow the disclosure of confidential information

- With the patient's consent.
- In the patient's interests.
- Court order.
- Statutory duty to disclose.
- In the public's interests.
- Police.
- Provisions within the Data Protection Act 1998.

*Source*: Adapted from Dimond, 2005.

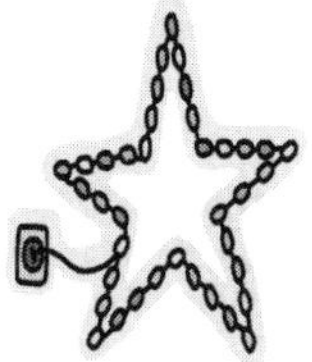

Martha is the nurse in charge of a gynaecology ward. One of her patients, Jean, has been admitted for a termination of pregnancy. Martha receives a telephone enquiry about Jean from a person saying he is Jean's father and asking how she is after the operation. Martha tells the caller that 'All went well.' He says he will be in later to pick her up and was it the gynaecology ward he needed to come to. Martha responds, 'Yes, the gynaecology ward on the third floor.' When Jean is fully awake Martha tells her that her father has called asking about her and that he will be in later to pick her up. Jean becomes very upset and tells Martha that she has no father and that her partner has threatened her if she goes ahead with the termination of pregnancy. Jean had told her partner she was away with her mother for a few days. Later it transpires that her partner had thought she would go ahead with the termination despite his objections and he had contacted several clinics and hospitals in the city.

Was confidentiality breached, as Martha only said that 'All went well', she did not say what the operation was for?

Confidentiality has been breached – unauthorised information has been given without Jean's consent. The nurse confirmed (unwittingly) what the partner had thought, that Jean was on the gynaecology ward. Acknowledgement that the patient is on a particular ward or unit, for example a psychiatric unit or a breast screening unit, could be deemed disclosure.

Martha should have checked with Jean whom she could disclose information to, if it became necessary. The ward or unit should have a policy in place to help Martha with regards to disclosure of any information.

**Disclosure in the Patient's Interests**

If information becomes known that would do the patient harm, then disclosure between the professionals involved in the patient's care would be justified. Dimond (2005) uses the problem of allergy to explain when disclosure in the patient's best interests may be permissible. For example, if the patient has told a doctor he/she has an allergy to a specific medication, then the nurse and pharmacist would need to be informed of this in order to prevent the administration of a drug that could potentially harm the patient.

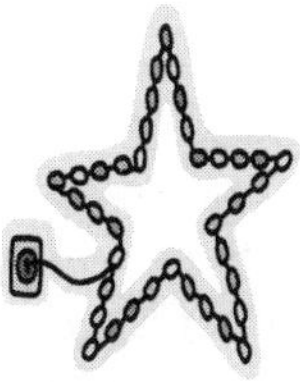

Jack is to undergo a right hip replacement. Jack has confided in you that he has a secret: he has hepatitis C and has not told the anaesthetist or the surgeon who have recently been to see him to talk about his operation tomorrow.

Having been given this information by Jack, whom, if anyone, might you tell – who needs to know?

Your answer to this question may be 'all those who care for him', or nobody as it has been told to you in confidence. The list of people you may tell could include:

- the surgeon
- the anaesthetist
- the theatre nurses and theatre staff
- the ward nurses

Would the following people also need to be informed?

- the staff who work in the pathology laboratory who may deal with Jack's body fluids
- the porter who transports his body fluids to the laboratory for analysis
- the domestic who cleans his room
- the phlebotomist who takes his blood for analysis

Those you do decide to tell (and you must only disclose in the patient's best interests) would also be bound by the duty of confidentiality. Disclosure of confidential information to others is justified if it is necessary to protect the health of the patient or the professionals who are to care for him/her. You must decide who they are and who truly needs to know, as opposed to those who may just be curious.

The response to this dilemma is difficult, as each case has to be considered on an individual basis. Each practitioner must decide on disclosure with regards to the specific circumstances (the context) associated with the individual case. Jack should have been told that information may be discussed and disclosed to other health-care professionals who care for him. The nurse should make every reasonable effort to persuade the patient to allow the information given to be disclosed to those who may need to know (Mason and McCall-Smith, 2005).

### Disclosure by Court Order

A court can demand a nurse to disclose information; this is known as a subpoena, and failure to disclose may render the nurse liable for contempt of court. There are, however, two grounds where the power of the court may fail to ensure disclosure and they are known as being privileged from disclosure. Public interest immunity is associated with national security and disclosure would be contrary to the public interest. Legal professional privilege is the second exception: this exception is associated with communications where litigation may occur or is taking place.

### Statutory Duty

There are statutory duties that will result in disclosure (regardless of the patient's wishes). Confidential information must be made known by law under the Acts detailed in Table 2.9.

### Public Interest

Disclosure is allowed if this is in the public interest. The major concern with disclosure under the heading of public interest is that there is no definition of public interest in law. Disclosure under this heading is referred to in the code of conduct (NMC, 2004) and exposure of information can only occur if there is a need to protect the patient or someone else from significant harm and the nurse acts for the good of society. Often disclosure would be justified if a serious crime has been committed, for example murder, child abuse or drug trafficking. Public interest has already been alluded to in the statutory duty to disclose in Table 2.9, for example the spread of infectious diseases.

### Disclosure to the Police

During a police investigation there may be instances where the police request a nurse to disclose information. There is no general legal duty to provide the police with information (apart from the issues described above; Dimond, 2005; Hendrick, 2004). It is, however, an offence to obstruct police investigations by providing false or misleading information. No offence will have been committed if the nurse refuses to answer questions posed by police providing the nurse has a lawful excuse for refusing; that is, their duty of confidentiality (Hendrick, 2004). A circuit judge can order that medical records be released

**Table 2.9** Statutory requirements to disclose

| Act | Requirement |
|---|---|
| Road Traffic Act 1988 | Any person is required to provide the police with information that is related to a road traffic accident that results in personal injury |
| Prevention of Terrorism Act 2005 | Any person who has information that he/she feels may be of assistance in the prevention of terrorism or apprehension of terrorists must make this known to the police |
| Public Health (Control of Diseases) Act 1984 | Any notifiable disease (e.g. plague, typhus, food poisoning), the name and the whereabouts of the person with the notifiable disease must be reported to the medical officer of the district |
| Abortion Act 1967 | Doctors must report to the Chief Medical Officer any information relating to termination of pregnancy |
| Births and Deaths Registration Act 1953 | Authorities must be notified of births and deaths |

to the police and the Coroner can ask to see the medical records of a dead patient (Hope et al., 2003).

**The Data Protection Act (1998) and Disclosure of Information**

Under the Data Protection Act 1998 every living person has the right to apply for access to their health records, including electronic and manual records (Hope et al., 2003). There are nine key principles associated with the Act, which aim to ensure that the data held is:

- accurate
- relevant
- held only for specific defined purposes for which the user has been registered
- not kept for longer than is necessary
- not disclosed to any unauthorised person

The Act allows data subjects (patients) to be:

- informed as to whether personal data is processed;
- provided with a description of the data held, the purposes for which it is processed and knowledge of the persons to whom the data may be disclosed;
- provided with a copy of the information constituting the data;
- given information on the source of the information.

There is also provision within the Act to allow a person to have the information rectified, to have inaccuracies corrected. As result of these inaccuracies, the patient may also have the right to receive compensation for the erroneousn entries that had been made.

A request, in writing, must be made by the patient to gain access to his/her records and a response to this request is then given to the patient within 40 days of the request being made. While provisions are made to enable the patient to gain access to medical records, certain information may be withheld in some circumstances. If it is deemed that the information could cause harm to the patient, access can be denied. Some of the circumstances are:

- potential physical or mental harm;
- if the request is made by some person other than the patient, e.g. a parent;
- if access would reveal the identity of another person, unless that other person has given their consent (this does not apply if the other person is a health-care professional who has been involved in the care of the patient, unless serious harm to that health-care professional's physical or mental health is likely to be caused by allowing access).

## INFORMED CONSENT

Any competent patient has the right to refuse any examination, any investigation or any proposed treatment. An adult patient can refuse any treatment, even if this treatment is considered to be 'life saving'. Every person has the right in law to consent to any touching of their person.

The concept of autonomy has already been considered from the nurse's and the patient's perspective. To uphold consent or to provide the patient with choice the issue of autonomy is central: the patient has the right to self-determination and what happens to his/her own body. Failure to comply with this principle may result in legal action (a charge of battery) by the patient and interference by the NMC, and furthermore should harm occur to the patient the nurse may also face a charge of negligence. There are situations where the law recognises that there are exceptions to the common-law requirement to obtain consent.

For consent to be valid there are three key principles that have to be satisfied (see Table 2.10).

**Table 2.10** Three key principles that have to be satisfied if consent is to be valid

| |
|---|
| • Consent is 'informed'. |
| • The patient is 'competent'. |
| • Consent is 'voluntary'. |

*Source*: Department of Health, 2001.

The patient needs to know in broad terms the nature and purpose of the procedure: failure to provide sufficient information would invalidate consent. The courts (*Sidaway* v. *Bethlam Royal Hospital Governors and Others* [1985]) have clearly demonstrated that when a competent individual has given consent (uncoerced) for a procedure to be performed, an action for trespass to the person cannot proceed. The patient should receive information about the procedure in general, for example how long it may take, what will happen as a result of the intervention/procedure, any alternatives and also information about specifics surrounding anaesthesia, for example will it be a general anaesthetic, regional or local anaesthesia. If the patient alleges that he/she was not given sufficient/significant information about the procedure, for example he/she was not told of the possible side effects and harm occurred, this may result in an action of negligence as opposed to battery. In order to ensure that the patient is provided with high-quality care, information is needed to help him/her consent to treatment. However this raises the question of how much information, and what information is needed.

There is no precise answer to the above question, however a general principle would be to expect the nurse to follow the reasonable standard of approved practice referred to as the Bolam test (*Bolam* v. *Friern Barnet HMC* [1957]). The Bolam test sets the standard that dictates how a nurse should practise in relation to other nurses; a nurse will be deemed negligent if he/she falls short of the standards expected of the 'reasonable' nurse. In summary, the nurse is judged against other reasonable nurses, how those reasonable nurses practise, and how they would act in the same or a similar situation. Below is an extract from the Bolam case that sets the expected standard:

> *The test is the standard of the ordinary skilled man exercising and professing to have that special skill. A man need not possess the highest expert skill at the risk of being found negligent . . . it is sufficient if he exercises the skill of an ordinary competent man exercising that particular art.*

Although this test concerns a doctor, the Bolam test is often used to judge the 'reasonableness' of any health-care professional's actions. It is now clear (Department of Health, 2001) that the final arbiter of what reasonable means will be the courts. However, what the NMC for example considers the standard of reasonable to be will remain influential.

One of the key reasons for providing the patient with information is to enable him/her to make a balanced judgement on whether to provide or withhold consent. The nurse is advised to provide the patient with any information that is 'material' or 'significant' (Department of Health, 2001) in relation to the risks he/she may take.

There may be some patients who do not wish to be informed of the treatment proposed, or only wish to know a little about it. In these cases the nurse should offer information and if the patient declines the offer this should be recorded in the patient's notes.

## PATIENT CAPACITY: IS THE PATIENT COMPETENT?

For a patient to be considered competent or to have the capacity to consent to treatment he/she must be able to comprehend and retain the information that has been given in order to make the decision. More importantly, he/she should understand the consequences of having or not having the proposed treatment. Having demonstrated an ability to do this he/she must then weigh this information in the decision-making process. Hence there are three elements associated with capacity:

- Comprehend and retain information.
- Understand the consequences of having or refusing the treatment.
- Weigh this information in the decision-making process.

All adults are said to have the capacity to consent. However, there may be situations where doubt exists and an assessment of capacity should be made. There may be some factors that might impinge on an individual's ability to understand, and therefore demonstrate the capacity to consent. These may include:

- shock/panic
- fear/anxiety
- pain
- the influence of medication (prescribed and nonprescribed)
- confusion

The nurse must take considerable care not to be influenced by his/her own feelings and beliefs. Some patients may be seen to be making irrational decisions regarding their treatment. Patients are entitled to make decisions based on their own beliefs and value system, even if this contradicts with the nurse's own system of beliefs.

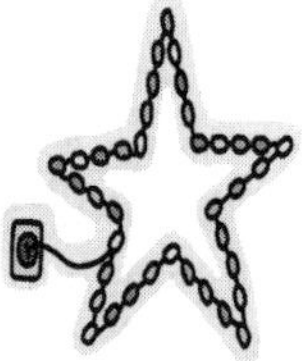

Jamie is a 22 year old who is suffering with anorexia nervosa. His physical condition is failing and he is losing a considerable amount of weight, he is very weak and unable to walk any more. He has been advised that tube feeding is the only alternative left to help his condition, but he is refusing. The team caring for Jamie has explained the situation and how seriously unwell he is.

How might you assess Jamie's capacity?

The three principles alluded to above must be assessed. Does Jamie understand the consequences of refusing to be tube fed? Can he comprehend and retain the information you have given him? Can he demonstrate to you that he has taken the information given to him and retained it? Does he understand the potential consequences and has he weighed this information in the decision-making process?

If Jamie is able to do this it would be difficult to consider him incapacitated or incompetent to refuse treatment.

The patient must be able to communicate his/her decision to the heath-care team. The nurse should never underestimate the patient's ability to communicate regardless of physical or psychological condition. For example, in the case of a patient with learning disabilities the nurse must make use of all resources available to facilitate communication, and this may include taking time to explain to the individual the issues in simple language, employing visual aids and if appropriate signing. It may be advisable for the nurse to engage the support of those who know the patient, for example the family, carers and staff from statutory and nonstatutory agencies.

## VOLUNTARY CONSENT

Consent must be given freely and voluntarily, without any pressure or undue influence being exerted on the patient. If the nurse feels the patient is being pressurised into agreeing to (or refusing) treatment by the family, for example, he/she should arrange to see the patient alone to ascertain if the decision is truly that of the patient.

Coercion invalidates consent. If a patient is being treated in an environment where he/she is being involuntarily detained, for example a psychiatric hospital, a psychiatric unit or a prison, care must be taken to ensure that the patient is not being coerced (Department of Health, 2001).

## CHILDREN AND YOUNG PEOPLE

For those under the age of 18 (the age of majority) the situation regarding consent and refusing treatment is different from the position for adults.

Those aged 16 to 17 years of age are entitled to consent to their own medical treatment (Family Law Reform Act 1969). Gaining consent from this age group will be the same as it is for adults. However, in this age group the refusal of treatment despite the person being aged over 16 years and competent can be overridden by a person with parental responsibility or the order of a court.

Those under 16 years of age who have sufficient understanding and intelligence to enable them to fully understand what is involved in the proposed intervention may have the capacity to consent to that intervention (Department of Health, 2001) Children who possess these abilities are said to be 'Gillick competent'. The term Gillick competent comes from a court case,

*Gillick* v. *West Norfolk and Wisbech Area Health Authority* [1985] 3 All ER HL. This concerned a teenage girl's right to consent to medical treatment without her parents' knowledge.

The child should be assessed to determine Gillick competence. Below are some questions that need to be asked:

- Does the child understand the proposed treatment, his/her medical condition, the consequences that may emerge if he/she refuses or agrees to treatment?
- Does he/she understand the moral, social and family issues involved in the decision he/she is to make?
- Does the mental state of the child fluctuate?
- What treatment is to be performed – does the child understand the complexities of the proposed treatment and potential risks associated with it?

## GIVING CONSENT

Consent can be gained in the following ways:

- written
- oral
- nonverbal

Written consent is thus only one way in which consent can be given. Written consent only serves as evidence of consent. A signature on a consent form does not in itself serve to say that the patient has consented to treatment if the consent did not meet the three elements of valid consent outlined in Table 2.10. A consent form related to a child is provided in Appendix 2.1.

Many aspects of nursing care are carried out with the patient orally agreeing to them. Oral consent lacks the written evidence as identified above, as it may be one person's word against another's (Dimond, 2005). Where any significant procedure (e.g. a surgical operation) is anticipated it is suggested that written consent be obtained (Department of Health, 2001).

Nonverbal or implied consent occurs in many situations and Dimond (2005) cites the case of the patient who when the nurse approaches him/her rolls up his/her sleeve for an injection, or the patient who sees the nurse coming towards him/her with a sphygmomanometer and rolls up his/her sleeve to have his/her blood pressure taken.

It is important to note that no one can give consent on behalf of an incompetent adult; however, treatment may still be given if it is considered to be in the patient's best interests. If the person you care for needs medical treatment, only he/she can agree to that treatment. No one can legally give or withhold consent to medical treatment on behalf of another adult.

Best interests go further than medical best interests and should include the patient's wishes and beliefs when he/she was competent. In some instances these best interests may have been made known in the form of an advanced directive.

## ADVANCED DIRECTIVES

Sometimes advanced directives are also known as living wills or advanced statements; these terms are often used interchangeably. The advanced directive is a legally binding statement in certain situations. Advanced directives allow people to state (in written form) what type of treatment they would or would not like carried out should they become unable to decide for themselves in the future.

Advance directives are a way for patients to communicate their wishes to family, friends and health-care professionals in order to avoid confusion later on, should they become unable to do so. Advanced directives can only be written by those who have reached the age of majority – 18 years (Fletcher and Buka, 1999).

Despite an increase in the number of advanced directives, their legal status remains ambiguous (Farsides, 2002; Burnard and Chapman, 2003). The patient must be deemed competent when making the advanced directive, and only clear refusals of specific treatments will be upheld. If any doubt exists as to the validity of the advanced directive, then a declaration may be obtained or treatment can be given in the patient's best interests. Refusal of the provision of basic care cannot be refused. Refusal of treatment that falls within the remit of the Mental Health Act 1983 treatment provisions cannot be refused by the use of an advanced directive.

## LEGAL PERSPECTIVES

Throughout the above aspect of this chapter the law and some legal perspectives have been discussed and how they impinge on nursing practice. A number of legal issues need to be considered by the nurse when working with patients in any setting. There are few areas of health care that are untouched by the law and involvement with the legal process may occur during the course of a nurse's career (Wall and Payne-James, 2004).

### THE LAW

Orderly behaviour in a collective society is governed by rules, and these rules are referred to in this context as laws. Wall and Payne-James (2004) state that the law is an official expression of the formal institutionalisation of the enforcement of these rules through:

- promulgation
- adjudication
- enforcement

The principal source of law is Parliament. The three points above are operated and organised through the system of the courts.

## SOURCES OF LAW

There are two primary forms of law that emanate through statute and common law:

- *Primary legislation* is established through Acts of Parliament, also known as statute. The law-making abilities are given to Parliament by society. There are various stages proposed and legislative law must pass through these prior to becoming enforceable. An Act of Parliament does not become statute until it has passed through both Houses of Parliament (the House of Commons and the House of Lords) and received royal assent. Secondary legislation is the making of regulation by statutory instruments.
- *Common law*, also known as case law or judge-made law, is law that is decided through the court system. This type of law comes into play when the courts cannot turn to a relevant statute. This may be because a particular Act of Parliament concerning the specific area of law under deliberation has not been made. In case law the courts look to precedent, considering previous cases to determine how a decision has been made and how statute has been interpreted.

The legal system is divided into:

- civil law
- criminal law

and a hierarchical court system exists where different courts administer the two kinds of law (see Table 2.11).

**Table 2.11** The criminal and civil courts

| | |
|---|---|
| **Civil law** | Concerned with the resolution of disputes between individuals (or in some instances organisations). Remedies in these courts are usually financial. |
| **Criminal law** | Associated with issues between the state and the individual. The outcome of a prosecution (if the seriousness of the offence warrants a prosecution) of an individual is usually in the form of a sentence or a fine – it is punitive. The outcome of the prosecution depends on the ability of establishing a standard of proof that is beyond reasonable doubt. |

**Table 2.12** The civil courts and their key functions

| Court | Key function |
|---|---|
| **House of Lords** | This is the final appellate court in the UK |
| **Court of Appeal (Civil Division)** | Will hear appeals on matters of law |
| **High Court** | Generally, hears the more complex cases and often the cases heard here are high monetary value cases. The High Court is divided into three divisions: |
| • **Chancery Division** | Specialises in matters such as company law |
| • **Family Division** | Specialises in matrimonial issues and matters associated with minors |
| • **Queen's Bench Division** | Concerned with issues of a general nature related to civil matters |
| **County Court** | Most civil cases are heard in the County Court |
| **Magistrates Court** | The lowest of the civil courts |

*Note*: Those under the age of 18 years are tried at special courts – youth courts.

**Table 2.13** The criminal courts and their key functions

| Court | Key function |
|---|---|
| **House of Lords** | This is the final appellate court in the UK. Often cases heard here are associated with important points of law |
| **Court of Appeal (Criminal Division)** | This court will hear appeals on matters of law |
| **Crown Court** | This court will hear the more serious or indictable offences. In the first instance it also hears any appeals from the Magistrates Court regarding points of law, conviction, or sentences passed |
| **Magistrates Court** | The lowest of the criminal courts. The majority of minor criminal cases are heard in this court |

*Note*: Those under the age of 18 years are tried at special courts – youth courts.

A lower court is bound by a decision of a higher court and is obliged to apply the principles of law set by that higher court. Tables 2.12 and 2.13 outline the civil and criminal courts' primary functions.

## EUROPEAN LAW

European law can also influence English law. In the past the greater part of European law was centred on free movement and economic activity; generally this is still the case. However, there are certain areas relevant to health care.

## THE HUMAN RIGHTS ACT 1998

The primary aim of this Act is to give the courts greater powers to protect some fundamental rights; it introduces the European Convention on Human Rights into British domestic law. Articles of the Act can be found in Appendix 2.2. All legislation must be compatible with the rights outlined in this Act. If incompatibility with primary legislation happens, then a declaration of incompatibility must be made.

The principles underpinning human rights apply to all nurses and they are to:

- maintain dignity
- promote and protect autonomy
- practise in a nondiscriminatory manner

## EUROPEAN DIRECTIVES

The European Union adopts legislation in the form of Directives and Regulations. European Directives require member states to implement their provisions for the benefit of Europe as a whole. Progammes for registration as an adult nurse must comply with the requirements of two European Directives, in particular 77/453/EEC and 89/595/EEC. These requirements are mandatory and require that awards (certificates and diplomas) be granted before registration. Article 1 of 77/453/EEC requires that the qualifications of adult nurses guarantee that the person has acquired:

- Adequate knowledge of the sciences on which general nursing is based, including sufficient understanding of the structure, physiological functions and behaviour of healthy and sick persons, and of the relationship between the state of health and physical and social environment of the human being.
- Sufficient knowledge of the nature and ethics of the profession and of general principles of health and nursing.
- Adequate clinical experience; such experience should be selected for its training value and should be gained under the supervision of qualified nursing staff in places where the number of qualified staff and the equipment are appropriate for the nursing care of patients.
- The ability to participate in the training of health personnel and experience of working with such personnel.
- Experience of working with members of other professions in the health sector.

This Directive also specifies that nursing programmes comprise a programme of three years with 4600 hours of training, with a balance between theory and practice. Practical instruction must include nursing in relation to:

- general and specialist medicine
- general and specialist surgery
- child care and paediatrics
- maternity care

- mental health and psychiatry
- care of the old and geriatrics
- home nursing

Directive 89/595/EEC makes clear the balance of theory and practice and dictates that this must be not less than one third theory and one half practice. The Directive also defines theoretical and clinical instruction. The NMC (2004), however, has dictated that a programme should contain 2300 hours of practice.

Both Directives cited are related to those students who embark on the adult branch of a pre-registration programme of study, regardless of whether the programme is offered at diploma or degree level.

## CONCLUSIONS

Ethical and legal issues will impinge on all aspects of physical and psychological care. Nurses are faced with ethical and legal challenges on a daily basis. It is therefore important that they have an understanding of the underlying principles associated with legal and ethical theory when applying this to nursing care.

This chapter has briefly described two ethical theories and various ethical principles associated with nursing practice. Key terms have been defined in order to promote a better and deeper understanding of the key issues. Most definitions of ethics include the term morals and suggest that ethics is the study of moral thinking. Ethics and morals can be broadly stated to be concerned with what is good or bad.

Confidentiality, the cornerstone of nursing practice, was discussed in detail. The close relationship between confidentiality and veracity was outlined, and trust and respect identified as two key features required by both the nurse and the patient if confidentiality is to exist. A patient has the right to expect that information given in confidence will be used only for the purpose for which it was given and will not be released to others without their permission. Patients permit nurses to perform intimate procedures on them and allow them to ask personal and probing questions in order to describe and reveal symptoms and problems they are experiencing. Without the element of trust this would not occur and could result in harm to the patient. Confidentiality is not an absolute principle – there are exceptions to the duty of confidentiality, seven of which were discussed. If confidentiality is to be breached then the nurse must consider the situation carefully in order to justify that decision.

Any competent patient has the right to refuse any examination, any investigation or any proposed treatment. If a nurse disregards this right then the patient may seek a remedy in law – a charge of battery. Consent is closely related to the ethical principle of autonomy and self-determination. Three key principles must be present if consent is to be valid: consent must be informed, the patient must be deemed competent and there must be no coercion associated with seeking consent (or refusal). There are separate rules for those who are aged less than 18 years of age. The person aged less than 16 years must be Gillick competent if he/she is to consent to treatment. Three key methods of providing consent were briefly outlined. The important point that no one can give consent on behalf of an incompetent adult was stressed, unless (in certain circumstances) there is an advanced directive or living will detailing what events should occur if the patient becomes unable to decide for him/herself in the future.

A brief overview of the English legal system was provided outlining the two primary sources of law – statute and common law. The impact of European legislation and the Human Rights Act 1998 was alluded to. Two particular European Directives were cited that impinge on the design and content of programmes of study associated with those students undertaking the adult branch.

## REFERENCES


Beauchamp, T.L. and Childress, J.F. (2001) (5th edn) *Principles of Biomedical Ethics*. Oxford University Press. Oxford.

Berlin, I. (1969) *Four Essays on Liberty*. Oxford University Press. Oxford.

Bolam *v.* Friern Barnet HMC [1957] 1 All ER 118.

Burnard, P. and Chapman, C.M. (2003) (3rd edn) *Professional and Ethical Issues in Nursing*. Balliere Tindall. London.

Cribb, A. (2002) 'The ethical dimension: Nursing practice, nursing philosophy and nursing ethics' in Tingle, J. and Cribb, A. (eds) (2nd edn) *Nursing Law and Ethics*. Blackwell. Oxford. Ch 2 pp 19–30.

Department of Health (1997) *The Caldicott Committee: Report on the Review of Patient Identifiable Information*. Department of Health. London.

Department of Health (2001) *Reference Guide to Consent for Examination or Treatment*. Department of Health. London.

Department of Health (2003) *Confidentiality: NHS Code of Practice*. Department of Health. London.

Dimond, B. (2005) (4th edn) *Legal Aspects of Nursing*. Longman. Harlow.

Dworkin, G. (1988) *The Theory and Practice of Autonomy*. Cambridge University Press. Cambridge.

Edwards, S.D. (1996) *Nursing Ethics: A Principle-Based Approach*. Palgrave. Basingstoke.

Farsides, B. (2002) 'An ethical perspective – Consent and patient autonomy' in Tingle, J. and Cribb, A. (eds) (2nd edn) *Nursing Law and Ethics*. Blackwell. Oxford. Ch 7b pp 121–130.

Fletcher, L. and Buka, P. (1999) *A Legal Framework for Caring: An Introduction to Law and Ethics in Health Care*. Palgrave. London.

Fry, S. and Johnstone, M.J. (2002) *Ethics in Nursing Practice: A Guide to Ethical Decision Making*. Blackwell. Oxford.

Fry, S. and Veach, M. (2000) *Case Studies in Nursing Ethics*. Jones and Bartlett. Sudbury.

Gastmans, C. (2002) 'A fundamental ethical approach to nursing. Some proposals for ethics education'. *Nursing Ethics*. Vol 9, No 5, pp 494–507.

Harkreader, H. and Hogan, M.A. (2004) (2nd edn) *Fundamentals of Nursing: Caring and Clinical Judgement*. Saunders. St Louis.

Hendrick, J. (2004) *Law and Ethics*. Nelson Thorne. Cheltenham.

Hope, T., Savulescu, J. and Hendrick, J. (2003) *Medical Ethics and Law: The Core Curriculum*. Churchill Livingstone. Edinburgh.

Husted, G.L. and Husted, J.H. (1995) (2nd edn) *Ethical Decision Making in Nursing*. Mosby. New York.

Kennedy-Schwarz, J. (2000) 'The "ethics" of instinct'. *American Journal of Nursing*. Vol 100, No 4, pp 71–73.

Kirby, C. and Slevin, O. (2003) 'Ethical knowing: The moral ground of nursing practice' in Basford, L. and Slevin, O. (eds) (2nd edn) *Theory and Practice of Nursing: An Integrated Approach to Caring Practice*. Nelson Thorne. Cheltenham. Ch 13 pp 209–254.

Mason, J.K. and McCall-Smith, R.A. (2005) (7th edn) *Law and Medical Ethics*. Oxford University Press. Oxford.

Mason, J.K., McCall-Smith, R.A. and Laurie, G.T. (2002) *Law and Medical Ethics*. Butterworth. London.

Mason, T. and Whitehead, E. (2003) *Thinking Nursing*. Open University Press. Milton Keynes.

McAthie, M. (1999) 'Ethical issues in nursing practice' in Linderman, C.A. and McAthie, M. (eds) *Fundamentals of Contemporary Nursing Practice*. Saunders. Philadelphia. Ch 9 pp 141–154.

*New Oxford Dictionary of English* (2001) Oxford University Press. Oxford.

Nursing and Midwifery Council (2004) *Standards of Proficiency for Pre-registration Nursing Education*. NMC. London.

Olsen, T.H. (2004) 'Ethical issues' in Daniels, R. (ed.) *Nursing Fundamentals: Caring and Clinical Decision Making*. Thompson. New York. Ch 9 pp 165–177.

Parker, M. and Dickenson, D. (2001) *The Cambridge Medical Ethics Workbook*. Cambridge University Press. Cambridge.

Royal College of Nursing (2003) *Confidentiality: RCN Guidance for Occupational Health Nurses*. RCN. London.

Royal College of Nursing (2004) *Research Ethics: RCN Guidance for Nurses*. RCN. London.

Rumbold, G. (1999) (3rd edn) *Ethics in Nursing Practice*. Bailliere Tindall. London.

Seedhouse, D. (2002) 'An ethical perspective – How to do the right thing' in Tingle, J. and Cribb, A. (eds) (2nd edn) *Nursing Law and Ethics*. Blackwell. Oxford. Ch 8b pp 150–158.

Sidaway *v.* Bethlam Royal Hospital Governors and Others [1985]1 All ER 643.

Stauch, M., Wheat, K. and Tingle, J. (2002) (2nd edn) *Source Book on Medical Law*. Cavendish Publishing. London.

Thiroux, J.P. (1995) *Ethics, Theory and Practice*. Prentice Hall. Englewood Cliffs.

Thompson, I.E., Melia, K.M. and Boyd, K.M. (2003) (4th edn) *Nursing Ethics*. Churchill Livingstone. Edinburgh.

Wall, I. and Payne-James, J. (2004) 'Legal institutions and the legal process' in Payne-James, J., Dean, P. and Wall, I. (eds) *Medico-Legal Essentials in Health Care*. Greenwich Medical Media. London. Ch 1 pp 1–9.

Whaite, I. (2002) 'Ethics' in Kenworthy, N., Snowley, G. and Gilling, C. (eds) (3rd edn) *Common Foundation Studies in Nursing*. Churchill Livingstone. Edinburgh. Ch 3 pp 77–112.

## APPENDIX 2.1 CONSENT FORM EXAMPLE

Department of Health

# [ANY HOSPITAL ANY TOWN]
# Consent form 2

## Parental agreement to investigation or treatment for a child or young person

**Patient details (or pre-printed label)**

Patient's surname/family name.................................

Patient's first names ..............................................

Date of birth ..........................................................

Age ......................................................................

Responsible health professional..................................

Job title ................................................................

NHS number (or other identifier)..................................

☐ Male ☐ Female

Special requirements ............................................
(e.g. other language/other communication method)

**To be retained in patient's notes**

**Patient identifier/label**

**Name of proposed procedure or course of treatment** (include brief explanation if medical term not clear)

..........................................................................................................

..........................................................................................................

..........................................................................................................

..........................................................................................................

**Statement of health professional** (to be filled in by health professional with appropriate knowledge of proposed procedure, as specified in consent policy)

I have explained the procedure to the child and his or her parent(s). In particular, I have explained:

The intended benefits

..........................................................................................................

..........................................................................................................

..........................................................................................................

Serious or frequently occurring risks

..........................................................................................................

..........................................................................................................

..........................................................................................................

..........................................................................................................

..........................................................................................................

Any extra procedures which may become necessary during the procedure

☐ blood transfusion..........................................................................

☐ other procedure (please specify)....................................................

..........................................................................................................

..........................................................................................................

I have also discussed what the procedure is likely to involve, the benefits and risks of any available alternative treatments (including no treatment) and any particular concerns of this patient and his or her parents.

☐ The following leaflet/tape has been provided.........................................

This procedure will involve:

☐ general and/or regional anaesthesia ☐ local anaesthesia ☐ sedation

Signed:.................................................. Date ..............................................

Name (PRINT) ........................................ Job title..........................................

**Contact details** (if child/parent wish to discuss options later)

**Statement of interpreter** (where appropriate)

I have interpreted the information above to the child and his or her parents to the best of my ability and in a way in which I believe they can understand.

Signed.................................................... Date ..............................................

Name (PRINT) ...........................................................................................

**Top copy accepted by patient: yes/no (please ring)**

**Statement of parent** **Patient identifier/label**

Please read this form carefully. If the procedure has been planned in advance, you should already have your own copy of page 2 which describes the benefits and risks of the proposed treatment. If not, you will be offered a copy now. If you have any further questions, do ask – we are here to help you and your child. You have the right to change your mind at any time, including after you have signed this form.

**I agree** to the procedure or course of treatment described on this form and **I confirm** that I have 'parental responsibility' for this child.

**I understand** that you cannot give me a guarantee that a particular person will perform the procedure. The person will, however, have appropriate experience.

**I understand** that my child and I will have the opportunity to discuss the details of anaesthesia with an anaesthetist before the procedure, unless the urgency of the situation prevents this. (This only applies to children having general or regional anaesthesia.)

**I understand** that any procedure in addition to those described on this form will only be carried out if it is necessary to save the life of my child or to prevent serious harm to his or her health.

**I have been told** about additional procedures which may become necessary during my child's treatment. I have listed below any **procedures which I do not wish to be carried out** without further discussion.........................................

.................................................................................................................

.................................................................................................................

.................................................................................................................

.................................................................................................................

Signature ..................................................... Date .............................................
Name (PRINT) .......................................... Relationship to child ....................

Child's agreement to treatment (if child wishes to sign)

I agree to have the treatment I have been told about.

Name ......................................................... Signature ......................................
Date ..........................................................................................................

**Confirmation of consent** (to be completed by a health professional when the child is admitted for the procedure, if the parent/child have signed the form in advance)

On behalf of the team treating the patient, I have confirmed with the child and his or her parent(s) that they have no further questions and wish the procedure to go ahead.

Signed:........................................................ Date ..............................................
Name (PRINT)........................................... Job title..........................................

Important notes: (tick if applicable)

☐ See also advance directive/living will (eg Jehovah's Witness form)
☐ Parent has withdrawn consent (ask parent to sign/date here)

*Source*: This is Crown copyright material which is reproduced with the permission of the controller of HMSO and the Queen's Printer for Scotland.

## APPENDIX 2.2 ARTICLES OF THE HUMAN RIGHTS ACT 1998

Article 2: Right to life

Article 3: Prohibition of torture

Article 4: Prohibition of slavery and enforced labour

Article 5: Right to liberty

Article 6: Right to a fair trial

Article 7: No punishment without law

Article 8: Respect for private and family life

Article 9: Freedom of thought, conscience and religion

Article 10: Freedom of expression

Article 11: Freedom of assembly and association

Article 12: Right to marry

Article 14: Prohibition of discrimination

# 3 Diversity and Culture

Every patient is a unique human being and is entitled to care that is provided in a fair and nondiscriminatory manner, acknowledging that there are differences in beliefs and cultural practices between patients and within patient groups. This chapter provides the reader with the knowledge with respect to diversity and culture when caring for patients from various communities and diverse circumstances, for example those patients with disability, however manifest.

The key aim of this chapter is to ensure that the student can act in such a way as to ensure that the rights of individuals and groups are respected and not compromised. It is important that the values, customs and beliefs of the patient are respected, and that the care provided is sensitive to the diverse needs of the patient the nurse is caring for.

Discrimination and disadvantage can obstruct the nurse's aim to provide care and have the potential to lead to inequality. Respecting and valuing the diversity of the people you work with, and the patients you care for, will help to ensure a quality service. In the *NHS Plan* (Department of Health, 2000) and the *National Service Framework for Older People* (Department of Health, 2001a) there is a clear message that age discrimination has no place in health-care delivery.

There are many differences that make us all unique, here are some of them:

- language
- religion
- race
- employment status
- class
- culture
- physical abilities

As a result of these differences it is important to recognise that a national, uniform service – a 'one-size-fits-all' approach to health care – cannot work and will fail to meet the needs of diverse populations (NHS Executive, 2000a).

The greater part of this chapter will focus on inequalities in health care and how to begin to tackle them. There remain striking inequalities in health care between groups and areas in the UK; one effect is that average life expectancy is the same today as the national average in the 1950s (Department of Health, 2002a).

## DEFINING KEY TERMS

In order to provide care that respects the patient, is inclusive and takes into account his/her individuality, the nurse will have to understand and be able to define key terms.

### CULTURE

Culture is a complex concept and has many facets associated with it. It can be summarised by saying that it describes patterns of learned human behaviour that are transferred from one generation to another (Hickerton, 2005). Culture is not transferred via biological mechanisms. Marsh (2000) suggests that culture is related to values, customs and accepted modes of behaviour that characterise a society or social groups within a society. Rodriguez (2004) believes culture to be associated with:

- knowledge
- beliefs
- ideas
- behaviours
- habits
- customs
- languages
- symbols
- rituals
- ceremonies
- practices

All of the above are unique to a particular group of people. Each person is culturally unique. Culture, like ethnicity, is fluid and dynamic. People may possess culturally predetermined values and beliefs, but these are subject to change and refinement as new information is gained.

Within particular cultural groups there is much diversity and the differences can come about as a result of individual practices and perspectives. The characteristics of culture, according to Rodriguez (2004), are the same for all cultures (see Table 3.1).

### ETHNICITY

The term ethnicity is highly contested and its precise meaning remains elusive. According to Ratcliffe (2004) the term in practice tends to be used loosely in the context of health. Ethnicity means a group that people belong to because of shared characteristics, including ancestral and geographical origins, cultural traditions, languages and skin colour. Bhopal (1997) suggests that ethnicity has become a euphemism for race.

**Table 3.1** Characteristics of culture

| |
|---|
| • Culture is learned and taught. |
| • Culture is shared. |
| • Culture is social in nature. |
| • Culture is dynamic, adaptive and ever changing. |

*Source*: Rodriguez, 2004.

Ethnicity is a fluid concept and the interpretation of it will depend on context. Self-assessment of ethnicity allows the individual to choose for him/herself. It can alter over time therefore: the person's original self-assessment of his/her chosen ethnic group can change depending on the interpretation at that time – and this is his/her privilege. Attempting to measure ethnicity with any degree of accuracy is therefore problematic (Ratcliffe, 2004). According to Giger and Davidhizar (2004) the most important characteristic of ethnicity is that the members of an ethnic group feel a sense of identity.

## RACE

While ethnicity can be described as a fluid concept, Malik (1996) considers race to be a floating signifier, implying that it has attached to it a variety of meanings that differ significantly to the biological notions associated with it. Humans are one species; there are no biological distinctions between them and little variation in genetic composition. When considering the term race in the pure sense of homogeneous populations, race does not exist in human species – there is only one human species. The term race is often used alongside ethnicity.

The concept of race is scientifically invalid, however race still retains a central position in contemporary society (Ratcliffe, 2004). Physical characteristics distinguishing races result from a small number of genes that do not relate closely to either disease or behaviour (Bophal, 1997). However, Giger and Davidhizar (2004) suggest that race can be related to biology. They suggest that members of a particular race share distinguishing physical features such as:

- bone structure
- skin colour
- blood group

For some, race may merely be a convenient set of descriptors; for others, it may have far more sinister connotations associated with it. The use of the term race can result in making a group feel inferior to the more dominant group, what Ratcliffe (2004) terms inferiorisation, in so far as it has the potential to be hierarchical.

### GENDER

Gender and gender roles are closely related to cultural context. Biological sex refers to male or female characteristics. Gender, however, refers to how we are expected to behave as men and women, how society expects men and women to 'be', and the way men and women are expected to be will differ between cultures (Nelson, 2005). Gender is a social construction; both men and women are gendered beings.

The media, schools and religion convey socially constructed meanings related to masculinity and femininity and these constructions can shape people's gender identities. Gender is that which cultural meaning has ascribed to such biological differences. It is a person's concept of him/herself as male or female. Physical appearance is likely to play a defining role (Rutter, 2000; Peate, 2004).

Gender can have an effect on the patient's physiological measurements – vital signs. Rayman (2004) states that women experience greater temperature fluctuations than men and this may be as a result of hormonal changes. Males in general have higher blood pressure than females of the same age. Vallerand and Polomano (2000) have reported that women in general have lower pain thresholds, a greater aptitude to distinguish painful sensations, higher pain ratings and a lower tolerance for pain than men.

### SPIRITUALITY

Fulton (2003) suggests that spiritual health relates to having a sense of meaning, hope and purpose in life. It is not only about having religious faith. Spirituality does not belong only to those who are dying or suffering, however it is often situated within the death and dying sections of some textbooks. Spirituality is an aspect of every part of our lives, what we do and how our bodies respond. When faced with illness (but not exclusively) our spiritual beliefs can be threatened. If this occurs the impact or the outcome can be harmful.

## VALUING DIVERSITY

### CULTURALLY COMPETENT NURSING CARE

The 2001 Census reported that the size of the UK minority ethnic population was 4.6 million; this is equivalent to 8 per cent of the total population. The data demonstrates that there has been an increase of 53 per cent based on the census of 1991 (Picker Institute Europe, 2003).

The code of professional conduct (2.2) (NMC, 2004) states:

> *You are personally accountable for ensuring that you promote and protect the interests and dignity of patients and clients, irrespective of gender, age, race, ability, sexuality, economic status, lifestyle, culture and religious or political beliefs.*

The crux of this statement is that nurses should not discriminate against any patient they care for; they should promote and protect each patient's diverse needs. Discrimination of any kind has no place in professional nursing care.

Culturally competent care has multidimensional facets associated with it. Mold et al. (2005) suggest that the provision of culturally competent care is a continuous challenge. Care provision should be built around the individual needs of individual patients. Some aspects of nursing care may be affected and even determined by issues such as religion or ethnic background. High-quality nursing care will recognise and respond in a sensitively effective, empathic and flexible manner, committed to ensuring that these needs are met – care should reflect the patient's life, beliefs and community.

Nurses should aim to preserve and accommodate the cultural beliefs, values and deep-rooted ideologies that some patients may have in this increasingly diverse society. Respecting these values and beliefs is true patient advocacy.

When managing diversity the nurse needs to focus on the care needs of people with differences and similarities in beliefs, values and cultures in order to provide culturally congruent, meaningful and beneficial health care (Leininger and McFarland, 2002). Nursing care should be provided in a multicultural environment that respects diversity.

The nurse must ensure that whatever social customs characterise the ethnic group being cared for, these customs are not neglected, but valued and facilitated. These customs may include:

- dietary practices
- religious practices
- dress
- social interactions within groups
- specific rituals enacted during periods of ill health, death and dying

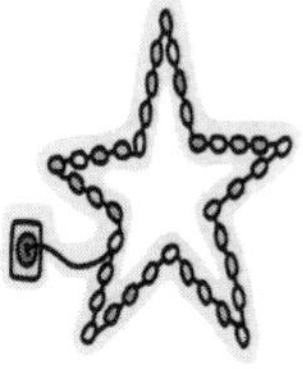

How would you typify the customs of someone who describes themselves as White English?

Your list may have included comments such as:

- stiff upper lip
- lover of fish and chips
- tea drinker
- celebrates Christmas
- goes to the pub

There may be some people who describe themselves as White English who may engage in all of the above, there may also be some who do not. Not all English people like tea, some White English people regard themselves as believing in the Christian God but may never go to church, they may be Jewish and go to the synagogue or could be atheist. Some may be vegans and not eat fish.

Britain is a multicultural and multifaith society. Developments in clinical practice will include cultural awareness regarding assessment, interpretation and information for patients and the public.

Improved patient care will emerge where there is an increasingly culturally competent workforce. This workforce will be more understanding and better informed about the cultural, economic and social aspects of disease (NHS Executive, 2000b). The next aspect of this chapter considers good practice in relation to culturally competent care and focuses on information regarding several ethnic and religious groups, including summaries of their beliefs and customs, along with health-care-related advice.

## GENERAL CONSIDERATIONS AND GOOD PRACTICE GUIDELINES

Every patient should be treated equally, regardless of gender, race or creed. They should have free access to religious support with the opportunity to practise their chosen religion while being cared for.

When first meeting the patient the nurse should establish the patient's ethnic identity and ascertain if he/she has a religious association (do not assume that if you have a religious faith others also have one). The information provided by the patient should be noted in the patient's case notes. Early on in the relationship anticipate with the patient if there are likely to be any issues that could arise during the examination, investigation, diagnosis, treatment or medication aspects of his/her care. Discuss with the patient how best you can help to have his/her religious/cultural needs met while caring for his/her. Ensure that the rest of the team caring for the patient are aware of these specific needs.

Admission to a mixed-sex ward may be problematic for members of some cultures where men and women are strictly segregated. Physical examination or investigation being carried out by a nurse of the opposite gender may be unacceptable. As far as possible the patient's needs and wishes should be met. Chaperones should be made available for all patients (RCN, 2002).

Appropriate information and interpretation are essential if the patient is to provide informed consent. Any information booklets or leaflets provided to patients explaining to them what to expect in hospital, or about a proposed investigation or examination, should be translated into several languages, particularly those that are most common in the local community. Translators may be needed if the nurse does not speak the patient's language. However, the use of family members may not always be ideal as they may be unfamiliar with the medical terminology, and both the patient and family member may be reticent about discussing sensitive information with older or younger relatives. Local liaison groups or the patient advisory liaison service may be able to recommend other resources to help translate.

When we are unable to communicate with patients because of language difficulties those patients are in danger of becoming disenfranchised. If the patient's first language is sign (British Sign Language) then the nurse may need to use interpreters, text telephones and telephone amplifiers. Televisions should have teletext subtitle provision.

Some patients may wish to fast in observing religious requirements and the nurse may need to make arrangements to have food available outside the fasting period. It may be acceptable to allow the patient's family, friends or community to bring in food, however the nurse must check hospital policy regarding this and ensure that if a medical diet is required this is adhered to. Always offer the patient choice, for example do not assume that a patient automatically takes milk in their drinks. Some Jews will not accept milk mixed with other liquids. Some foods may be prohibited and there may be requirements concerning the way other foods are prepared. Avoid using local names for food: some people may not know what is meant by 'Welsh rarebit' or 'Irish stew'.

Table 3.2 provides an overview of some ethnic groups and information the nurse may find helpful when providing culturally competent nursing care. Care and sensitivity are needed when caring for all patients. The nurse must ensure that he/she preserves the modesty of the patient at all times and, when possible, provide space for the patient to worship as he/she sees fit. Furthermore, the nurse should consult with the patient, and if appropriate the family, when addressing needs at a time when there may be much pain and suffering, for example as the patient is dying and when the patient has died. Religious and cultural views must be upheld while caring for the dying person (Department of Health, 2001b). The nurse is advised to seek advice and help from the appropriate religious organisation if he/she has any queries regarding the patient's cultural needs.

## MEASURING SOCIAL INEQUALITIES

Since 1911 in the UK the most popular method of measuring inequalities has been through occupation. This method, the Registrar General's scheme, was developed originally to construct the 1911 census. It was the head of the household – the male – whose occupation was used to determine the social class membership of that household. Oakley (1974) makes three points about methods of defining social stratification using the 1911 system:

- The family is the unit of social stratification.
- The social position of the family is determined by the status of the man in it.

**Table 3.2** An overview of some ethnic groups and information the nurse may find helpful when providing culturally competent nursing care

| | Introduction | Health care | Death and dying | Food | Notes |
|---|---|---|---|---|---|
| **Buddhism** | Buddhism is a way of life as opposed to an organised religion; it is intended to be a collection of ways to help individuals seek betterment and enlightenment, it is not a set of ritualistic practices. The Buddha means the Enlightened One. | There are no strict dress codes for Buddhists unless they are nuns or priests.<br><br>If possible a separate room should be made available so the Buddhist patient can meditate or chant in private, and without disturbing other patients. | **At the moment of death**<br>Tibetan Buddhism explains the process of death in eight clear stages. At the fourth stage, when breathing stops (when the air element dissolves), death has not yet occurred because it is felt that consciousness still exists for up to three days.<br><br>**After death and preparation of the body**<br>As death does not occur for up to three days, the body (if in hospital) should be moved to an empty room. Death has occurred when heat is no longer emitted from the heart, the body begins to emit an odour and a small amount of fluid leaves the sexual organs or the nostrils. Mantras can be chanted and prayers read. If the body needs to be touched in order to move it then the crown of the head or the hair on the crown should be touched or pulled. Once this has happened other body parts can be touched. | Many Buddhists are vegetarians or vegans as they should not be responsible for the death of any other living organism.<br><br>Buddhists do not condone the consumption of recreational drugs or the use of alcohol. | At any stage of the patient's stay or death a Buddhist priest should be contacted to help guide and support care. |

**Table 3.2** *Continued*

| | Introduction | Health care | Death and dying | Food | Notes |
|---|---|---|---|---|---|
| **Buddhism continued . . .** | | | Post mortem examination is usually acceptable to Buddhists. However, a post mortem occurring within three days of death should be avoided.<br><br>Organ donation can be discussed with the family of the deceased. There is much debate about organ donation and therefore the nurse should consult a priest.<br><br>It is normal for cremation to take place several days after the body has lain in state.<br><br>It is not a Buddhist trait to grieve after a person has died.<br><br>The body may be donated to science, so long as time has been allowed for the consciousness to be dispersed (normally three days).<br><br>Suicide is not forbidden but is deeply regretted by the Buddhist community.<br><br>Termination of a pregnancy is believed to be unethical by many Buddhists. Most Buddhists would regard the decision to undergo a termination of pregnancy a very serious one. | | |

**Table 3.2** *Continued*

| | Introduction | Health care | Death and dying | Food | Notes |
|---|---|---|---|---|---|
| **Church of England** | The Church of England is the established or state church in England. As the Church of England is the established church, many nonpractising Christians cite it as their religion, some as a matter of course, and may or may not seek comfort from it during times of illness.<br><br>Some members of the Church of England may wish to receive Holy Communion when they are in hospital, and possibly the sacrament of the sick. | There are no strict dress codes for Christians unless they are nuns or priests. | A dying patient may request to see a member of the clergy before death and receive the sacrament of the sick. They, or their visitors, may wish to have prayers at their bedside. Routine last offices are appropriate for a dying Christian. More prayers may be said after someone has died.<br><br>After death, a Christian should be wrapped in a sheet with their arms and hands placed at their sides. They may be buried or cremated, in accordance with their wishes.<br><br>Christians do not usually have any religious objections to organ donation and post mortems.<br><br>Most Christians view suicide as a rejection not of life itself, but of a particular life, and as a cry for help.<br><br>The Church of England is opposed to abortion. | Some Christians may not eat meat on Fridays. They should therefore be offered a fish or vegetarian alternative. | |

**Table 3.2** *Continued*

| | Introduction | Health care | Death and dying | Food | Notes |
|---|---|---|---|---|---|
| **Hinduism** | Hinduism has developed over thousands of years; it includes a diverse range of customs and beliefs.<br><br>It is difficult to generalise about Hinduism due to its diversity. | Generally female Hindus adhere to dress codes. A sari is a common item of clothing. Most Hindu patients would prefer to be examined by health-care staff of the same gender as themselves. A chaperone should be provided; family members may act as chaperones. Young men and boys are often chaperoned by their father or brother and young women and girls by their mother or sister. A married woman may be chaperoned by her husband or sister-in-law.<br><br>Specific care must be taken with any sacred objects the patient is wearing, for example jewellery, threads or *bindi* (the holy | As with most other religious groups Hindus have last rites and religious ceremonies to perform. Often the immediate and extended family make every effort to pay their last respects to a family member who is in the final stages of dying. Most Hindus would prefer to die at home. A dying Hindu may request to be nursed on the floor in order to be as close to Mother Earth as possible.<br><br>The family of the dead patient may prefer to prepare the body. A clean white sheet should be used to wrap the body. There are many rituals that may need to be observed.<br><br>Hindus prefer to cremate the dead body as soon as possible.<br><br>Generally, there is no objection to organ donation. If a post mortem is required this should be conducted as soon as possible so that arrangements can be made for the cremation to take place. | Most Hindus are strict vegetarians or vegans. The cow is considered to be a sacred representation of the bounty of the gods. It is important to ensure that all medication is free from beef products such as gelatin.<br><br>Hindus are not permitted to eat meat, drink alcohol or smoke. As with any religion some Hindus may vary in their adherence to such rules. | Many Hindus have strong beliefs in Ayurvedic medicines. They may wish to continue using Ayurvedic medicines and prescribed medications. |

**Table 3.2** *Continued*

| | Introduction | Health care | Death and dying | Food | Notes |
|---|---|---|---|---|---|
| **Hinduism continued . . .** | | dot is an auspicious makeup worn by young Hindu females on their forehead). If a man's sacred thread needs to be removed prior to surgery the nurse must ensure it is never placed on the floor, close to the feet or shoes or any place where it may become contaminated by body fluids.<br><br>A toothbrush is generally used to clean the teeth but the patient may also use a 'U' wire tool to clean his/her tongue. | | | |

**Table 3.2** *Continued*

| | Introduction | Health care | Death and dying | Food | Notes |
|---|---|---|---|---|---|
| **Christian Scientists** | Christian Science is a Christian religion. Christian Scientists do not believe in medical intervention and are likely to be in hospital for child birth only, for the setting of broken bones or involuntarily. | It is not uncommon for Christian Scientists to be cared for and treated by practitioners or nurses who are themselves Christian Scientists, who would only provide food, cleansing and prayer or religious reading.<br><br>Dental care is permitted but it must be performed without any pain relief.<br><br>Christian Scientists are opposed to all medications and this will include pain relief. | When a Christian Scientist is dying no medical intervention is permitted and when a Christian Scientist dies, no rituals or rites need to be performed.<br><br>A dead female body should be handled by female staff.<br><br>Cremation is often preferred to burial; however the choice is up to each individual.<br><br>Unless it is legally required a Christian Scientist is unlikely to consent to a post mortem. | Usually no particular diet is followed; however Christian Scientists do not use alcohol or tobacco, and may not drink tea or coffee. | All health-care decisions are up to the individual, some parents may agree to their children receiving life-saving medical intervention. |
| **Jehovah's Witnesses** | Jehovah's Witnesses believe in the teachings of the Bible, using | Jehovah's Witnesses are opposed to taking blood or blood products into the body, preferring | There are no particular rites and rituals associated with death and dying. A dying Witness patient may request a visit from one of the elders of their | Issues concerning blood or blood products are also related to food. Anything that | Jehovah's Witnesses worship in Kingdom Halls as often as five times per week, and at large |

**Table 3.2** *Continued*

| | Introduction | Health care | Death and dying | Food | Notes |
|---|---|---|---|---|---|
| **Jehovah's Witnesses continued . . .** | their own translation. Jehovah's Witnesses do not use the symbol of the cross because they believe it to be of pagan origin. | to use alternative treatments. For example, bloodless surgery does not involve the use of blood or blood products. | faith.<br><br>Individuals can opt for burial or cremation.<br><br>Termination of pregnancy is unacceptable to Jehovah's Witnesses.<br><br>It is unlikely that a Jehovah's Witness will object to a post mortem.<br><br>Jehovah's Witnesses may not wish to donate their organs as another person's blood would flow through them. In organs that do not involve blood flow, for example corneas, this is acceptable. | contains blood or blood products is unacceptable, as is meat from an animal that has been strangled, or shot and not bled properly. Some Jehovah's Witnesses do not eat meat at all.<br><br>It is believed that tobacco and other recreational drugs are incompatible with Jehovah's Witness principles. Drinking alcohol is allowed but drunkenness is not condoned. | gatherings three times a year. Bone-marrow transplants may be acceptable to some individuals, as may be albumin, immuno globulin or clotting factors – each patient must be assessed individually.<br><br>Vaccination is acceptable.<br><br>A special card is carried by most Jehovah's Witnesses that identifies them as such, and directs staff to avoid using blood or blood products in their treatment. |
| **Catholics** | The Catholic Church (also known as the Roman Catholic Church) is one of the major Christian | There are no strict dress codes for Catholics unless they are nuns or priests. | A priest should always be called when a Catholic patient is dying. Routine last rites are appropriate for all Christians.<br><br>It is unlikely that a Catholic will have any religious objections | Some Catholics may not eat meat or drink alcohol on Fridays and on Ash Wednesday. | There are many rituals associated with the Catholic Church.<br><br>The Catholic Church is opposed |

**Table 3.2** *Continued*

| | Introduction | Health care | Death and dying | Food | Notes |
|---|---|---|---|---|---|
| **Catholics continued . . .** | churches in the UK.<br><br>Patients may request to take regular holy communion and arrangements may also have to be made for them to make a confession. | | to organ donation and the same relates to post mortem examinations.<br><br>The Catholic Church has always condemned the termination of pregnancy. | | to artificial contraception and sterilisation. |
| **Sikhism** | Sikhism is prevalent in Indian society. There are five signs that Sikhs must wear at all times, known as the five Ks:<br><br>**Kesh**: Uncut beard and uncut hair.<br>**Kangha**: A wooden comb.<br>**Kara**: A steel bracelet worn around the right wrist.<br>**Kirpan**: A sharp knife with a double-edged blade.<br>**Katchera**: Specially made | Running water is the preferred method of maintaining hygiene. If a shower is not available then a bowl and jug are acceptable.<br><br>The combing of the hair on a regular basis with the kangha is important for Sikhs and they may need help from the nurse to do this.<br>Unless the patient has given you permission do not touch or remove any of the five Ks. If any of the | Prior to touching the body of a dead Sikh the nurse must wear gloves to avoid direct contact. The nurse should not wash the body as the family may wish to carry out this task. Never remove any of the five Ks. The body should be wrapped in a clean white sheet.<br><br>There is no Sikh ruling against post mortem examination or the donation of organs.<br><br>The decision to bury or cremate the body is left up to individual choice.<br><br>Suicide is a grave offence and the deceased is expected to serve great penance in a later life.<br><br>Termination of pregnancy is considered taboo. | Sikhs generally do not eat meat, most are vegetarian and some are vegan. | The place of worship for Sikhs is called a Gurdwara. It is also seen as a community centre, a teaching room and a kitchen. |

**Table 3.2** *Continued*

| | Introduction | Health care | Death and dying | Food | Notes |
|---|---|---|---|---|---|
| **Sikhism continued** . . . | long underpants. | items are removed they should be treated with respect and never placed on the floor or close to a person's feet. If the turban or head scarf is removed provide the patient with alternative hair covering such as a theatre cap. If hair needs to be removed, for example prior to surgery, then ask the patient for permission and determine if he/she would like it to be returned after it has been removed. | | | |
| **Judaism** | The followers of Judaism are diverse. It is a religion, a way of life and a culture, and because of this it is difficult to | Some Jews may need help from the nurse with ritual washes they have to perform prior to eating and praying.<br><br>The nurse should | Death occurs according to the Halakhic definition when the body is without heart beat or breath.<br><br>If possible always stay with the body after death until help arrives. It is considered | Jewish patients should be offered Kosher food. Kashrut rules apply equally to both foods and medicines. When available a Kosher | Each Jewish community can have different ways of interpreting the laws of the religion. It is divided into three |

**Table 3.2** *Continued*

| | Introduction | Health care | Death and dying | Food | Notes |
|---|---|---|---|---|---|
| **Judaism continued** ... | define Judaism. | bear in mind that there may be some restrictions placed on the Jewish patient on the Sabbath and other holidays.<br><br>Some Jewish holidays may require the patient to fast. These holidays do not have a fixed date each year and the nurse needs to bear this in mind when caring for the patient. | disrespectful to leave the body alone or in the dark before burial. A light should always be left on.<br><br>Prior to touching the body of a dead Jew the nurse must wear gloves to avoid direct contact.<br><br>Ideally the body should be buried within 24 hours of death.<br><br>The nurse should leave catheters, drains and tubing in position, they should be buried with the patient – as they are considered a part of the body.<br><br>As a general rule post mortem examinations are not permitted under Jewish law unless this is legally required.<br><br>Organ donation may be permitted where a transplant is vital to save a life.<br><br>Generally cremation is forbidden by Jewish law and burial is the preferred method of body disposal.<br><br>Suicide is condemned and forbidden in Jewish law. | alternative should be made available. | major categories:<br>Orthodox<br>Reform<br>Liberal/progressive<br><br>The nurse should seek the help and advice of a rabbi if there are concerns regarding the care of the Jewish patient. |

*Source*: Adapted from Akhtar, 2002; Baxter, 2002; Christmas, 2002; Collins, 2002; Gill, 2002; Jootun, 2002; Northcott, 2002; Papadopoulos, 2002; Simpson, 2002.

- Only in rare circumstances is the social position of women not determined by that of the men to whom they are attached by marriage or family of origin.

Using such an approach denied acknowledgement of women's occupations and as such they did not receive their own social class position. The focus when undertaking measurement therefore considered occupation in isolation, neglecting other kinds of social difference.

The system employed may have been appropriate then and possibly did reflect the characteristics of the population at the time. However, in the twenty-first century that may not be the case as it neglects to consider the many social and economic changes that have occurred over the years, for example the increase in the number of women who are employed and the decline of manual work. The old system has undergone modification and was renamed in 1990 as the Social Class Based on Occupation System, but it continues to be used to describe data regarding health. Table 3.3 outlines the current system.

**Table 3.3** Social class based on occupations

| Social class | Occupation |
|---|---|
| **I** Professional | Accountants, engineers, doctors |
| **II** Managerial and technical/intermediate | Nurses, marketing and sales managers, teachers, journalists |
| **IIIN** Non-manual skilled | Clerks, shop assistants and cashiers |
| **IIIM** Manual skilled | Carpenters, goods van drivers, cooks, joiners |
| **IV** Partly skilled | Security guards, machine tool operators, farm workers |
| **V** Unskilled | Building and civil engineering labourers, other labourers, cleaners |

*Source*: Drever and Whitehead, 1997.

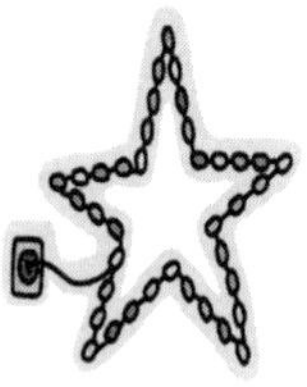

Did you expect to see nurses in social class II? You may have expected the nursing profession to be in social class I alongside doctors, or conversely you might have thought that nurses should be situated within social class IIIN, since nursing is often described as a hands-on profession.

In the grouping scale described above, where might you place or think that the following occupations should be placed:

- police officers
- university lecturers
- hairdressers
- publicans
- undertakers
- librarians
- social workers

Think about those people who have never had paid work, as result of disability for example, what category would they fall into?

The current schema to some extent captures some of the important features of social inequality (Department of Health, 2003). As a person moves up the class ladder, standards of living improve alongside educational attainment, employment prospects and health.

There are a number of other issues that will impinge on social differentiation such as ethnicity, gender, sexuality, age, area, community and religion (Anthias, 1992; Bhopal, 1997; Department of Health, 2003). These are outlined in Figure 3.1.

Determinants of health include all of the nongenetic and biological influences on health (Department of Health, 2003) and, as such, would include individual risk factors such as smoking. These determinants must also be considered as they have the potential to impinge on a person's health and can modify life chances. Nazroo (2003) notes that socioeconomic disadvantage is a major contributor to the health of African-Caribbean, Bangladeshi and Pakistani groups of people. Racial discrimination can also take its toll on the health of these communities.

While the current occupation approach scheme used to measure social inequalities, health experiences and patterns of mortality has some valid purpose, a concerted effort must be made to produce a measure that encompasses and embraces all of the factors (and more) described in Figure 3.1.

## HEALTH INEQUALITIES

Equality was the founding principle of the NHS (Ross, 1952). Since its foundation there has been an era of extraordinary progress in many fields, people are living longer and are more prosperous than ever before, and new treatments that could never have been thought possible a generation ago are saving thousands of lives each year (Department of Health, 2003). Britain is now collectively healthier than it has ever been (Health Development Agency, 2004). Yet there are sections of our society who are still treated unequally in respect to health-care provision.

The cost of these inequalities to individuals, communities and the nation is huge. People who are affected by the inequalities die at a younger age and are likely to spend more of their lives suffering ill health.

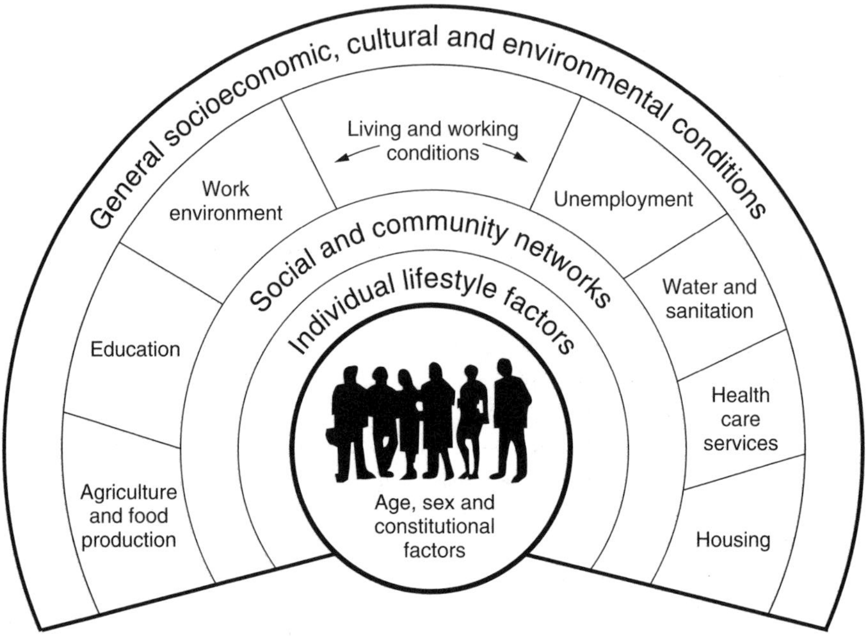


**Figure 3.1** Factors that have the potential to modify health and impinge on a person's life chances
*Source*: Acheson, 1998. This is Crown copyright material which is reproduced with the permission of the Controller of HMSO and the Queen's Printer for Scotland.

Addressing the various problems and inequalities faced by a diverse nation means that we must recognise that the problems are a result of diverse and complex causes. While at a distance the health inequalities appear to be similar they are not. This means that they will require diverse solutions, as opposed to identical approaches, to tackle local needs experienced by the most disadvantaged in our society. A mix of national standards and local services is required to meet a diversity of local needs: local solutions for local health inequality problems. Local communities know best what their problems are and how to handle them. The Department of Health (2003) suggests that health inequalities are stubborn, persistent and difficult to change. There is a need to address both the short-term consequences of avoidable ill health and the longer-term causes.

Health and wellbeing are influenced by several factors, including past and present behaviours, the type of health provision available to treat illness and injury, and provision of care for those with disabling conditions, as well as social, cultural and environmental factors. Income, education, employment, housing and lifestyle must also be considered. Wanless (2004) asserts that some of these issues have traditionally been considered outside of the health domain. However, it is impossible to devise policy and provide meaningful health care if they are not included in the health provision equation.

When health analysts measure health inequalities they use data that demonstrates that, when measured by occupation, there is a marked difference in health. They do this using a top-to-bottom occupational hierarchy (Acheson, 1998). Using the evidence generated by analysis of the data provides others (for example governments) with the information to produce policies that will help to reduce the inequalities in health care. The key aim is to enhance health and decrease health differences between groups occupying unequal positions within society (Graham, 2004a).

Having determined that there are inequalities in health, a response is required to address and tackle these inequalities. Those responsible for the formulation of policy must take into account those members of society:

- who find themselves in the poorest circumstances
- with the poorest health
- who are most socially excluded
- with the highest risk factors
- who are difficult to reach

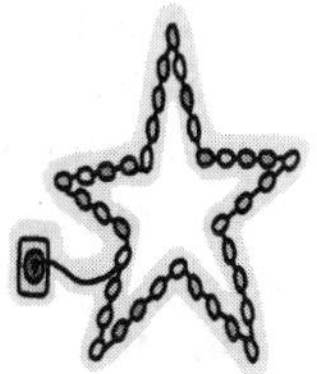

Can you think of who some of those people may be?

You might have a list that resembles that in Table 3.4.

## SOCIAL POSITION

Social position is related to the position people find themselves at in the social hierarchy. People occupy many social positions, for example a black gay woman in a managerial occupation or a heterosexual white man in a manual occupation. The Department of Health (2003) suggests that many health researchers regard social position as lying at the root of how healthy a person is.

Social position encompasses a person's educational level and their employability and the work they do. For example, this links directly to risk factors they are exposed to affecting or impacting on their health, such as workplace hazards, damp housing and poor diet (Department of Health, 2003). Graham (2005) states that there is an enduring association between socioeconomic position and health, both over time and across major causes of death. This is marked even further in children and adults with learning disabilities, as they

**Table 3.4** Some members of society who should be given particular consideration when policy and approaches to addressing and tackling inequalities in health are being proposed and formulated

| Those at risk | Example |
|---|---|
| Those who find themselves in the poorest circumstances | Socially and educationally deprived individuals |
| Those with the poorest health | People with long-term conditions such as HIV, diabetes mellitus |
| The most socially excluded | The elderly<br>The disabled<br>People with learning disabilities |
| Individuals with the highest risk factors | People who smoke<br>Those who do not exercise<br>Some people with specifically genetically inherited diseases |
| Those who are difficult to reach | The homeless<br>People in prison<br>Individuals who do not have English as their first language |

are disproportionately represented among the poorer and less healthy sections of society. Figure 3.2 demontrates how the key health determinants are interconnected and result in the wellbeing of the person.

The association between socioeconomic position and health has endured over the years. In contemporary society changes have occurred, for example chronic disease has replaced environmentally transmitted infections (Department of Health, 2003). Table 3.5 demonstrates how the association between socioeconomic position and health over the years has changed but still continues.

The following discussions will briefly outline some of the inequalities faced by individuals and communities. The reader is encouraged to consult other key texts for a deeper understanding and insight related to inequality and health care.

## CHILDREN AND HEALTH INEQUALITIES

In childhood the effects of poverty and disadvantage begin before birth (in utero). For example, a mother's poor nutritional status will have an effect on her unborn child who will be undernourished and vulnerable, potentially leading to serious long-term disease in adult life. Graham and Power (2004) have highlighted how an adult's socioeconomic position (as lawyer or unskilled worker, for example) is impressively shaped by the socioeconomic status of the parents. An increase in child poverty has profound implications for health inequalities in both current and future generations (Graham, 1999).

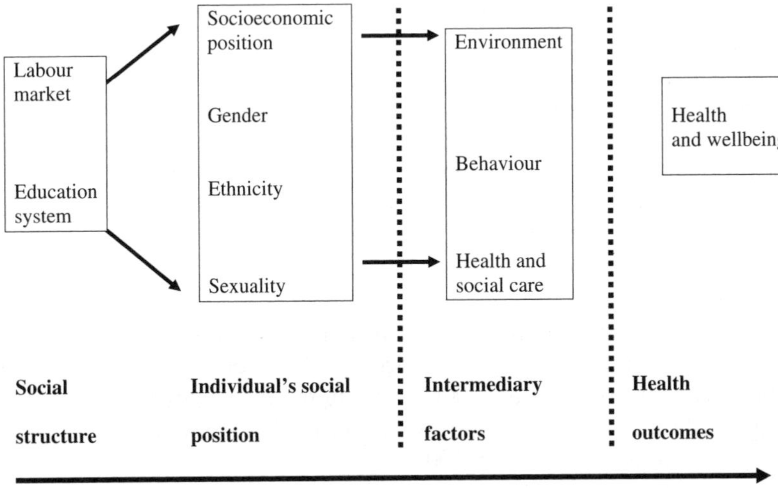


**Figure 3.2** Key health determinants and the association they have with health outcomes
*Source*: Graham, 2005.

**Table 3.5** Socioeconomic position and health outcomes

| Period of time | Health outcome | Social position | Rates |
|---|---|---|---|
| 1911 | **Infant mortality** by father's occupation | Higher nonmanual occupations<br>Semi and unskilled labourers | 42 deaths per 1000 births<br>171 deaths per 1000 births |
| 1959–63 | **Death rates from suicide** by social class (men aged 15–64 years) | Social class I<br>Social class V | 91 deaths per 100 000 person years<br>184 deaths per 100 000 person years |
| 1997–1999 | **Death rates from ischaemic heart disease** by social class, men and women aged 35–64 years | Social class I and II<br><br><br>Social class IV and V | Men<br>90 deaths per 100 000 person years<br>167 deaths per 100 000 person years<br>Women<br>22 deaths per 100 000 person years<br>50 deaths per 100 000 person years |

*Source*: Registrar General, 1913; Reid, 1977; White et al., 2003.

Every child is exposed to the possibility of injury as part of their everyday life. However, the burden is not evenly distributed: injury affects some children more than others. Variations occur in injury mortality and morbidity. These variations reflect a child's age, social and economic factors, gender, culture, ethnicity and the place where they live (Health Development Agency, 2005). Socioeconomic gradients are also apparent in birth weight, cognitive and physical development and range of adult diseases (Kuh et al., 2003). Children and adolescents who come from poorer families are more likely to experience mental health problems such as emotional, behavioural and hyperkinetic problems than those who come from better-off families (Meltzer et al., 2000). In one study, in families with a gross income of less than £100 per week mental health problems among boys affected 22 per cent, compared with 7.1 per cent of those boys who lived in a family whose income was over £770 per week (Meltzer et al., 2000).

Families who have a child with learning disabilities are significantly economically disadvantaged when compared with other families with a child (Disability Rights Commission, 2004). Among families living with a child with learning disabilities 44 per cent are living in poverty, compared with 30 per cent of other families (Emerson, 2003).

The inequalities specifically associated with children, as with other groups, cannot be explained by one single set of risk factors such as smoking or poor diet. The environment in which the child has been raised and family relationships, for example, can also impinge on health outcomes for the child (Disability Rights Commission, 2004).

## INEQUALITIES RELATED TO PEOPLE WITH LEARNING DISABILITY AND MENTAL HEALTH

While it has been noted that opportunities for good health are not equally distributed among all people, people with a disability are affected by the broader issues associated with inequality, and also specific issues that disability brings with it. Living with illness and impairment can make economic hardship hard to avoid. Issues such as persisting health difficulties and discrimination increase the risk of unemployment, dependency and poverty (Maughan et al., 1999).

In the Disability Discrimination Act 1995 disability is defined as:

> *A physical or mental impairment which has a substantial and long-term adverse effect on a person's ability to carry out normal day-to-day activities.*

Impairment covers both physical and mental impairments. These include:

- physical impairments affecting the senses, such as sight and hearing;
- mental impairments including learning disabilities and mental illness (if it is recognised by a respected body of medical opinion).

The term 'substantial' means more than minor, for example:

- Inability to see moving traffic clearly enough to cross a road safely.
- Inability to turn taps or knobs.
- Inability to remember and relay a simple message correctly.

Consideration must also be given to the term 'long-term'. This means that the condition will have lasted at least 12 months or is likely to last at least 12 months or for the rest of the life of the person affected.

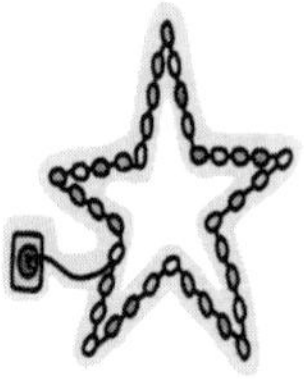

Can you list some of the conditions that may be covered by the Act?

Did you remember to consider conditions experienced by those with mental health problems and learning disabilities as well as physical conditions? For example:

- cancer
- HIV infection
- multiple sclerosis
- muscular dystrophy

The Department of Health (1999) has acknowledged that there are higher levels of mental health problems associated with being worse off financially. It is estimated that 10 per cent of neurotic disorders in the UK can be attributed to a low standard of living (Lewis et al., 1998).

Those with a mental illness are expected to have higher than average rates of physical illness (Seymour, 2003). In particular, the greater prevalence of smoking-related fatal disease among people with schizophrenia results in higher death rates (Joukamaa et al., 2001).

Despite the fact that GP consultations are three to four times higher for people with mental health problems than the general population (Seymour, 2003), people who use psychiatric services are less likely to be offered health-promotion interventions such as smoking-cessation assistance or blood-pressure checks (Cohen and Hove, 2001).

A learning disability is defined in *Valuing People* (Department of Health, 2001b) by the presence of both:

- A significantly reduced ability to understand new or complex information, to learn new skills (impaired intelligence).
- A reduced ability to cope independently (impaired social functioning), which started before adulthood, with a lasting effect on development.

People with learning disabilities have an increased risk of early death when compared with the population in general and those with severe impairments have higher mortality rates (NHS Scotland, 2004).

In a study confined to two districts in London, it was estimated that the risk of dying under the age of 50 years between 1982 and 1990 was almost 58 times higher than in the general population. Hollins et al. (1998) reported that this risk was significantly associated with:

- cerebral palsy
- incontinence
- mobility impairments
- residence in a hospital

The key cause of death for those with a learning disability is respiratory disease associated with pneumonia, dysphagia and gastro-reflux disorder. These are followed by coronary heart disease; almost half of the people with Down's syndrome have congenital heart problems (NHS Scotland, 2004; Elliot et al., 2003).

Those with learning disabilities have a greater variety of health-care needs. However, these needs go unmet or unrecognised compared with the general population (Kerr, 2004). Unrecognised or poorly managed medical conditions, according to Elliott et al. (2003) and Kerr (1998), include:

- hypertension
- obesity
- coronary heart disease
- abdominal pain
- respiratory disease
- cancer
- gastrointestinal disorders
- diabetes mellitus
- chronic urinary tract infections
- oral disease
- musculoskeletal conditions
- visual and hearing impairments

There is much inequality among people with learning disability, for example issues concerning the availability and uptake of cervical and breast screening need further investigation. Uptake of immunisations against tetanus, poliomyelitis and influenza, according to NHS Scotland (2004), is lower than among the general population. Lack of uptake of influenza immunisation is a concern, as it has already been stated that people with learning disability have a high prevalence of respiratory infection associated with premature deaths as a result of pneumonia.

## OLDER PEOPLE AND HEALTH INEQUALITIES

There is a substantial body of research on inequalities in the health of the population as a whole and among working-age people. Much less research is available on health inequalities in the older population, particularly concerning people in late old age. Mortality data associated with social class in older people (those aged 65 years or over) is limited as occupation is not recorded at all on death certificates of men and women who are aged over 75 years (Acheson, 1998).

When using alternative measures of social classification, for example housing tenure, it is noted that compared to the national average the mortality rates for those aged 60 to 74 years who had been living in local authority rented accommodation showed a 16 per cent excess, whereas those who had been living in owner-occupied accommodation showed a 13–14 per cent deficit (Smith and Harding, 1997).

Life expectancy at 65 years is 2.6 years greater in men (2 years greater in women) from social classes I and II compared to men from social class IV and V (Hattersley, 1997). Grundy and Holt (2000) have demonstrated that those older people who have followed more disadvantaged pathways throughout their adult lives, for example long periods of unemployment, earlier age at marriage and more children, were more likely to report ill health and experience longstanding illness. Other life events such as the death of a child and getting fired from work were also seen as risk factors for poorer health. Those older people who reported lack of social support also had worse health (Grundy and Holt, 2001).

## GENDER INEQUALITIES

Many boys and girls have similar experiences throughout childhood, however they are exposed to different risks. As the boy and girl become man and woman they are yet again exposed to risks, but different risks associated with the labour market and home circumstances.

Men on average die four years younger than women (Cooper, 2001). There is a vast amount of data available for the poor state of men's health when compared to women's. Table 3.6 outlines some of those inequalities.

Mortality in males is greater at all ages. From 1 to 14 years the higher mortality rates are in boys and they are more likely to die from:

- poisoning and injury
- motor vehicle accidents
- fire and flames
- accidental drowning and submersion

As the boy ages the gender differences in mortality widen, so that by the time the boy reaches 15 years he will have a 65 per cent higher potential mortality than girls (Botting, 1997).

The majority of suicides now occur in young males. In men under 35 years of age suicide is the most common cause of death. There are many factors associated with suicide and they include (Department of Health, 2002b):

**Table 3.6** Some data comparing certain health outcomes for men and women

| Health outcome | Men | Women |
|---|---|---|
| Life expectancy at birth – years (UK, 1997) | 74.6 years | 79.6 years |
| Life expectancy at birth by social class – years (England and Wales, 1987–91) | | |
| Classes I and II | 74.9 years | 80.2 years |
| Classes IV and V | 69.7 years | 76.8 years |
| Heart disease – death rates per 100 000 from ischaemic heart disease (England, 1998) | 251.3 | 203.9 |
| Cancer – death rates per 100 000 from all cancers (England, 1998) | 273.2 | 242.6 |
| Suicide – death rates per 100 000 from suicide (England, 1998) | 15.5 | 4.8 |
| Weight problems – % of adults considered overweight or obese (England, 1997) | | |
| Overweight | 45 | 33 |
| Obese | 17 | 20 |
| Smoking – % of adults who smoke (UK, 1998) | 28 | 26 |
| Alcohol consumption – % of adults consuming above recommended levels (UK, 1998) | 27 | 15 |
| GP visits – % of adults who visited GP in previous two weeks (UK, 1998–99) | 12 | 18 |

- social circumstances
- biological vulnerability
- mental heath problems
- life events
- access to means of support

Women also have serious health problems that are gender specific. Employing an unrefined analytical approach that compares men's health with women's health can mask inequalities for both men and women. Women have more morbidity from poorer mental health, particularly that related to anxiety and depressive disorders. Psychosocial health in women is strongly influenced by socioeconomic status. Lone mothers have particularly poor psychosocial wellbeing (Acheson, 1998). Owen and Milburn (2001) report that fewer women are in receipt of specialist mental health services than men. They comment that women are a minority group whose needs are often overlooked.

## ETHNICITY AND INEQUALITY

The numbers and proportions of older people from black and minority ethnic communities have risen rapidly, from 60 000 in 1981 to 350 000 in 2001. Black and minority ethnic older people are more likely to face a greater level of poverty, live in poorer-quality housing and have poorer access to benefits and pensions than white older people (John Rowntree Foundation, 2004).

Acheson (1998) recognises that there are variations between ethnic populations:

- People in black (Caribbean, African and other) groups and Indians have higher limiting longstanding illness than white people. Those of Pakistani or Bangladeshi origin have the highest rates.
- There is an excess mortality among men and women born in Africa and men born on the Indian subcontinent.
- Among mothers who were born in countries outside the UK, those from the Caribbean and Pakistan have infant mortality rates about double the national average. Perinatal mortality rates have also been consistently higher than for babies and mothers born outside the UK. The differences between the group have not decreased over the last 20 years.

Coronary heart disease is moderately higher in South Asian groups than the population as a whole, and the poorest groups of Bangladeshis and Pakistanis have the highest rates. Mortality ratios for men and women from Scotland and Ireland are also elevated. The prevalence of diabetes mellitus in South Asians and Caribbeans is high (Aspinall and Jacobson, 2004). Indian, Bangladeshi and Chinese ethnic groups are less likely to receive in-patient service (Morris et al., 2004).

The Maternity Alliance (2004) has identified that ethnic women are twice as likely to die during or immediately after the birth of a child as white women. Poor-quality maternity care is delivered to one fifth of mothers who die during this period.

## ADDRESSING HEALTH INEQUALITIES

The reasons for health inequalities are various: there is a link between poverty and illness and the health of those who are worse off; there are differences between those who are better off and those who are poor; a health gap exists between those who are worse off in society and those who are better off; advantages and disadvantages exist right across the social spectrum. The Health Development Agency (2004) has identified three broad ranges of causes of health inequalities:

- poor health of poor people
- health gaps
- health gradient

A continued improvement in the constituents of socioeconomic provision occurred from 1970 to 2000: average income rose and the proportion of the population with educational qualifications and in higher nonmanual groups also rose. Nevertheless, policies that had been devised to produce the above results failed to reduce inequalities in socioeconomic position. In higher education, for example, participation widened, as was the case in access to secure well-paid occupations and in income (Nickell, 2003; Shepherd, 2003).

Objectives have been set by the government to tackle the major determinants of health and health inequalities (Wanless, 2004). Understanding what the determinants are that have the potential to influence health outcomes can help address and reduce health inequalities, for example being aware of the need to raise educational standards, improve living standards and reduce risk factors (e.g. smoking and obesity).

Improving the health of poorer groups, reducing the health differences between poorer and better-off groups and raising the levels of health across the socioeconomic hierarchy to those closer to those at the top must be given careful consideration at a local and national level (Graham, 2004b).

Improving the health of poor people requires concerted efforts to achieve positive changes in the poorest of groups. Social conditions and life chances need to be improved; changes must be made in risk-taking behaviours. Attention needs to be focused on the groups of people who have missed out in the general rise in living standards and life expectancy, for example the unskilled manual group where life expectancy is yet to reach the level achieved by the professional groups. Social inclusion and regeneration of communities, which may help to ensure life chances and health opportunities of poorer groups, should be promoted.

Targeting specific groups, such as disadvantaged groups including the mentally ill or those with a learning disability, with specific targets to achieve positive health outcomes may have an impact on health outcomes. What must be remembered is that health inequalities affect every member of society; they do not and should not only concern those who suffer most – the disadvantaged.

There is a health gap between the best off and the worst off. Addressing health gaps means that the health of the poorest needs to be raised fastest (Milburn, 2001). In an attempt to raise the health of the poorest fastest, there is a need to improve the health of the poorest at a rate that outstrips that of the wider population (Health Development Agency, 2004). Evaluation of policy imposed to reduce the health gaps must demonstrate that the rate of improvement in disadvantaged groups is greater than in the comparison (the advantaged) group. A faster rate of improvement is the vital measure of effectiveness.

At each step up the socioeconomic ladder health improves – health gradients occur. There are health gradients associated with disability and chronic illness as well as most major causes of death, such as coronary heart disease and lung cancer (Health Development Agency, 2004).

The Department of Health (2003) has highlighted the actions that are likely to be needed in order to have the greatest impact on the health gap:

- Improvements in early-years support for children and families.
- Improved social housing and reduced fuel poverty among local vulnerable populations.

- Improved educational attainment and skills development among disadvantaged populations.
- Improved access to public services in disadvantaged communities in urban and rural areas.
- Reduced unemployment and improved outcomes among the poorest.

The above actions are to be achieved by the implementation of a programme for action that will aim to reduce health inequalities by 2010. Twelve government departments are involved in achieving the programme for action, pointing to the fact that a one-size-fits-all approach will not work. The nurse therefore will not be working in isolation; he/she must consider the wider context and other factors that can impinge on health outcomes.

The founding principle of the World Health Organisation is that the highest standard of attainable health is a fundamental right (World Health Assembly, 1998). The standards of health of the better off should be attainable by all. This is implied in the World Health Organisation's Constitution (World Health Organisation, 1948): there should be no distinction for race, religion, political belief, economic or social condition – good health for all.

## CONCLUSIONS

Every person is an individual and this therefore extends to every patient, who is also an individual. The nurse must respect and recognise the diversity of the population. The provision of culturally competent care will promote equality and therefore enhance the quality of nursing care.

The nurse can and must act in such a way as to ensure that the rights of individuals and groups are respected and not compromised. The values, customs and beliefs of the patient should be given due consideration and the care that the nurse provides ought to be sensitive to the diverse needs of the patient being cared for.

Discrimination and disadvantage have the powerful potential to hinder the nurse's aim – to provide care – and can lead to inequality. Respecting and valuing the diversity of the people you work with and patients you care for will help to ensure a quality service.

This chapter provided definitions of the following key terms:

- culture
- ethnicity
- race
- gender

It was acknowledged that when attempting to define these terms difficulties arose. They are often fluid terms and can change depending on the context in which they are being used.

The UK is a multicultural society and care provision should be built around the individual needs of individual patients, acknowledging that some aspects of nursing care may be affected and even determined by issues such as religion or ethnic background. A one-size-fits-all approach, it was suggested, does not work and if used will result in inequality and discrimination.

An overview of eight ethnic groups was presented, including information that the nurse may find helpful when providing culturally competent nursing care. Issues surrounding death and dying, dietary requirements and specific material relating to the provision of nursing for these groups were provided in outline format.

Since 1911 the most common method of measuring inequalities in the UK has been through occupation; a similar method is still used today. Despite all of the advances in nursing care and medical technology, there are still members of our society who are treated unequally in respect to health-care provision. There are many factors that have an affect on health outcomes and the most appropriate approach to begin to address these problems is to devise methods that recognise the complexities of the causes and the diversity of the population. Diverse solutions as opposed to identical approaches are advocated, seeking to engage the local population to address local needs.

Social position is seen by some researchers as the root cause influencing health. There are various key determinants that interact and result in health and wellbeing. Inequality and socioeconomic position will determine health outcomes. Inequalities were discussed and highlighted. The nurse is in an ideal position to identify and address the inequalities, working not in isolation but with others considering the wider context.

## REFERENCES


Acheson, D. (1998) *Independent Inquiry into Inequalities in Health: Report.* The Stationery Office. London.

Akhtar, S. (2002) 'Nursing with dignity: Part 8: Islam'. *Nursing Times.* Vol 98, No 16, pp 40–42.

Anthias, A. (1992) 'Connecting race and ethnic phenomena'. *Sociology.* Vol 26, pp 421–438.

Aspinall, P.J. and Jacobson, B. (2004) *A Focused Review of the Evidence and Selected Examples of Good Practice.* London Health Observatory. London.

Baxter, C. (2002) 'Nursing with dignity: Part 5: Rastafarianism'. *Nursing Times.* Vol 98, No 13, pp 42–43.

Bhopal, R. (1997) 'Is research into ethnicity and health racist, unsound, or important science?' *British Medical Journal.* Vol 314, pp 1751–1756.

Botting, B. (1997) 'Mortality in childhood', in Drever, F. and Whitehead, M. (eds). *Health Inequalities: Decennial Supplement: DS Series no 15.* The Stationery Office. London.

Christmas, M. (2002) 'Nursing with dignity: Part 3: Christianity I'. *Nursing Times.* Vol 98, No 11, pp 37–39.

Cohen, A. and Hove, M. (2001) *Physical Health of the Severe and Enduring Mentally Ill: A Training Pack for GP Educators.* Sainsbury Centre for Mental Health. London.

Collins, A. (2002) 'Nursing with dignity: Part 1: Judaism'. *Nursing Times.* Vol 98, No 9, pp 33–35.

Cooper, Y. (2001) 'Campaigning for better health for all', *Men's Health Journal*, Vol 1, No 1, p 3.

Department of Health (1999) *Saving Lives: Our Healthier Nation.* The Stationery Office. London.

Department of Health (2000) *The NHS Plan: A Plan for Investment, A Plan for Reform.* Department of Health. London.

Department of Health (2001a) *National Service Framework for Older People.* Department of Health. London.

Department of Health (2001b) *Valuing People: A New Strategy for Learning Disability for the 21st Century.* The Stationery Office. London.

Department of Health (2001c) *Care Homes for Older People: National Minimum Standards.* Department of Health. London.

Department of Health (2002a) *Tackling Health Inequalities: 2002 Cross-Cutting Review.* Department of Health. London.

Department of Health (2002b) *National Suicide Prevention Strategy for England: Consultation Document.* Department of Health. London.

Department of Health (2003) *Tackling Health Inequalities: A Programme for Action.* Department of Health. London.

Department of Health (2004) *Choosing Health? A Consultation on Improving People's Health.* Department of Health. London.

Disability Rights Commission (2004) *Equal Treatment: Closing the Gap.* DRC. Stratford-upon-Avon.

Drever, F. and Whitehead, M. (1997) *Health Inequalities: DS No 15.* Office for National Statistics. London.

Elliot, J., Hatton, C. and Emerson, E. (2003) 'The health of people with learning disabilities in the UK: Evidence and implications for the NHS'. *Journal of Integrated Care.* Vol 11, No 3, pp 9–11.

Emerson, E. (2003) 'Mothers of children and adolescents with intellectual disability: Social and economic situation, mental health status, and the self assessed social and psychological impact of the child's difficulties'. *Journal of Intellectual Disability Research.* Vol 47, pp 385–399.

Fulton, C.E. (2003) 'The critically ill patient' in Alexander, M.F., Fawcett, J.N. and Runciman, P.J. (eds) (2nd edn) *Nursing Practice: Hospital and Home: The Adult.* Churchill Livingstone. Edinburgh. Ch 29 pp 873–892.

Giger, J.N. and Davidhizar, R.E. (2004) (5th edn) *Transcultural Nursing: Assessment and Intervention.* Mosby. St Louis.

Gill, B.K. (2002) 'Nursing with dignity: Part 6: Sikhism'. *Nursing Times.* Vol 98, No 14, pp 39–41.

Graham, H. (1999) 'Inquiry into inequalities of health', *Health Variations.* Vol 3, pp 2–4.

Graham, H. (2004a) 'Social determinants and their unequal distribution: Clarifying policy understandings'. *Millbank Quarterly*, Vol 82, pp 1010–1124.

Graham, H. (2004b) 'Tackling health inequalities in England: Remedying health disadvantage, narrowing gaps or reducing health gradients'. *Journal of Social Policy.* Vol 33, pp 115–131.

Graham, H. (2005) 'Socioeconomic inequalities in health: Patterns, determinants and challenges'. *Journal of Applied Research on Intellectual Disabilities.* Vol 18, No 2, pp 101–111.

Graham, H. and Power, C. (2004) *Childhood Disadvantage and Adult Health: A Life-course Framework.* Health Development Agency. London.

Grundy, E. and Holt, G. (2000) 'Adult life experiences and health in early old age in Great Britain'. *Social Science and Medicine.* Vol 51, pp 1061–1074.

Grundy, E. and Holt, G. (2001) 'Health inequalities in the older population'. *Health Variations.* No 7, pp 4–5.

Hattersley, L. (1997) 'Expectation of life by social class' in Drever, F. and Whitehead, M. (eds) *Health Inequalities: Decennial Supplement: DS Series no 15.* The Stationery Office. London.

Health Development Agency (2004) *Health Inequalities: Concepts, Frameworks and Policy.* HDA. London.

Health Development Agency (2005) *Injuries in Children Aged 0–14 Years and Inequalities.* HDA. London.

Hickerton, M. (2005) 'Women with special needs and concerns'. in Andrews, G. (ed.) (3rd edn) *Women's Sexual Health.* Elsevier. Edinburgh. Ch 6, pp 113–140.

Hollins, S., Attard, M.T., von Fraunhofer, N. and Sedgwick, P. (1998) 'Mortality in people with learning disability: Risks, causes and death certification findings in London'. *Developmental Medicine Child Neurology.* Vol 40, pp 50–56.

John Rowntree Foundation (2004) *Black and Minority Ethnic Older People's Views on Research Findings.* John Rowntree Foundation. York.

Jootun, D. (2002) 'Nursing with dignity: Part 7: Hinduism'. *Nursing Times.* Vol 98, No 15, pp 38–40.

Joukamaa, M., Heliovaara, M., Knekt, P., Aromaa, A., Raitasalo, R. and Lehtinen, V. (2001) 'Mental disorders and cause-specific mortality'. *British Journal of Psychiatry.* Vol 179, pp 498–502.

Kerr, M. (1998) 'Primary health care and health gain for people with a learning disability'. *Tizard Learning Disability Review.* Vol 3, No 4, pp 6–14.

Kerr, M. (2004) 'Improving the general health of people with learning disabilities', *Advances in Psychiatric Treatment.* Vol 10, pp 200–206.

Kuh, D., Ber-Schlomo, Y., Lynch, J., Halqvist, J. and Power, C. (2003) 'Life course epidemiology', *Journal of Epidemiology and Community Health*, Vol 57, No 10, pp 778–783.

Leininger, M. and McFarland, M. (2002) (3rd edn) *Transcultural Nursing.* McGraw Hill. New York.

Lewis, G., Bebbington, P., Brugha, T., Farrell, M., Gill, B., Jenkins, R. and Meltzer, H. (1998) 'Socioeconomic status, standard of living, and neurotic disorder'. *Lancet.* Vol 352, pp 605–609.

Malik, K. (1996) *The Meaning of Race.* Macmillan. London.

Marsh, I. (2000) (2nd edn) *Sociology: Making Sense of Society.* Prentice Hall. Harlow.

Maternity Alliance (2004) *Experiences of Maternity Services: Muslim Women's Perspectives.* Maternity Alliance. London.

Maughan, B., Collinshaw, S. and Pickles, A. (1999) 'Mild mental retardation: Psychological functioning in adulthood'. *Psychological Medicine.* Vol 29, pp 351–366.

Meltzer, H., Gatward, R., Goodman, R. and Ford, T. (2000) *The Mental Health of Children and Adolescents in Great Britain.* Office for National Statistics. London.

Milburn, A. (2001) 'Breaking the Link Between Poverty and Ill Health'. *Long-term Medical Alliance Conference.* Royal College of Physicians. London.

Mold, F., Fitzpatrick, J.M. and Roberts, J.D. (2005) 'Caring for minority ethnic older people in nursing care homes.' *British Journal of Nursing.* Vol 14, No 11, pp 601–606.

Morris, S., Sutton, M. and Gravelle, H. (2004) *Inequity and Inequality in the Use of Health Care in England: An Empirical Investigation.* Centre for Health Economics. University of York.

Nazroo, J.Y. (2003) 'The structuring of ethnic inequalities in health: Economic position, racial discrimination and racism.' *American Journal of Public Health.* Vol 92, pp 277–284.

Nelson, S. (2005) 'Women's sexuality' in Andrews, G. (ed.) (3rd edn) *Women's Sexual Health.* Elsevier. Edinburgh. Ch 1 pp 3–14.

NHS Executive (2000a) *The Vital Connection: An Equalities Framework for the NHS.* NHSE. London.

NHS Executive (2000b) *Positively Diverse.* NHSE. London.

NHS Scotland (2004) *People with Learning Disabilities in Scotland: Health Needs Assessment Report.* NHS Scotland. Glasgow.

Nickell, S. (2003) *Poverty and Worklessness in Britain.* Centre for Economic Performance, London School of Economics. London.

Northcott, N. (2002) 'Nursing with dignity: Part 2: Buddhism'. *Nursing Times.* Vol 98, No 10, pp 36–38.

Nursing and Midwifery Council (2004) *Code of Professional Conduct. Standards for Conduct, Performance and Ethics.* NMC. London.

Oakley, A. (1974) *The Sociology of Housework.* Blackwell. Oxford.

Office for National Statistics (2001) *Living in Britain: Results from the 2000 General Household Survey.* The Stationery Office. London.

Owen, S. and Milburn, C. (2001) 'Implementing research findings into practice: Improving and developing services for women with serious enduring mental health problems'. *Journal of Psychiatric and Mental Health Nursing.* Vol 8, pp 221–231.

Papadopoulos, I. (2002) 'Nursing with dignity: Part 4: Christianity II'. *Nursing Times.* Vol 98, No 12, pp 36–37.

Peate, I. (2004) *Men's Sexual Health.* Whurr. London.

Picker Institute Europe (2003) *Improving Patients' Experience: Sharing Good Practice.* Picker Institute Europe. Oxford.

Ratcliffe, P. (2004) *'Race', Ethnicity and Culture.* Open University Press. London.

Rayman, S.M. (2004) 'Health assessment' in Daniels, R. (ed.) *Nursing Fundamentals: Caring and Clinical Decision Making.* Thompson. New York. Ch 27 pp 545–650.

Reid, I. (1977) *Social Class Difference in Britain.* Open Books. London.

Registrar General (1913) *Registrar General's 74th Annual Report 1911.* Registrar General's Office. London.

Rodriguez, D.A. (2004) 'Culture and ethnicity' in Daniels, R. (ed.) *Nursing Fundamentals: Caring and Clinical Decision Making.* Thompson. New York. Ch 5 pp 90–112.

Ross, J. (1952) *The National Health Service in Great Britain.* Oxford University Press. Oxford.
Royal College of Nursing (2002) *Chaperoning: The Role of the Nurse and the Rights of the Patient: Guidance for Nursing Staff.* RCN. London.
Rutter, M. (2000) 'Becoming a sexual person' in Wells, D. (ed.) *Caring for Sexuality in Health and Illness.* Churchill Livingstone. Edinburgh. Ch 9 pp 151–170.
Seymour, L. (2003) 'Not all in the mind. The physical health of mental health service users'. *Radical Mentalities – Briefing Paper 2.* Mentality. London.
Shepherd, A. (2003) *Inequality Under the Labour Government: Briefing Note 33.* Institute for Fiscal Studies. London.
Simpson, J. (2002) 'Nursing with dignity: Part 9: Jehovah's Witnesses'. *Nursing Times.* Vol 98, No 17, pp 36–37.
Smith, J. and Harding, S. (1997) 'Mortality of women and men using alternative social classifications' in Drever, F. and Whitehead, M. (eds). *Health Inequalities: Decennial Supplement: DS Series No 15.* The Stationery Office. London.
Vallerand, A.H. and Polomano, R.C. (2000) 'The relationship of gender to pain'. *Pain Management Nursing.* Vol 1, No 3, pp 8–15.
Wanless, D. (2004) *Securing Good Health for the Whole Population: Final Report.* Her Majesty's Stationery Office. London.
White, C., van Galen, F. and Chow, Y.H. (2003) 'Trends in social class differences in mortality by cause 1986 to 2000'. *Health Statistics Quarterly.* Vol 20, pp 25–37.
World Health Assembly (1998) *World Health Declaration, Health-For-All Policy for the 21st Century.* WHA. 51.7. Fifty First World Health Assembly. Geneva.
World Health Organisation (1948) *Constitution of the World Health Organisation.* WHO. London.

# II Care Delivery

# 4 Therapeutic Relationships

In order to provide an effective therapeutic relationship in a mutually therapeutic environment, it is vital that the nurse uses appropriate communication and interpersonal skills. Effective communication, according to Elton (2003), is central to the effective delivery of health care.

The thrust of this chapter is to convey to the reader the importance of effective communication skills, for example processes and forms of communication, and the importance of establishing, maintaining and disengaging from professional care relationships with patients. In addition, there will be discussion concerning barriers to communication.

Caring for well or sick people is complex and the nurse needs to liaise and communicate with a range of health- and social-care professionals from various statutory and voluntary agencies. This chapter will describe some of those health- and social-care professionals and the various agencies that may be encountered in practice, exploring the skills required to participate effectively as a member of the multidisciplinary team.

Working together as a team for the benefit of the patient has been stressed in *The NHS Plan* (Department of Health, 2000b) and *Shifting the Balance of Power* (Department of Health, 2001b). Teamworking has the potential to enhance the quality of care; furthermore, a growing body of evidence suggests that teamworking can have a major impact not only on the quality of care but also on the efficient use of resources, and on staff satisfaction (Department of Health, 2001b).

## COMMUNICATING WITH HEALTH-CARE PROFESSIONALS

Communicating effectively with other health-care professionals can be difficult; there are many health-care professionals that the nurse and the patient may come into contact with. To act as a patient's advocate it is important to understand your own role and the role others play in health-care delivery.

The Nursing and Midwifery Council (2004b) requires that all nurses work in a collaborative manner with the patient and other health-care professionals to enhance and promote high-quality care.

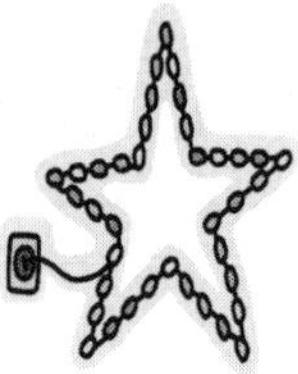

In the following situation, can you list the health-care workers that Carole and her family may come into contact with?

> Carole is a 26 year old who was born with Down's syndrome. She has recently had a chest infection but her condition has worsened and she now has pneumonia. Carole smokes approximately 20 cigarettes a day. She has been living at home with her father and her brother Thomas until this recent admission to hospital.
>
> Carole now requires much nursing support provided by her father and various health-care professionals. Over the last two weeks her condition has deteriorated and she was admitted to the ward (an acute care ward) after she had been diagnosed with pneumonia.

Carole and her family will have come into contact with many health-care professionals, including various nursing staff prior to and on admission. You might have thought about the health-care professionals listed in Table 4.1.

**Table 4.1** Some health-care professionals Carole and her family may have come into contact with

| | |
|---|---|
| • Nursing staff | • Various medical staff |
| • Health visitor | • Speech therapist |
| • Community nurses | • Occupational therapist |
| • Physiotherapists | • Social worker |
| • Domestic and portering staff | • Social services |
| | • Technicians |
| • General practitioner | • Dietician |
| | • Pharmacist |

The following is a list of nursing and medical staff employed within the NHS. You should familiarise yourself with their various roles and responsibilities:

**Nursing staff**

- Chief Nursing Officer
- nurse consultant

- ward sister/charge nurse
- staff nurse
- student nurse
- health-care assistant

**Medical staff**

- Chief Medical Officer
- consultant
- general practitioner
- registrar general practitioner
- specialist registrar
- senior house officer
- house officer
- medical student

Faulkner (1998) has suggested that if professionals fail to communicate effectively with each other they are less likely to be effective when they interact with patients and carers. Despite this, some nurses find interacting with colleagues more of a challenge than interacting with the patient (Fallowfield et al., 2001). Mullally (2000) suggests that the reason for this may be related to:

- power differences
- role confusion
- variations in communication styles
- variations in philosophies of care

There are several ways in which these differences may be addressed and the nurse should reflect on the way in which they communicate. Faulkner (1998) advocates team meetings in order to enhance inter-professional communication, thus reducing stress and confusion for both staff and patients.

## BOUNDARIES IN PROFESSIONAL RELATIONSHIPS

The only appropriate professional relationship between a patient and a nurse is one that focuses exclusively on the needs of the patient. There is a potential power differential (an imbalance of power) in this relationship which the nurse must be aware of. This is generated by the patient's need for care, assistance, guidance and support. McQueen (2000) states that nurses and patients cannot enjoy totally equal relationships. This is the result of the contractual relationship the nurse and patient are engaged in: it is an encounter of necessity, not choice. Both patients and nurses, according to Ronayne (2001), must acknowledge these inequalities but implicitly value each other's competencies. At all times the nurse must maintain appropriate professional boundaries within this relationship.

Setting boundaries defines the limits of behaviour that allow a patient and a nurse to engage safely in a therapeutic caring relationship. The boundaries are based on:

- trust
- respect
- the appropriate use of power

The relationship between the nurse and the patient is a therapeutic relationship, which has the key aim of focusing on and meeting the health and care needs of the patient. This relationship should not be established in order to build on personal or social contacts for the nurse. An unacceptable abuse of power occurs when the focus of care is moved away from meeting the patient's needs towards meeting the nurse's own needs.

All professional relationships are capable of producing conflicts of interest. There may be occasions when nurses develop strong feelings for a particular patient or family. There is nothing abnormal or wrong with these feelings in themselves, but compromising of the professional relationship occurs if the practitioner acts on them in an improper manner. On occasions personal or business relationships may pre-exist prior to the professional relationship and there may be instances where dual relationships exist, for example the nurse may already be a personal friend of a patient. The nurse has the responsibility of ensuring that each relationship stays within its own appropriate boundary.

An essential aspect of the therapeutic relationship will involve physical contact. When providing reassurance to a patient for example, supportive physical gestures are essential in helping that patient. Appropriate supportive physical contact should be maintained in the nurse–patient relationship.

However, abuse can occur within the privileged nurse–patient relationship. Often this is the result of a misuse of power between the nurse and the patient, which the nurse ought to know and would result in physical or emotional harm to the patient. For example:

- a betrayal of trust
- a betrayal of respect
- intimacy between the nurse and the patient

There are many different forms of abuse; these may be:

- physical
- psychological
- verbal
- sexual
- financial and/or material
- neglect

Patients themselves may identify that they are being abused by the nurse and in some instances suspicion may be raised by the patient's carers, family members, advocates or other health-care professionals.

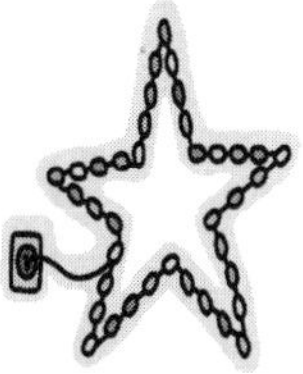

What would you do if you suspected that a patient was being abused by a nurse or other health-care professional?

Every incident or allegation of suspected abuse requires a thorough and careful investigation, which must take full account of the circumstances and the context of the abuse. It is the NMC which is charged with this responsibility. Should you have any suspicions you must make these known to your immediate superior or line manager in order for the allegation(s) to be dealt with in the most appropriate manner. If the issues concern a doctor it is the General Medical Council (GMC) that deals with these matters; any other issue concerning another health-care professional is dealt with by the Health Professions Council (HPC). Go back to Chapter 1 and revisit the section that dealt with allegations of misconduct.

## PHYSICAL ABUSE

Any physical contact that harms patients or is likely to cause them unnecessary and avoidable pain and distress can be deemed physical abuse. For example:

- Handling the patient in a rough manner.
- Giving medication inappropriately.
- Poor application of manual handling techniques.
- Unreasonable physical restraint.

Physical abuse may also cause the patient psychological harm or distress.

## PSYCHOLOGICAL ABUSE

This type of abuse occurs when any verbal or nonverbal behaviour happens that demonstrates disregard for the patient and could be emotionally or psychologically damaging. Some examples might include:

- mocking
- ignoring

- coercing
- threatening to cause physical harm
- denying privacy

## VERBAL ABUSE

Verbal abuse is any remark that is made to or about a patient that may reasonably be perceived to be:

- demeaning
- disrespectful
- humiliating
- intimidating
- racist
- sexist
- homophobic
- ageist
- blasphemous

Some examples of verbal abuse might include:

- Making sarcastic remarks.
- Using a condescending tone of voice.
- Using excessive and unwanted familiarity.

## SEXUAL ABUSE

Forcing, inducing or attempting to induce the patient to engage in any form of sexual activity is sexual abuse. Both physical behaviour and remarks of a sexual nature made towards the patient are included here. The following are some examples of sexual abuse:

- Touching a patient in an inappropriate manner.
- Engaging in sexual discussions that have no relevance to the patient's care.

## FINANCIAL AND/OR MATERIAL ABUSE

Financial and/or material abuse is not only associated with illegal acts such as stealing a patient's money or property, it is also related to the inappropriate use of a patient's funds, his/her property or resources. Examples can include:

- Borrowing property or money from a patient or a patient's family member.
- Inappropriate withholding of a patient's money or possessions.
- Inappropriate handling of, or accounting for, a patient's money or possessions.

NEGLECT

Neglect is the refusal or failure on the part of the nurse to meet the essential care needs of a patient. For example:

- Failure to attend to a patient's personal hygiene.
- Failure to communicate adequately with the patient.
- The inappropriate withholding of food, fluids, clothing, medication, medical aids, assistance or equipment.

All nurses have a duty and a responsibility to protect all patients from all forms of abuse.

## THERAPEUTIC NURSING INTERVENTIONS

Therapeutic nursing interventions are nursing actions carried out to offer holistic nursing care. Holistic nursing care considers all aspects of the patient – body, mind and spirit – and the nurse using the nursing process in relation to individuals, their families, groups of people and communities. Holistic nursing has been explored many times over the years (Narayanasamy, 1999). Therapeutic nursing interventions have at their heart the caring relationship. The nurse uses a professional approach when delivering therapeutic nursing interventions. The essence of nursing is reflected in the therapeutic relationship the nurse and patient develop. It is, however, difficult to define and evaluate the impact of therapeutic nursing as the emotional labour often remains hidden (Ronayne, 2001).

To provide effective nursing care the nurse must communicate effectively with the patient, the patient's family (however he/she defines this) and other health-care professionals. Effective communication incorporates effective use of your interpersonal skills. Chapter 3 was concerned with the diverse needs of the patient and it pointed out how diverse the population is; the nurse will meet many patients from various backgrounds and will have to employ interpersonal skills to ensure that effective two-way communication takes place. This next section of the chapter is concerned with the content and the process of communication.

## INTERPERSONAL SKILLS

Allender and Spradley (2005) suggest that there are three types of interpersonal skills that build on sending and receiving skills. These interpersonal skills go beyond the simple exchange of messages. To be able to demonstrate a therapeutic partnership with the patient the nurse must show that he/she possesses the following three skills:

- respect
- rapport
- trust

## RESPECT

Showing respect means that the nurse must demonstrate a genuine interest in the patient and his/her needs. Addressing the patient in a manner that is respectful, listening carefully without interrupting the patient while he/she is telling his/her story (providing you with his/her history), showing concern for the patient's condition, preserving modesty and promoting dignity are all ways in which the nurse can demonstrate respect. The correct way to address a person is important, for instance using the courtesy titles of Ms, Mrs or Mr until the patient has given you permission to address him/her in any other manner. Expressing a sincere desire to understand the patient, showing kindness and being concerned for any fears or discomfort are also ways of expressing respect to the patient and the patient's family.

## RAPPORT

Establishing a rapport with the patient or his/her family can be confirmed by showing respect as described above. Possessing communication skills that are effective can instil in the patient a sense of confidence, competence and trust that will validate rapport (Meredith, 2000). See Table 4.2 for ways of establishing rapport.

## TRUST

Trust must be earned by the nurse; trust generates trust. Often patients will resist expressing their true feelings if they do not trust the nurse. The nurse

**Table 4.2** Examples of ways in which the nurse may establish rapport with the patient

| |
|---|
| • Provision of an open channel of communication. The nurse should endeavour to ensure that he/she has face-to-face interaction with the patient. |
| • Jargon and technological terminology should be avoided and the patient's educational level, culture and any communication impairments should be catered for. |
| • Subtly mirroring the patient's posture can make the patient feel more at ease and helps to establish rapport, e.g. leaning forwards when the patient does. |
| • Be aware of your and the patient's body language. |
| • Use paralanguage – the rate of speech, the tone of voice. This approach is powerful and can communicate emotional information to both the patient and the nurse. |

*Source*: Adapted from Meredith, 2000.

can lay down solid foundations for trust building, by enhancing this he/she demonstrates that he/she respects and has a rapport with the patient. Trust, like respect, is associated with an ability to provide the patient with genuine interest and care. Meredith (2000) suggests that gaining the trust of the patient can be achieved in the following ways:

- Admitting your limitations and seeking appropriate assistance when help is needed.
- Remaining nonjudgemental and objective.
- Taking the patient's fears and apprehensions seriously.
- Maintaining the patient's sense of comfort, dignity and privacy.
- Acting as the patient's advocate as needed.
- Demonstrating genuine empathy and kindness.
- Behaving in a professional manner.

Trust is developed by providing an open, honest and patient-focused approach (Allender and Spradley, 2005). As trust develops and grows, so too will free-flowing communication.

### EMPATHY

Empathy is another interpersonal skill. Allender and Spradley (2005) define empathy as the ability to communicate understanding and vicariously experience the feelings and thoughts of others. The British Association for Counselling and Psychotherapy (2002) defines empathy as the ability to communicate understanding of another person's experience from that person's perspective. The nurse demonstrates empathy by reflecting another person's feelings and expressing those feelings to another person. The reflections should be done by using the same terms and phrases the other person has used.

Empathising with a patient sends him/her the message that you are seeking validation of the messages/issues that have been communicated to you: 'This is how it seems to me' or 'Did I get that right?' The nurse must continue to seek validation in order to ensure that the message received is correct. By empathising the nurse focuses on the patient and this aims to reduce their anxieties and fears. The patient should feel that he/she is being listened to and that his/her participation is valued.

## EFFECTIVE COMMUNICATION SKILLS

Effective communication involves the use of many different skills. The Department of Health (2001a), in its benchmark statement concerning communication, states that all practicable steps must be taken to communicate effectively with patients and their carers. The effectiveness of communication is mediated by intrapersonal, interpersonal and other factors. Interpersonal skills are skills that are often learnt early on in life, during childhood for example, and as we grow we tend to refine these skills. When practising nursing, however, these skills can mean the skills or techniques used by nurses in an attempt to produce therapeutic benefit during professional interactions with patients and others, as described above.

Irurita (1996) has identified elements that are present within the helping relationship that patients value and these include:

- genuineness
- respect
- being available
- being honest
- listening actively
- being able to empathise

A person cannot *not* communicate (Smith et al., 2004). Communication is the process of sending and receiving messages via symbols, words, signs, gestures or other actions such as cues.

Figure 4.1 provides a diagrammatic representation of how the process of communication can work. Using a model to describe communication is helpful, but it is also limited in its value as it does not include, and indeed cannot include, the context of care. There are many factors that can enhance/impinge on the nurse's ability to communicate effectively with his/her patient.

The person sending the message is called the sender; in some models of communication he/she is referred to as the source encoder (Sherman, 1994). The

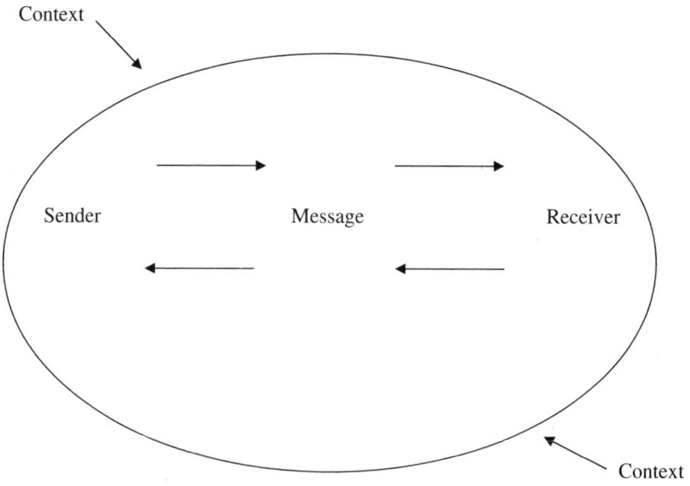


**Figure 4.1** A model of communication

source is concerned with the idea or the event; the receiver, or in some models the decoder, is the person receiving the message and he/she can receive this message through sight, sound or touch. Be aware, however, that the message sent may not be the message received. The three media mentioned here – sight, sound and touch – are also known as the channels through which the message is transmitted. Messages can contain overt and covert communications; while the sender may be aware of the overt meaning of the message he/she may not be aware of the covert meaning within it.

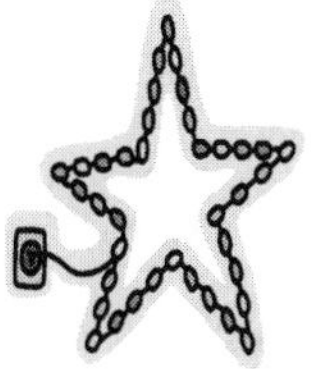

Take some time to think about the ways in which people communicate with you and how you communicate with them. Think particularly about the gestures and symbols used.

What message is being given to you when a person kisses you? This gesture is usually associated with kindness.

The messages sent and received can have the potential to define the relationship between the various parties. Communication is required in order to fulfil defined goals, for example to transmit facts, feelings and meanings.

Most people would suggest that they can communicate, but in reality that may not be true. The test comes when one word is placed in front of the word communication – 'effectively'. Communication is a process that we undertake on a daily basis; we often do it without thinking and feel that we are successful at both understanding others and being understood. However, most people, including nurses, fail to communicate effectively. Communication appears easy when it is done well. It requires engagement, empathy and the ability to listen to and respond; it also requires time.

Many health-care workers do communicate effectively, although some patients are unhappy about the information they are given and the manner in which it is given (NHS Scotland, 2003). When the nurse uses his/her communication skills effectively, both the nurse and the patient may benefit (Maguire and Pitceathly, 2003; see Table 4.3).

Effective communication is an essential requirement in nursing. All aspects of the nurse–patient relationship involve some form of communication. For example:

- Providing health education to a young person with anorexia.
- Listening to the concerns of a worried parent.
- Performing a nursing procedure with a patient who has profound learning disabilities.

**Table 4.3** The benefits of effectively communicating with the patient

- Patients' problems are identified more accurately.
- Patients are more satisfied with their care and can better understand their problems.
- Patients are more likely to comply with treatment or life style advice.
- Patients' distress and their vulnerability to anxiety and depression are lessened.
- The overall quality of care is improved by ensuring that patients' views are taken into account.
- The nurse's own wellbeing is improved.
- Fewer clinical errors are made.
- Patients are less likely to complain.

*Source*: Adapted from Maguire and Pitceathly, 2003.

The modes or forms of communication are varied and include both verbal and nonverbal communication. Some of these are described in the next sections. Effective communication is affected by various factors, including the intrapersonal framework of the person, the relationship between participants and the purpose of the interaction. The communication process is very complex: it is often what you say and how you say it that will have most impact. In order to assess a patient's needs effectively the nurse must employ many skills including:

- communication
- observation
- measurement

When assessing a patient's needs the nurse should employ the skills associated with interviewing, for example listening, talking, recording and documenting. Although listening may appear to be a very passive skill, it is indeed also very complex.

Becoming a better listener means that the nurse listens not only with his/her ears but with his/her whole body. Listening means that you should avoid talking about yourself or your own opinions, keep quiet – listen. There are five fundamental actions the nurse can take to ensure that he/she actively listens – summed up by the acronym SOLER (Egan, 2002):

**S**it squarely, facing the patient: the nurse should adopt a position whereby the patient feels he/she is being listened to.

**O**pen posture: avoid adopting a defensive position, e.g. arms folded.

**L**ean towards the other person: the nurse when leaning towards the patient will demonstrate that he/she is actively listening.

**E**ye contact should be maintained: avoid excessive eye contact or limited eye contact, you should aim to strike a balance.

**R**elax as much as possible: demonstrating that you are relaxed may encourage the patient to relax.

## VERBAL COMMUNICATION

The word 'verbal' would suggest that communication in this sense is linguistic; that is, it is spoken or said. Effective verbal communication will depend on issues such as the tone and the pitch of a person's voice. Just as important is the use of language, which is very important in achieving an understanding between the person sending the message and the individual receiving it. According to Sidtis (2004), expression of speech is important and statements used on an everyday basis through slang, sayings, clichés and conventional expressions become a large part of a speaker's competence. Messages only transmitted through a verbal means of communication have to be much clearer than ones that are sent with the aid of other means of communication, in order for the recipient to receive them effectively. Speakers (the people sending the message) have the potential to control the interaction through the language they choose to use. Nurses may do this unconsciously by using jargon with the patient.

## OPEN AND CLOSED QUESTIONS

Most of our daily conversation involves either asking or answering questions; we use questions every day. There are a variety of questioning styles available to the nurse and depending on the context of the interaction, this will result in the nurse choosing one approach over the others in order to have the most impact. The choice of technique will impinge on the efficacy of information gathering.

The use of open questions invites the respondent to elaborate on his/her responses, as opposed to closed questions. When using open questions the nurse aims to understand more specifically what the patient means. Using clarification techniques provides the patient with the opportunity to expand and amplify his/her previous comment (Buckman, 2001). Ryrie and Norma (2004) cite the following as open questions:

- What are your feelings about that experience?
- What thoughts did you have at the time?
- Could you say a little more about what that means for you?

Open questions are designed to give information; they begin with words such as:

- How . . .
- Why . . .
- When . . .
- Where . . .
- What . . .
- Who . . .
- Which . . .

Closed questions can be recognised as they start with words such as:

- Do . . .
- Is . . .
- Can . . .
- Could . . .
- Will . . .
- Would . . .
- Shall . . .
- Should . . .

Closed questions allow the respondent to reply with a single categorical answer to the question posed, for example when looking for a straight 'Yes' or 'No'. This type of question can be useful, for instance if the patient is short of breath you would not seek elaboration to a question as this may exhaust or exacerbate the patient's condition.

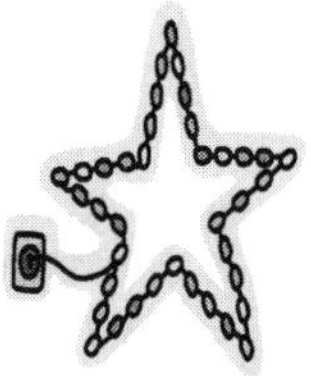

With another colleague, ask him/her a question beginning with 'How', 'Why' or 'When'. You may have found it was difficult for him/her to respond with a simple 'yes' or 'no'. That is because you began the question with an 'open' word.

Figure 4.2 demonstrates how, by using various approaches to asking questions, it is possible to filter data down in order to gather the information that is being sought.

## NONVERBAL COMMUNICATION

Abercrombie (1968) states that we may well speak with our vocal organs, but we converse with our whole body. Hargie et al. (2004) note that much emphasis is placed on the verbal aspects of communication, for example the words used, their sequencing and structure. Nonverbal communication or body language is often unconscious and therefore spontaneous and candid.

Messages can be relayed to others in different ways as well as when we speak, for example through the following channels:

- glances
- gestures
- facial expressions
- posture

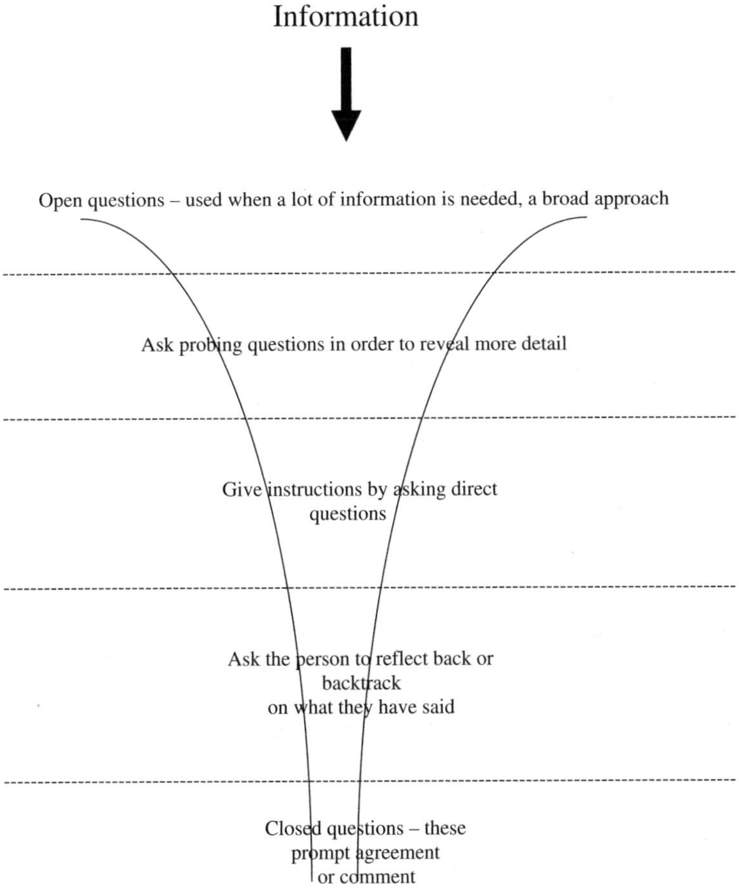
Information
Open questions – used when a lot of information is needed, a broad approach
Ask probing questions in order to reveal more detail
Give instructions by asking direct questions
Ask the person to reflect back or backtrack on what they have said
Closed questions – these prompt agreement or comment

**Figure 4.2** The information funnel

- tone of voice
- dress
- body orientation
- silence

These modes of communication are known as nonverbal communication and they sometimes do not get noticed when we converse with each other. It is often nonverbal communications that are crucial in the transmission of information and are the prime ways in which we judge or make opinions about others (Smith et al., 2004). Communication is very often a mixture of both verbal and nonverbal messages, sometimes known as metacommunication.

Nonverbal communications have many functions within the communication process. They have the ability to regulate and influence the processes associated

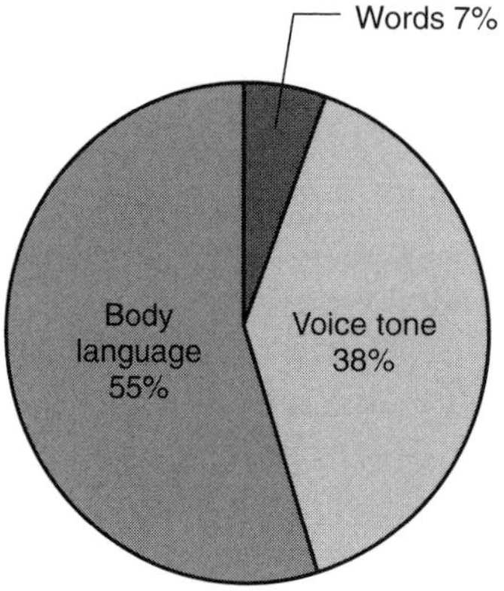


**Figure 4.3** The elements of communication

with human interaction; they can also support or replace communications that are verbalised.

It is suggested that approximately 7 per cent of messages transmitted between people are attributed to words. The other 93 per cent are nonverbal messages (Sherman, 1994). Of this 93 per cent, 38 per cent are transmitted through vocal tones and the remaining 55 per cent are through facial expressions; see Figure 4.3.

There are nine types of nonverbal communication:

- paralanguage
- kinesics
- occulesics
- appearance
- proxemics
- haptics
- olfactics
- chronemics
- facial expressions

**Paralanguage**

Paralanguage is the vocal cues that accompany language, the way we say words. Hargie et al. (2004) include features such as speech rate and intensity; pitch, modulation and quality of the voice; articulation and rhythm control. The faster a person speaks the more competent he/she may appear; soft-spoken speakers may be considered timid or shy. Young children (infants) do not understand words and rely on nonverbal communication for information. A raised voice to a child may result in an alteration in the child's behaviour.

### Kinesics – Body Movements

Kinesics is the study of nonverbal communication through facial or body movements. Knapp and Hall (1997) have identified five categories associated with kinesics:

- *Emblems* – these are body gestures that translate directly into words or phrases, for example the thumbs-up sign for 'a good job'.
- *Illustrators* – these types of nonverbal communication often accompany the verbal message. Generally people illustrate with their hands, however other parts of the body can be used, such as the head. Illustrators can also communicate the shape or size of the objects that you are talking about.
- *Regulators* – regulators are behaviours that have the ability to monitor, coordinate, control or maintain the speaking of another person. An example may be when the head is nodded during conversation, which gives the speaker the signal to continue speaking.
- *Display of feelings* – sometimes also known as affect display. This is associated with movements of the face or body, for example a frown or raising of the eyebrows, which often conveys emotional meaning.
- *Adaptors* – an example of an adaptor might be tapping a pen or twisting the hair. Hargie et al. (2004) refer to adaptors as self-manipulative gestures.

### Occulesics

Occulesics are associated with eye movements and messages conveyed by the eyes. There are many cultural rules associated with eye movements and gaze. There is a balance between how long you engage in eye contact: too long may be threatening, too short a time may convey timidity or shyness.

Eye contact or gaze can play several important roles in face-to-face interaction (Knapp and Hall, 1997), for example:

- initiate contact
- define the relationship
- regulate the flow of conversation
- monitor feedback
- coordinate discussion

### Appearance

The human body reveals much about the person. Tall people are said to be paid more than for the same job done by a shorter person. Attractiveness can also be seen as an artifact. Those who are deemed physically attractive are considered more personable, popular, confident, persuasive, happy, interesting and outgoing (Guerrero et al., 1999). Attractive people fare better in all walks of life, for example they do better at school and are more preferred as work mates (Burgoon et al., 1996).

The way an individual dresses can also influence the ability to communicate effectively. People make inferences about the way you dress. Issues relating to clothing can include uniforms and occupational attire, the style and type of leisure clothes and the colour of the clothes worn.

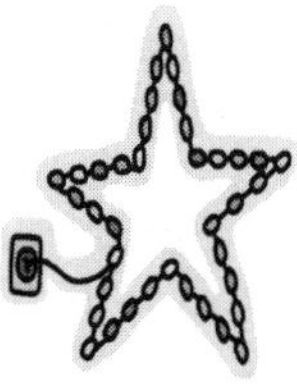

Think about the clothes people around you are wearing. Are there people in leisure clothing, office smart clothing, uniforms? Could you place them in a socioeconomic group, judge the amount of money they earn based only on the clothing they wear?

Often people really do 'judge a book by its cover' and the clothing we wear (regardless of whether we have chosen to wear that particular type of clothing or it is a requirement of our job) is our 'cover'. Think for example about the inferences people will make about you if you wear, or do not wear, a wedding ring.

### Proxemics

Proxemics or interpersonal space concerns the distance people maintain while interacting with others. Hargie et al. (2004) point out that there are many factors that shape interpersonal distance:

- culture/background
- gender
- personality
- interpersonal relations
- age
- topic of conversation
- physical features of the other
- physical/social setting

Proxemic distances can be measured in relation to the purpose of the encounter; see Table 4.4.

### Haptics

The study of touch is known as haptics. Ritualistic touching occurs throughout the day and this can be in the form of handshaking, hugging or kissing. Touch can be seen as an intimate way of communication. Touch can convey

**Table 4.4** Interpersonal space and distances

| Relationship | Distance | |
|---|---|---|
| Intimate relationship | Approximately 45 cm | Usually reserved for very close friends or family |
| Personal/casual relationship | From about 45 cm to 1.30 m | Used during informal/ casual conversations/ discussions with friends and associates |
| Social relationship | 1.30 m to approximately 4 m | Used for impersonal business dealings |
| Public relationship | Over 4 m but within the range of sound and vision | Conferences, large meetings, formal gatherings |

*Source*: Adapted from Brody, 2004.

many messages: it can communicate positive feelings, reassure patients and comfort them. There are some patients who do not like to be touched because of personal desires or as a result of cultural norms.

### Olfactics

Olfactics is the study of smell or in this context olfactory communication. People relate to or disengage with others as a response to smell, for example the smell of another person's breath or their aftershave/perfume. Smell is a very powerful memory aid; often it is possible to recall an event that occurred months or years ago when a similar smell is encountered again.

### Chronemics

This is the study of time or temporal communication. It is associated with the way people organise and react to time. The communication process is often hindered because of the challenges associated with time.

### Facial Expressions

As children we learn how to manage facial expressions. For example, sometimes it is considered rude to yawn openly, so often people attempt to suppress a yawn; we may frown when we are given bad news. Humans have 80 facial muscles that can create in excess of 7000 facial expressions.

There are six main types of facial expression that can be found in all cultures (see Table 4.5).

**Table 4.5** Facial expressions that can be found in all cultures

| Expression | Manifestation |
|---|---|
| Happiness | Round eyes, smiles, raised cheeks |
| Disgust | Wrinkled nose, lowered eyelids and eyebrow, raised upper lip |
| Fear | Round eyes, open mouth |
| Anger | Lowered eyebrow and intense stare |
| Surprise | Raised eyebrow, wide open eyes, open mouth |
| Sadness | Area around mouth and eyes lowered |

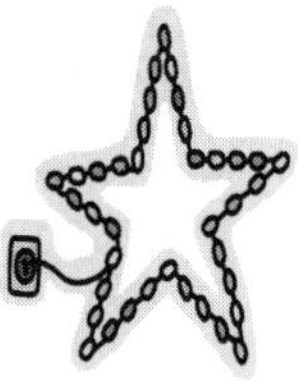

If you were a patient, without using any verbal communication, how might you try to express the following to a nurse who is caring for you:

- I am in pain.
- I need a bedpan.
- I am scared.
- You are not listening to me.

You may have come up with many ways of expressing your needs in the above situations. You might have used the expressions outlined in Table 4.5.

## COMMUNICATION SKILLS, COUNSELLING AND COUNSELLING SKILLS

Nurses support and give advice to patients in a variety of ways in their everyday work. Nurses are not counsellors, however the nurse should aim to provide the patient with an opportunity to offer his/her support, as well as allowing the patient to refuse that support, and when appropriate giving them an opportunity to work through complex issues relating to their health needs. Providing the patient with information may enable him/her to do this.

It should be noted that there are close relationships between:

- counselling
- communication skills
- counselling skills

**Table 4.6** The variety of activities related to counselling

| Guidance | Advice | Counselling |
|---|---|---|
| • Highly directive<br>• Highly structured<br>• The counsellor determines, the client accepts<br>• Closed – addresses specific issues<br>• Information content high<br>• Demands competence in communication skills | • Moderately directive<br>• Semi-structured<br>• The counsellor determines with the client's agreement<br>• Flexible – issues broadly agreed<br>• Information content moderate<br>• Demands competence in interpersonal skills | • Highly nondirective<br>• Mainly unstructured<br>• The client determines, the counsellor facilitates<br>• Open – addresses emerging issues<br>• Information content low<br>• Demands competence in relational skills |
| Counsellor is a guide | Counsellor is an adviser | Counsellor is a therapist |

*Source*: Slevin, 2003.

When the nurse uses counselling skills in an appropriate manner they are providing the patient with an opportunity to become more self-aware, and in so doing Sully (2003) suggests that the patient gains the ability to make more informed choices.

Slevin (2003) provides another approach to differentiating the variety of counselling activities. He suggests that there is a selection of counselling activities, ranging from guidance, a highly directive and structured approach, to counselling where the approach could be said to be nondirective and unstructured (see Table 4.6).

In order to avoid confusion with key terms, Russell (2002) prefers to use the term therapeutic communication as opposed to counselling.

Nurses can develop and use their therapeutic communication and therapeutic nursing interventions to help the patient identify his/her own problems and seek resources to deal with these problems.

The nurse may also be required to communicate with and counsel the patient over the telephone. NHS Direct operates a 24-hour nurse advice and health information service, providing confidential information on:

- What to do if you or your family are feeling ill.
- Particular health conditions.
- Local health-care services, such as doctors, dentists or late-night-opening pharmacies.
- Self-help and support organisations.

There may be other reasons why the nurse needs to communicate with the patient over the telephone, for example to provide them with information or instructions, or they may need to speak with other health-care professionals to obtain blood results.

If face-to-face communication is not possible and a telephone call is required, then remember that telephone conversations can be overheard, and confidentiality rules still apply. A telephone call from the patient must be returned as soon as possible. The purpose, content and outcome of the telephone conversation must be documented.

## GUIDELINES FOR RECORDS AND RECORD KEEPING

Most encounters the nurse has with the patient will potentially involve recording the information that has been exchanged between the two parties. Local policies are in place that will guide the nurse regarding records and record keeping. Guidelines have been provided by the NMC (2004a) concerning records and record keeping. Record keeping is a fundamental aspect of nursing care. Despite the fact that the NMC (2004a) provides guidance, it does not determine the content, nor does it offer a rigid framework for the content of records or record keeping. Ultimately what to include, exclude and the format used is left up to the accountable practitioner and his/her professional judgement.

When the nurse keeps and maintains good records he/she is protecting the interests of the public (NMC, 2004a) by:

- Promoting high standards of nursing care.
- Ensuring continuity of care.
- Providing enhanced communication and dissemination of information between other members of the inter-professional health-care team.
- Maintaining a correct description of treatment, care planning and delivery.
- Offering the ability to reveal problems, such as a change in the patient's circumstances, at an early stage.

There may be occasions when a patient's records (or notes) may be called as evidence before a court of law by the Health Service Commissioner, or at a local level to look into a complaint. The records may also be requested by the Nursing and Midwifery Council when the Fitness to Practice Committees are investigating complaints made about nurses. In this instance the records may include:

- care plans
- diaries
- anything that makes reference to the patient

Records must show that the nurse has acted professionally and in the best interests of the patient (see Table 4.7).

Errors do occur in record keeping and Table 4.8 highlights some of these.

**Table 4.7** Elements associated with documentation, demonstrating that nurses have taken into account their duty of care to the patient

- A full account of the assessment, the care planned and what has been implemented.
- Relevant information about the patient's condition at any given time and any measures that have been taken in response to patient needs.
- Evidence that the nurse has understood and honoured the duty of care owed to the patient, that all reasonable tasks have been taken to care for the patient and that any actions or omissions have not compromised patient safety in any way.
- A record of any arrangements that the nurse has made for the continuing care of the patient.

*Source*: Adapted from NMC, 2004a.

**Table 4.8** Some common mistakes recorded in patient records

- Time not included.
- Handwriting that is impossible to read.
- Use of abbreviations that were vague/unclear.
- Use of correction fluid to cover up errors.
- Signature omitted.
- Inaccuracies, particularly relating to the dates.
- Delays in completing the record.
- Record completed by a person who did not care for the patient.
- Inaccuracies relating to name, date of birth and address.
- Unprofessional terminology, e.g. 'dull as a door step'.
- Meaningless phrases, e.g. 'nice person'.
- Opinion mixed up with facts.
- Subjective as opposed to objective comments, e.g. 'slept well'.

*Source*: Adapted from Dimond, 2005a.

## THE USE OF ABBREVIATIONS

The NMC has stated that the use of abbreviations in health care is unacceptable (NMC, 2004a). However, abbreviations may be used to save time, for example often nurses use the abbreviations T for temperature, BP for blood pressure and P for pulse; if they did not use them then much more time would be needed for record keeping. If abbreviations are used then it may be advisable for NHS Trusts to compile a list of approved abbreviations and acceptable symbols in order to reduce the risk of misinterpretation and misunderstanding.

Uncertainty can arise when abbreviations are used, which can lead to confusion resulting in danger to the patient. Dimond (2005b) provides a list of common abbreviations that are sometimes used that may have different meanings (see Table 4.9).

Good record keeping is the hallmark of a skilled, competent, confident and safe practitioner and can result in effective communication. However, the

**Table 4.9** Some abbreviations with different meanings

| Abbreviated form | Possible meaning |
|---|---|
| **PID** | Pelvic inflammatory disease **OR** Prolapsed intervertebral disc |
| **DOA** | Dead on arrival **OR** Date of admission |
| **Pt** | Patient **OR** Physiotherapist **OR** Part time |
| **NFR** | Not for resuscitation **OR** Neurophysiological facilitation of respiration |
| **NAD** | Nothing abnormal discovered **OR** Not a drop |
| **FBC** | Fluid balance chart **OR** Full blood count |

*Source*: Adapted from Dimond, 2005b.

message being communicated will only be as good as the nurse who is recording the information. Other health-care workers may depend on the information contained in the records you make and, as a result of what you have documented (or omitted to document), may act on this (Peate, 2005).

It is the registered nurse who is professionally accountable for any duties that they choose to delegate to any other member of the inter-professional health-care team, for example the student nurse. This includes the delegation of record keeping to pre-registration nursing students or health-care assistants. It is imperative that these members of the team are appropriately supervised and that they are capable of carrying out the task. The registered nurse should countersign any such entry and bear in mind that they are professionally accountable for the consequences of such an entry. It is deemed bad practice to use initials in any record; the full signature should be used with the name written alongside it.

## OBSTRUCTIONS TO EFFECTIVE COMMUNICATION: CAUSES OF COMMUNICATION FAILURE

There are many ways in which the message being transmitted never reaches the recipient and messages can become blocked for many reasons. Barriers to communication can occur if the recipient has failed to convey the meaning or the importance of the message.

If sender breakdown occurs, the person transmitting the message may send too much information and as a result the recipient can miss key points. Conversely, too little information can also be a cause of sender breakdown (Kozier et al., 2004). The language or the use of jargon can be difficult for the recipient and sender to understand, or the sender may have limited knowledge concerning the message being sent (Brody, 2004). The information being transmitted may be the wrong information. The nurse's attitude can covey the message that he/she is not interested in the information. In some instances the sender may be making false assumptions about the recipient (Taylor et al., 2005).

Or there may be recipient breakdown, when the recipient deliberately makes a choice to misinterpret or refuse to accept the transmitted message. This can be for a variety of reasons. For some the breakdown may be due to reasons beyond the recipient's control, for example:

- a speech defect/dysphasia
- deafness
- poor sight
- developmental level
- poor cognitive skills
- facial injuries/disorders/dysarthria

Physical reasons may be only one aspect of communication breakdown. Emotional aspects can also impinge on effective communications (Taylor et al., 2005):

- perceptions
- prejudice
- aggression
- threat

Other problems with communication could be related to the following:

- There may be a long chain of command. The message gets passed on to many different people before reaching the recipient, making the process long and offering the possibility that the message may change.
- The reason for the message may be vague, e.g. lacking in detail, more explanation being needed.
- The recipient may be confused or demented.
- The medium used to transmit the message may be inappropriate, for example inappropriate written or verbal form.
- Actions can be delayed as a result of the late arrival of the message.
- The status of the two parties, e.g. the patient and the nurse, has the potential to intimidate either party because of their gender, age and knowledge base.
- Distraction, e.g. through pain and anxiety, can cause communication channels to break up.

Generally to reduce the possibility of communication breakdown the nurse should:

- Actively listen to the patient.
- Speak slowly.
- Ask one question at a time and avoid multiple questioning.
- Provide only one piece of information at a time – avoid information overload.
- Use simple language.
- Consider using gesture.

- If possible reduce noise pollution, e.g. from background noise.
- Check to see if the patient has any aids he/she uses to enhance communication, such as a hearing aid or spectacles.
- Not shout.
- Think about using the written word if appropriate.

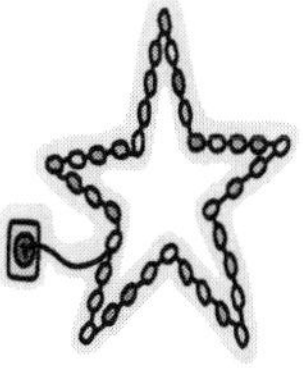

How might you attempt to reduce noise pollution on a busy children's ward when you wish to communicate with the parents of a sick child?

To maintain confidentiality, first you would want to conduct the conversation in private if possible, which offers one way in which you can eliminate background noise and interference. However, private areas may not always be available, therefore you could ensure that communications take place when the ward is less busy, for example avoiding meal times, ward rounds or when the ward is being cleaned.

## DEALING WITH PATIENTS' COMPLAINTS

Often complaints arise as a result of poor communication (Taber, 2003). Complaints can range in severity from dissatisfaction about food to concerns arising as a result of allegations of professional misconduct or inappropriate or incorrect surgical intervention.

Patients who complain about the care or treatment they have received have a right to expect a prompt, open, constructive and honest response. This will include an explanation of what has happened and, where appropriate, an apology. The nurse must never allow a patient's complaint to prejudice the care or treatment provided for that patient.

The Department of Health does not deal with individual complaints. Complaints are dealt with through the NHS complaints procedure. Complaints that arise if the patient is a private patient paying for his/her treatment are directed to the independent providers complaints procedure, which is a requirement under the Care Standards Act (2000).

When making a complaint about treatment or services offered by the NHS the patient (or his/her representative) should be encouraged to contact the patients' advisory service (PALS). PALS have been set up in all NHS Trusts and primary care trusts. The creation of PALs was as a result of the NHS Plan (Department of Health, 2000a). PALS are intended to enable patients and the public to access information and raise concerns with their Trust, and the service provides 'on-the-spot' help. While the work of PALS is growing, the adequacy of existing resources with regards to children, young people and parents needs to be given further deliberation (Heaton and Sloper, 2003). PALS are not a part of the complaints procedure, however they may be able to help resolve the problem informally, or offer the patient advice regarding other routes/ways to make a complaint.

The National Health Service (Complaints) Regulations 2004 (the 'Complaints Regulations') came into force on 30 July 2004. These regulations demand that each NHS body must make arrangements for the handling and consideration of complaints. The arrangements that have been made must be accessible to ensure that complaints are dealt with speedily and efficiently, and that patients are treated courteously and sympathetically and, as far as possible, involved in decisions about how their complaints are handled and considered. There must be a copy of the arrangements available in writing and when requested a copy must be given, free of charge, to any person who requests one.

Every NHS body is required to appoint a complaints manager who is obliged to manage the procedures for handling and considering complaints. Where a person wishes to make a complaint he/she may make it to the complaints manager or any other member of the staff of the NHS body that is the subject of the complaint. A complaint may be made orally or in writing (and this includes electronically). If the complaint is made orally, the complaints manager must make a written record of the complaint, which includes:

- The name of the patient.
- The subject matter of the complaint.
- The date on which it was made.

There are time limits for making a complaint. The complaint must be made within six months of the date on which the matter occurred or six months of the date on which the matter came to the notice of the patient. If the complaint is made after the expiry of the period mentioned above, the complaints manager may investigate it if he/she is of the opinion that:

- Having regard to all the circumstances, the patient had good reasons for not making the complaint within that period.
- It is still possible to investigate the complaint effectively and efficiently even though the time has elapsed.

The complaints manager must send to the patient a written acknowledgement of the complaint within two working days on which the complaint was made. If the complaint was made orally, an acknowledgement is also required as above with an invitation to the patient to sign and return it. Any person identified in the complaint must receive a copy of the complaint. The patient has to be informed about his/her right to assistance from the independent advocacy services.

It is the responsibility of the complaints manager to investigate the complaint to the extent and in the manner that he/she feels is necessary in order to resolve it speedily and efficiently. If the complaints manager thinks it would be appropriate, he/she could make arrangements for conciliation, mediation or other assistance, but only if the patient agrees with this. The complaints manager must take such steps as are reasonably practicable to ensure that the patient is informed about the progress of the investigation.

A written response to the patient by the complaints manager must be prepared. This must:

- Summarise the nature and substance of the complaint.
- Describe the investigation.
- Summarise its conclusions.

The chief executive of the NHS body must sign the response. The patient has to receive the response within 20 working days from the date on which the complaint was made or as soon as reasonably practicable. Included in that response the patient must be notified of his/her right to refer the complaint to the Healthcare Commission. Copies of the response must also be sent to any other person identified in the complaint.

The remit of the Healthcare Commission (an independent body) is to carry out a review of the complaint made by the patient if he/she is dissatisfied by the outcome of the investigation conducted by the complaints manager. When a complaint is received by the Healthcare Commussion an initial review is conducted to determine if it is possible or appropriate for the complaint to be looked at further by the Healthcare Commission. If the patient is unhappy with the outcome of the initial review, he/she has the right to complain about the decision made by the Healthcare Commission to the Health Service Ombudsman.

The Health Service Ombudsman undertakes independent investigations into complaints about the National Health Service. The results of selected investigations are published in public bi-annual reports.

It is clear that complaints made about services or the care provided by the NHS can be dealt with locally or, if appropriate, can go though various processes to ensure that the patient's complaint is addressed fairly and fully. The nurse should always seek advice when providing the patient with details concerned with making a complaint, as it can be a long and tortuous process for all parties.

## DEALING WITH COMPLIMENTS

Just as complaints are received, so too are compliments given. Compliments, as with complaints, should help people learn and therefore enhance the quality of care. Compliments should also be recorded. Often compliments are given in writing in the form of thank-you cards or gifts such as chocolates or sweets.

The nurse may be offered gifts, favours or hospitality from patients during the course of or after a period of care or treatment. The code of conduct (NMC, 2004b) states that the nurse must refuse any gift, favour or hospitality that could be interpreted, now or in the future, as an attempt to obtain preferential consideration from the nurse. The underlying principle is not that the nurse must never receive gifts or favours, but that they must never be interpreted as being given by the patient to the nurse in return for preferential treatment.

## DISENGAGING FROM A PROFESSIONAL RELATIONSHIP

The final aspect of this chapter deals with leaving or breaking away from a professional relationship. This is in contrast to the preceding aspects of the chapter where the formation and maintenance of the relationship have been promoted. Just as the nurse needs to concentrate on engaging with the patient, he/she must also invest time and energies in leaving the relationship. The nurse may need to consider planning to end the relationship even before it has begun, in order to prepare him/herself for this potentially upsetting experience. Preparing for the expected outcomes could help to make disengagement easier.

Varcarolis (2002) suggests that ending meaningful relationships that have been created during the time the nurse has spent with the patient can sometimes be difficult as it may evoke feelings of sadness, fear or uncertainty at saying goodbye.

The reason for the termination of the relationship may be a consequence of several things; it may be permanent or temporary:

- The patient has recovered enough to be discharged.
- The patient has deteriorated and may need to be discharged to another unit/institution.
- The nurse may be leaving his/her job.
- The patient may have died.

When disengaging from a therapeutic relationship the nurse should be encouraged to reflect on the experience in order to learn and develop. There may be feelings of pleasure – having achieved goals, aims and objectives with the patient and his/her family. There may also be feelings of sadness as a result of having to leave a relationship that had flourished or the deterioration of the patient's health and even his/her death.

Support can be given in the form of facilitative discussion networks at work or the place of study. Opportunities can and should be made for the nurse to speak about his/her feelings.

Ending a therapeutic relationship must be given much thought as the patient may have become reliant on the nurse for many things. Termination of a relationship may leave the patient feeling abandoned and thus vulnerable, so suitable arrangements must be made for the continuation of care/therapy/ treatment where appropriate.

The beginning and the ending of a relationship with a patient or the staff with whom you have worked can provoke many feelings, both positive and negative.

## CONCLUSIONS

Communication with patients and their families should never be seen as an optional extra, it is a fundamental clinical skill that all nurses, regardless of grade or level, should possess (Wilkinson, 1999). This chapter has focused on establishing, maintaining and disengaging from professional relationships. Fallowfied and Jenkins (1999) have demonstrated that effective communication with patients has the potential to:

- improve satisfaction
- foster compliance and control pain
- reduce anxiety
- establish trust and rapport
- support and educate the patient
- establish a plan for treatment

Caring for people is a complex activity that requires skill. In order to provide a therapeutic relationship with the patient at the centre of the affiliation, the nurse has to work within a team. This chapter has explored the concept of teamworking and outlined some of the health-care professionals who may be involved in patient care. Effective teamworking has positive outcomes for patient care.

The nature of the nurse–patient relationship means that this can never be a completely equal relationship. The inequalities should be acknowledged by both patient and nurse; both parties ought to value each other's competencies. The relationship evolved through mutual trust and respect. Abuses of power can and do occur. This is often the result of a shift in the focus of care, for instance the needs of the nurse supersede the needs of the patient. These potential abuses were described in this chapter.

Therapeutic nursing interventions aim to provide holistic nursing care in relation to individual aspects of the body, mind and spirit. Caring is central to therapeutic nursing care. The nurse needs to develop and build on his/her interpersonal skills in an attempt to provide a therapeutic partnership; that is, respect, rapport and trust. By enhancing skills associated with communication the nurse may then be able to form more elaborate and effective relationships with the patient and other health-care professionals. Applying these skills in an accomplished manner can provide a therapeutic lift to the patient.

To use communication skills effectively there are many competencies that must be brought into play, such as respect, honesty and empathy. There was much discussion in this chapter concerning communication methods. For instance, active listening is a complex skill that not only includes the use of the ears but the whole body. Verbal and nonverbal communications were detailed. Verbal communication accounts for 7 per cent of the messages transmitted between people, with 55 per cent related to the use of body language as a communication medium and the remaining 38 per cent associated with the tone of voice.

Much communication between the nurse and other health-care professionals occurs through the written word – the patient record. Many encounters the nurse has with the patient will involve some form of recording the encounter, recording the information that has been exchanged. The NMC (2004a) has provided advice to the nurse regarding records and record keeping. Good record keeping is the hallmark of a skilled, competent and safe nurse.

Communication processes are complex and because of this there is the potential for obstructions to occur that will impede effective communications. Some of the causes of communication failure were described.

Despite striving to maintain open, honest and effective communication, complaints can and do occur. Complaints are commonly associated with poor communications. Complaints can range in severity from dissatisfaction about the cleanliness of toilets to allegations of professional misconduct. If complaints do arise they are dealt with (when appropriate) at a local level adhering to local policy. The NHS Complaints Procedure is used to help arrive at a satisfactory explanation of the cause of the complaint. The aim is to deal with the complaint speedily and efficiently, courteously and sympathetically. Advice should always be sought when a complaint has been made, as it can be a long and tortuous process for all concerned.

Compliments are also received by the nurse from the patient. If gifts are given, the principle is not that the nurse must never receive gifts or favours, but that they should never be interpreted as being given by the patient to the nurse in return for preferential treatment.

While much effort is put into initiating and maintaining a professional relationship, there are skills that are needed to disengage from that professional relationship. Time and energy must be invested into planning the end of the relationship. The reasons for the termination of the relationship are varied, for example the patient fully recovers or he/she may die. Ending the relationship can result in feelings of being abandoned and vulnerable and both parties may need to take part in facilitative discussions in order to deal with and acknowledge these feelings.

## REFERENCES


Abercrombie, K. (1968) 'Paralanguage'. *British Journal of Disorders of Communication*. Vol 3, pp 55–59.

Allender, J.A. and Spradley, B.W. (2005) (6th edn) *Community Health Nursing: Promoting and Protecting the Public's Health*. Lippincott. Philadelphia.

British Association for Counselling and Psychotherapy (2002) *Ethical Framework for Good Practice in Counselling and Psychotherapy*. British Association for Counselling and Psychotherapy, Rugby.

Brody, M. (2004) 'The nurse–client relationship' in Daniels, R. (ed.) *Nursing Fundamentals: Caring and Clinical Decision-Making*. Thompson. New York. Ch 4 pp 68–89.

Buckman, R. (2001) 'Communication skills in palliative care: A practical guide'. *Neurological Clinics*. Vol 19, No 4, pp 989–1004.

Burgoon, J.K., Buller, D.B. and Woodall, W.G. (1996) (2nd edn) *Nonverbal Communication: The Unspoken Dialogue*. McGraw-Hill. New York.

Department of Health (2000a) *The NHS Plan: A Plan for Investment: A Plan for Reform*. Department of Health. London.

Department of Health (2000b) *The NHS Plan*. Department of Health. London.

Department of Health (2001a) *Essence of Care: Patient Focused Benchmarking for Healthcare Practitioners*. The Stationery Office. London.

Department of Health (2001b) *Shifting the Balance of Power Within the NHS: Securing Delivery*. Department of Health. London.

Dimond, B. (2005a) (4th edn) *Legal Aspects of Nursing*. Pearson. Harlow.

Dimond, B. (2005b) 'Abbreviations: The need for legibility and accuracy in documentation'. *British Journal of Nursing*. Vol 14, No 12, pp 665–666.

Egan, G. (2002) *The Skilled Helper: A Problem Management and Opportunity Approach to Helping*. Cambridge Brookes/Cole. Pacific Grove.

Elton, J. (2003) 'Care delivery: The needs of the mature adult' in Hinchliff, S., Norman, S. and Schober, J. (eds) (4th edn) *Nursing Practice and Health Care*. Arnold. London. Ch 10 pp 223–243.

Fallowfield, L. and Jenkins, V. (1999) 'Effective communication skills are the key to good cancer care'. *European Journal of Cancer*. Vol 35, No 11, pp 1592–1597.

Fallowfield, L., Saul, J. and Gilligan, B. (2001) 'Teaching senior nurses how to teach communication skills in oncology'. *Cancer Nursing*. Vol 24, No 3, pp 185–191.

Faulkner, A. (1998) 'The ABC of palliative care: communication with patients, families and other professionals'. *British Medical Journal*. Vol 316, No 7125, pp 130–132.

Guerrero, L.K., DeVito, J.A. and Hecht, M.L. (1999) (2nd edn) *The Nonverbal Communication Reader*. Waveland Press. Illinois.

Hargie, O., Dickson, D. and Tourish, D. (2004) *Communication Skills for Effective Management*. Palgrave. Basingstoke.

Heaton, J. and Sloper, P. (2003) *Access to and Use of Patient Advice and Liaison Services (PALS) by Children, Young People and Parents – A National Survey*. Social Policy Research Unit. University of York.

Irurita, V. (1996) 'Preserving integrity: A theory of nursing' in Greenwood, J. (ed.) *Nursing Theory in Australia: Development and Application*. Harper. Sydney.

Knapp, M. and Hall, J. (1997) *Nonverbal Communication in Human Interaction*. Harcourt Brace. Orlando.

Kozier, B., Erb, G., Berman, A. and Snyder, S. (2004) (7th edn) *Fundamentals of Nursing: Concepts, Process and Practice*. Prentice Hall. New Jersey.

Maguire, P. and Pitceathly, C. (2003) 'Key communication skills and how to acquire them'. *British Medical Journal*. Vol 325, pp 697–700.

McQueen, A. (2000) 'Nurse–patient relationships and partnership in hospital care'. *Journal of Clinical Nursing*. Vol 9, pp 723–731.

Meredith, P.V. (2000) 'Essentials of professional communication' in Meredith, P.V. and Horan, N.M. (eds) *Adult Primary Care*. Saunders. Philadelphia. Ch 7 pp 91–110.

Mullally, S. (2000) 'The annual Robert Tiffany Memorial Lecture: June 2000'. *European Journal of Cancer Care*. Vol 9, No 4, pp 186–190.

Narayanasamy, A. (1999) 'A review of spirituality as applied to nursing'. *International Journal of Nursing Studies*. Vol 36, pp 117–125.

National Health Service Scotland (2003) *Talking Matters: Developing the Communication Skills of Doctors*. NHS Scotland. Edinburgh.

Nursing and Midwifery Council (2004a) *Guidelines for Records and Record Keeping*. NMC. London.

Nursing and Midwifery Council (2004b) *Code of Professional Conduct: Standards for Conduct, Performance and Ethics*. NMC. London.

Peate, I. (2005) *Manual of Sexually Transmitted Infections*. Whurr. London.

Ronayne, S. (2001) 'Nurse–patient partnerships in hospital care'. *Journal of Clinical Nursing*. Vol 10, pp 591–592.

Russell, P. (2002) 'Social behaviour and professional interactions' in Hogston, R. and Simpson, P.M. (eds) (2nd edn) *Foundations of Nursing Practice: Making the Difference*. Palgrave. Basingstoke. Ch 11 pp 343–370.

Ryrie, I. and Norman, I. (2004) 'Assessment and care planning' in Norman, I. and Ryrie, I. (eds) *The Art and Science of Mental Health Nursing: A Textbook of Principles and Practice*. Open University. Milton Keynes. Ch 7 pp 183–207.

Sidtis, D.V.L. (2004) 'When novel sentences spoken or heard for the first time in the history of the universe are not enough: Toward a dual-process model of language'. *International Journal of Language and Communication Disorders*. Vol 39, No 1, pp 1–44.

Sherman, K.M. (1994) *Communication and Image in Nursing*. Delmar. New York.

Slevin, O. (2003) 'Therapeutic intervention in nursing' in Basford, L. and Slevin, O. (eds) (2nd edn) *Theory and Practice of Nursing*. Nelson Thornes. Cheltenham. Ch 30 pp 533–568.

Smith, S.F., Duell, D.J. and Martin, B.C. (2004) *Clinical Nursing Skills: Basic to Advanced Skills*. Pearson. New Jersey.

Sully, P.C. (2003) 'Communication in adult nursing' in Brooker, C. and Nichol, M. (eds) *Nursing Adults: The Practice of Caring*. Mosby. Edinburgh. Ch 3 pp 39–56.

Taber, S.M. (2003) 'Managing risk in a health care organization' in Hinchliff, S., Norman, S. and Schober, J. (eds) (4th edn) *Nursing Practice and Health Care*. Arnold. London. Ch 15 pp 345–368.

Taylor, C., Lillis, C. and LeMone, P. (2005) (5th edn) *Fundamentals of Nursing: The Art and Science of Nursing Care*. Lippincott. Philadelphia.

Varcarolis, E.M. (2002) 'Developing therapeutic relationships' in Varcarolis, E.M. (ed.) (4th edn) *Foundations of Psychiatric Mental Health Nursing: A Clinical Approach*. Saunders. Philadelphia. Ch 6 pp 221–239.

Wilkinson, S. (1999) 'Communication: It makes a difference'. *Cancer Nursing*. Vol 22, No 1, pp 17–20.

# 5 Health Promotion

Understanding the key concepts associated with health promotion will enable the nurse to apply these theories and principles in order to provide high-quality health promotion. Health promotion plays a major part in helping the population maximise their health.

It is not possible in a chapter of this size to address all of the complex issues associated with health promotion, so this chapter only begins to address the key issues. The reader is advised and encouraged to delve deeper and become immersed in the topic in order to hone and build on current knowledge and skills.

There are several ways in which the nurse can promote the health and well-being of patients, and one way of doing this is by helping patients gain access to health promotion information. A discussion is provided on how to provide health information in an accessible and effective manner.

One aspect of the nurse's role in relation to health promotion is to support patients. This can be achieved by attempting to empower and educate them, to protect them from illness and to promote and maintain their health; this chapter provides the reader with the knowledge to put this aspect of the nurse's role into action. There are a variety of health promotion models that are discussed in this chapter and the definitions of a range of key terms are provided.

Developing an awareness of the key concepts related to health promotion may allow the nurse to apply these theoretical principles to practice in an attempt to provide patients with opportunities to promote their health. Several government policies have been produced that aim to improve health, for example *Making a Difference* (Department of Health, 1999a), *The NHS Plan* (Department of Health, 2000), *Shifting the Balance of Power* (Department of Health, 2001a) and *Choosing Health* (Department of Health, 2005a).

The NMC (2004) stipulates that the nurse must ensure that he/she promotes the interests of patients and clients. There are many ways in which this can occur and one way is by helping patients gain access to information that will enhance or promote their health – health promotion information. The NMC (2004) states that the nurse should acknowledge and respect the role of the patient as a partner in his/her care and the contribution he/she can make to it. This points out that the patient, where appropriate, should be involved in all aspects of his/her care.

Approaches to health promotion and health promotion developments have been given new status in recent years. There is an increasing focus on health outcomes and investments in the determinants of health through health promotion activity (Department of Health, 2005b). The roots of health promotion and disease prevention are deep. For example, the ancient Egyptians recorded examples of public health practice such as sewage disposal and how to distribute excess grain to feed the poor. Sigerist (1946) noted nearly 60 years ago that health is promoted among other things by providing a decent standard of living and working conditions. The foundations had been laid down even then to consider health promotion from a holistic perspective.

The nurse's role with regard to health promotion is to support patients by endeavouring to empower and educate, for example to protect from infection. There are many characteristics that are shared with good nursing practice and health promotion, for example the patient is central and health promotion activities are based on an individual assessment of individual needs, respecting and valuing the patient's own views. When working with the patient and the community the nurse spends time listening to, and talking with, the patient, empowering him/her to make decisions for his/her own health.

## DEFINING KEY TERMS

The definitions below provide a useful function in clarifying meaning and relationship between the various terms that are in common usage, as well as helping in practical application. These core definitions are central to the concepts and principles associated with health promotion. The use of the terms defined is often situation specific and guided by social, cultural and economic circumstances. The reader must bear in mind that definitions by their very nature can be restrictive and can only provide a summary of complex ideas and activities. Despite these restrictions and limitations, definitions can help when attempting to understand fundamental ideas and concepts associated with health promotion activities.

The key terms that are associated with health promotion are:

- health
- health education
- health promotion
- public health
- disease prevention

## HEALTH

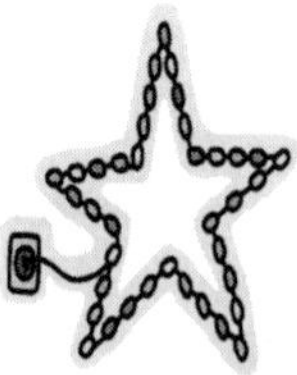

How would you define health? Make a list of the things you would include in your definition of health.

There are no right or wrong answers to this question. Your response may have included things such as:

- free from disease
- the ability to function, e.g. go to university or work and function effectively
- clean water to drink
- availability of health services
- achieving your hopes and ambitions
- a good quality of life

Your list might have focused on the physical aspects of health, but do not forget that health is about the whole person, mind and body, and often it even extends to the whole community. The way you define health could have been guided or influenced by your own personal experiences (Melling et al., 2004). We often use the term health, but when asked to define it, it may mean different things to different people. Think how a person who lives on the street may define health – do you think it might be different to your definition?

The term health is therefore complex and there are various definitions available (Forster et al., 1999). Health is seen as a fundamental human right, regardless of race, religion, political belief, economic or social condition (WHO, 1986). Many issues will impinge on and influence health (Hampson, 2002):

- personal behaviour
- environment
- politics
- social and genetic factors

A popular definition of health that has not been amended since 1948 is provided by the World Health Organisation (1948). It is:

> *A state of complete physical, mental and social wellbeing and not merely the absence of disease or infirmity.*

Health in this definition can be regarded as a positive resource that is used in everyday life. This definition will allow the nurse to consider the person from three distinct and, at the same time, interrelated perspectives (see Figure 5.1).

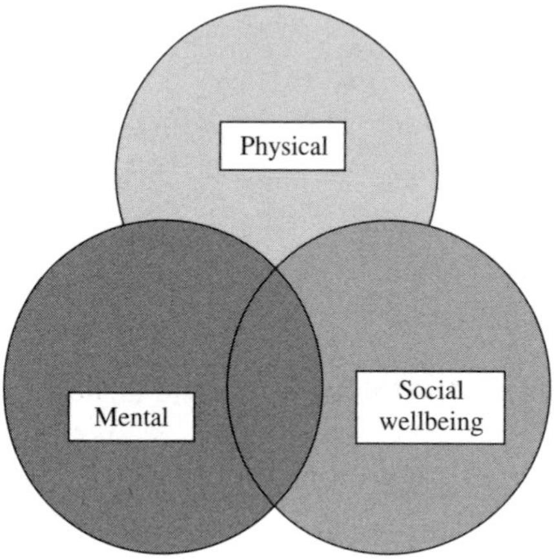


**Figure 5.1** The three interrelated aspects associated with the definition of health

For the fundamental right to health to become a reality, the Ottawa Charter (WHO, 1986) maintains that particular prerequisites must be in place:

- peace
- adequate economic resources
- food and shelter
- stable ecosystem
- sustainable resource use

Accepting these prerequisites to health demonstrates the inextricable link between social and economic conditions, the physical environment and individual lifestyles and health. The links described will enable the nurse to develop a holistic approach to understanding health, which is at the core of health promotion.

Viewing health as a positive concept encompasses social and personal resources as well as the individual's physical capability. All systems that govern health, including social and economic conditions, should be taken into account and given due consideration when devising and developing health promotion activities.

## HEALTH EDUCATION

Health education is one of the three overlapping spheres of activity making up health promotion:

- health education
- health protection
- ill health prevention

Health education can be seen as a communication activity with the key focus aimed at enhancing wellbeing and preventing ill health through positively influencing the knowledge, beliefs, attitudes and behaviour of the community (Tannahill, 1985). An example of health education might be the promotion of breast-feeding skills.

Health protection includes the policies and various codes of practice designed to prevent ill health or positively enhance wellbeing. An example of codes of practice that might be designed to prevent ill health might be related to cervical and breast-screening programmes.

Prevention refers to the initial occurrence of disease and also to its progress and, consequently, the final outcome. Preventive activities could be related to no-smoking policies in the workplace and at leisure venues.

While the communication of health information is important, health education is also concerned with fostering the motivation, skills and confidence needed to take action to improve health. It is associated with the conscious construction of opportunities for learning, with the aim to improve health literacy, knowledge and life skills (WHO, 1998). Health literacy is associated with more than the ability to read health education materials, it encompasses an individual's ability to use the information effectively in order to empower. Life skills are the skills that consist of personal, interpersonal, cognitive and physical skills that can help people to control and direct their lives, for example decision-making and problem-solving skills (Tones, 2001).

Any measure taken in a planned and premeditated way that aims to enhance health and an individual's awareness of health, leading to empowerment of that individual or the community through learning, can be deemed to be health education. There are many activities the nurse can use to enhance health and health awareness (Long, 2003).

## HEALTH PROMOTION

Health promotion is the process whereby people are empowered and enabled to strengthen the control they have over the determinants of health, and in so doing improving their health. It is a political and social process that has the potential to strengthen the skills and the capabilities of individuals and communities. The process can lead to changes in social, environmental and economic conditions, alleviating their impact on public and individual health (WHO, 1998). Health promotion, therefore, can be influential on many fronts.

Four key health promotion values feature in health promotion practice:

- empowerment
- social justice and equity
- inclusion
- respect

Determinants of health are defined as:

> *A range of personal, social, economic and environmental factors which determine the health status of individuals or populations.* (WHO, 1998)

These factors are both numerous and interactive. Health promotion has the ability to address the full range of determinants of health that are modifiable and these include the individual's actions, such as lifestyle and chosen health behaviours, as well as working conditions and access to appropriate health services. The determinants of health alone and/or in combination will have an impact on health; changes in the determinants of health will ascertain health status. It follows, therefore, that those who encounter inequalities in health may also experience an impact on their health as a result of the disparity (Chapter 3 discussed determinants of health inequalities in more detail).

There are several definitions of health promotion available. One definition offered by the World Health Organisation (1998) is:

> *the process of enabling people to increase control over, and to improve their health. Health promotion represents a comprehensive social and political process, it not only embraces actions directed at strengthening the skills and capabilities of individuals, but also action directed towards changing social, environment and economic condition so as to alleviate their impact on public and individual health.*

## PUBLIC HEALTH

As with all of the other definitions provided above, the definition of public health will mean different things to different people (Hayes, 2005) depending on their:

- affluence
- health status
- the environment
- educational standing
- social, political and cultural contexts

The description offered by Acheson (1988) is:

> *Public health is the science and art of preventing disease, prolonging life and promoting physical health through the organised efforts of society.*

Public health is concerned with protecting, maintaining and improving health through organised effort in the community. Health and illness are studied in the context of the community as a social group (Sarafino, 2006).

The purpose of public health, according to Hayes (2005), has four essentials associated with it:

- Improve the health and wellbeing of the population.
- Prevent disease and minimise its consequences.
- Prolong valued life.
- Reduce inequalities in health.

Public health draws on a variety of issues, such as environmental movements, political parties and international agencies, including the United

Nations (Naidoo and Wills, 2000). Public health is as diverse as the public it addresses.

### DISEASE PREVENTION

Many advances in health over the years are a result of efforts to prevent illness and of improvements in diagnosis and treatments (Sarafino, 2006). Recurring themes within current health policy have given increased attention to disease prevention (Wright, 2001). Naidoo and Wills (2000) suggest that the dominance of the medical model is responsible for health promotion being seen as disease prevention, addressing individuals who have 'high-risk' factors associated with the development of a specific disease. Disease-prevention activities often identify individuals or communities who exhibit identifiable risk factors, for example monitoring the health of those people who undertake hazardous activities as a part of their job (Lisle, 2001).

Primary prevention of disease is aimed at preventing the initial occurrence of a disease or disorder and focuses on risk factors and risk conditions. Secondary prevention methods are directed at arresting or slowing down the progression of existing disease, prior to medical intervention. Reducing the occurrence or relapse of a disease or disorder is associated with tertiary prevention (Sarafino, 2006). Early detection and appropriate treatment are approaches used to detect and prevent disease (Naidoo and Wills, 2000; WHO, 1998).

## HEALTH PROMOTION THEORIES AND MODELS

There are a number of significant theories and models that underpin the practice of health promotion, all with the aim of improving health and wellbeing. When attempting to promote health in an effective way for various individuals, groups and communities, the nurse needs to use multiple, complementary strategies and these interventions must be sensitive to the patient's particular needs. Stand-alone approaches may not be as effective as using multiple methods, therefore a complementary approach may be more effective.

Nutbeam (2000) and Colquhoun and Kellehear (1996) suggest that there are three main categories in which health promotion models can be placed, infrastructure, policy and practice. Five influential health promotion approaches or models have been considered by Ewles and Simnett (2003) and Naidoo and Wills (2000):

- medical or preventive
- behaviour change
- educational
- client centred or empowerment
- societal change

The model or approach chosen will depend on the health promotion strategy that is being considered. Table 5.1 outlines, in brief, five approaches to health promotion. All five models/approaches and the elements associated with them are not mutually exclusive; frequently all five approaches can and are used together and interchangeably. All approaches use different means to achieve their goals, however they all aim to uphold good health and diminish or avoid the effects of ill health.

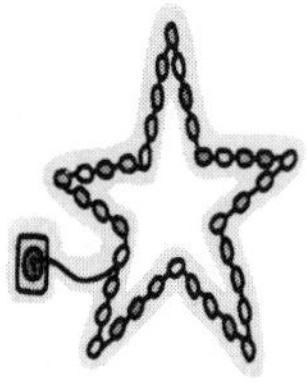

Are there any groups of patients who you think may be responsible for their own ill health?

You might have listed the following:

- Smokers.
- People who do not exercise or eat a balanced diet, resulting in obesity.
- Those who drink more than the recommended amount of alcohol.
- People who have contracted a sexually transmitted infection because they have engaged in unsafe sexual activity.
- Those who use intravenous drugs recreationally.

Think about what impact this 'blaming' attitude may have on the therapeutic relationship you have with these patients and your role as health promoter. Your attitude may be different if, for example, you are a smoker or you engage in unsafe sexual activity.

While making people aware of their own health and health needs can be seen as a positive approach to empowering them, it may also have negative connotations. Stroebe (2000) and Russell (2005) note that making people responsible can also lead to engendering a culture of blame. Examples of blame culture are often argued and debated within the HIV/AIDS arena, for example: 'I have practised safer sex and I am healthy, you have failed to practise safer sex and the reason you have HIV is your own fault.'

In delivering health promotional activities or carrying out health promotion, Ewles and Simnett (2003) suggest that the nurse needs to possess or to develop some key competencies:

- managing, planning and evaluating
- education
- communicating
- facilitating and networking
- marketing and publicity
- influencing policy and practice

**Table 5.1** An outline of five models/approaches to health promotion

| Model/ approach | Principles/characteristics | Comments |
|---|---|---|
| **Medical** | Health is seen as the absence of illness or disease. The traditional view held by many health-care professionals is that health is the 'normal' state, similar to that of a well-adjusted or well-oiled machine (the mechanical metaphor).<br>There are several practical advantages associated with the medical model. Most of the advances in medical science have been made by scientists who have viewed the human body as a series of systems that follow physical laws. The model takes on the view that there is a mind–body dualism and disease is the result of a disorder that has occurred within the machine (the body). The medical model is closely linked to medical practice and in particular the domain of biomedicine. Power and authority in the form of medical paternalism are a result of the medical model; medicine dominates. Individuals do not think of their own health in simple terms, such as the presence or absence of physical symptoms. The mental, emotional or social health of the individual can be just as important. Nurses should keep in mind that these things are important to their patients also.<br>When applied to health promotion the medical model emphasises prevention and, in particular, primary prevention. This can result in victim blaming and risk. This model tends to ignore the environmental and socio-political factors that impinge on health. The health-care professional becomes the expert and the contribution and responsibility of the individual and community are eroded, which leads to disempowerment. The medical model has much power and those in authority (health-care professionals) are often deferred to, reinforcing this dominance and power. | The model does not always correspond to an individual's subjective perception of their own health. There is an over-reliance on an idea of 'normality' that is far from universally applicable.<br>Other aspects of health may be ignored that the individual sees as equally, or even more, important to them. Focusing on the machine (the body) and the times it goes wrong could encourage a reactive, as opposed to a proactive, role for the health promoter.<br>In many instances, health promotion activity that follows and subscribes to the medical model is in danger of viewing interventions as being done to people and communities as opposed to for them. Working in partnership and involving communities, as opposed to being passive recipients of health-care services, will fail to take into account what the expert (the patient) needs. It also has the potential to disempower and to fail to work with the patient and community as an equal partner. |

**Table 5.1** *Continued*

| Model/ approach | Principles/characteristics | Comments |
|---|---|---|
| | The model is dominated by qualitative, objective fact in contrast to accepting patients' subjective feelings and experiences. The model is always searching for a causative link to ill health. The medical model remains a popular model. | |
| **Behavioural change** | Models of behavioural change take into account the individual's own attitudes towards health issues and their own health. Individuals contribute to their own health (and the health of others) by avoiding health-damaging behaviours, such as smoking, or by adopting health-enhancing behaviours, for example taking regular exercise.<br>The model encourages individuals to adopt healthy behaviours and attitudes towards a healthier lifestyle. This may sound simplistic, but making health-related decisions is a multifaceted process. Health is seen as belonging to individuals – they own it. Individuals make the decision to change their behaviour based on its feasibility and the pros and cons associated with it. The decisions individuals make are often dependent on whether they feel threatened by the consequences of not taking a health action, if they feel a change would be beneficial and if they feel competent to carry it out. There must be a perceived susceptibility to disease and a perceived seriousness of disease if people are to make a change in their behaviour or attitude. For example, persuasive education is used in order to promote a change in behaviour, such as in smoking-cessation approaches.<br>In industrialised societies it has been noted that much of the mortality and morbidity is predominantly associated with individual patterns of behaviour, for example unsafe sex activities. Interventions that are used to modify risky behaviour such as poor diet must be aimed at changing or | Changing attitudes, values and beliefs require the nurse to be highly skilled and knowledgeable. The focus of this model is on the individual, and it could be suggested that it fails to take into account the complexity surrounding health choices and how these choices may be constrained by social factors.<br>The underlying principle of this model is that individuals are rational beings. This is a limitation and it fails to take into account that sometimes individuals do not make rational decisions; they may be fearful or in denial. Being frightened can lead to denial and avoidance of the message.<br>As the model's underlying premise is that the individual is a rational being, it also relies on the provision of information regarding risk and health hazards. Not all individuals can access or make use of the information often offered through the mass media. The approach appears to use a 'top-down' approach and this may be at odds with community norms, values and practices.<br>This model could be seen as embracing a victim-blaming philosophy. |

| | | |
|---|---|---|
| | influencing lifestyle. The approach chosen will be most successful if it is adapted to individual, specific needs.<br>While the focus is on behavioural change other changes, such as an increase in knowledge, are also valid indicators of this model's effectiveness. | |
| **Educational** | This model aims to offer advice and information to encourage the patient to make informed decisions. The fundamental objective of the educational model is to increase autonomy. The information provided relates to the cause and effects of factors that hinder good heath.<br>Individuals have a right to choose when they have all the information required to help them make a judgement. The role of the nurse is to assess the needs of the individual. The nurse is seen either as the leader (authority figure) or facilitator (negotiator) who when appropriate provides educational content.<br>There are several models that define health promotion as a range of interventions, e.g. health persuasion and personal counselling. There are a range of approaches that can make up a programme or intervention and the approach depends on many issues, e.g. views about health as well as power and control. | As with other approaches assumptions are being made with this model, for example does the individual have the capacity or the inclination to learn and take on board the advice given?<br>Furthermore, the model assumes that the nurse or health-care practitioner has the skills and knowledge to implement health education programmes. There are other factors that need to be taken into consideration, for example external factors that influence a person's ability to choose and become autonomous. |
| **Client centred** | Self-empowerment is at the centre of this model and is used to describe health-promotion strategies. The strategies are based on counselling and use nondirective, patient-centred approaches with the key objective to increase people's control over their lives. Nurses are often engaged in patient-centred work; they are concerned with facilitating patient autonomy. It is the patient who sets the agenda and the nurse's role is to facilitate, guide, support and empower the patient to make informed choices. | This approach is laudable, however factors outside the control of the patient or the nurse may impinge on fully engaging in client-centred work, e.g. material and human resources.<br>Be aware that the patient may have the intention to carry out a specific behaviour but that intention may not lead to action. For example, a patient who is overweight or |

**Table 5.1** *Continued*

| Model/ approach | Principles/characteristics | Comments |
| --- | --- | --- |
| | The nurse works with the patient on the patient's own terms. The issue(s) that patient feels are pertinent are addressed, for example what choices the patient has and what actions he/she may wish to take (or not). The patient determines what it is he/she wishes to know. In this relationship the patient and nurse are equal partners. | obese may intend to diet but may not actually do so. |
| **Societal change** | This approach attempts to address the socio-economic and environmental causes of ill health. Individuals group together in order to change their physical and social environments and act collectively. The model recognises that there is a close relationship between an individual's health and the social and material circumstances they encounter. The social and material aspects become the target for change. Self-empowerment, a part of social action, becomes the channel for collective action.<br>The community acts collectively to make attempts to change and challenge determinants that influence ill health, e.g. health inequalities, often based on class, race, gender and geography. The model attempts to empower communities. Examples of collective community action may be seen in work that is carried out with those who use intravenous drugs; in this example community outreach approaches are used to achieve sub-cultural changes in reducing HIV infection by the implementation of needle exchanges.<br>The health-promotion agent must develop skills related to lobbying, policy planning, negotiation and implementation. The remit becomes political in some respects. | The key principle underpinning this approach is the notion of 'community' and what this means. Making change occur has cost repercussions and implications related to the accessibility of the proposed changes.<br>The proposed changes have to be supported by the whole community, who need to be convinced of their importance.<br>There may be an element of social regulation associated with this approach. |

*Source*: Adapted from Bridle et al., 2005; Naidoo and Wills, 1998, 2000, 2001, 2005; Russell, 2005; Tones and Green, 2004; Dunkley, 2000; Montazeri et al., 1998; Beattie, 1991; Tannahill, 1985; Illich, 1976; Becker, 1974.

Despite the competencies being individually listed above they are, and should be, used together to achieve the desired outcomes. The nurse will have to develop and draw on pre-existing skills and knowledge and adapt these to meet the individual needs of the patient who may be in a particular environment, for example in a prison.

## THE OTTAWA CHARTER FOR HEALTH PROMOTION: A FRAMEWORK FOR PRACTICE

A world-wide approach to health promotion has been taken up, led by the World Health Organisation. In 1986 the Ottawa Charter was published under the auspices of the WHO (WHO, 1986). The Charter built on the progress made through the Declaration on Primary Health Care at Alma Ata (WHO, 1978).

The Ottawa Charter for Health Promotion (WHO, 1986) is a framework that can be used successfully by nurses in many health-care settings. The primary aim of the Ottawa Charter is to bring about positive long-term changes to the health of communities. The potential role of workplaces, neighbourhoods and schools in improving people's health and reducing health inequalities was deliberated in *Saving Lives: Our Healthier Nation* (Department of Health, 1999b). *The Health of the Nation* (Department of Health, 1992) cited cities, schools, workplaces, homes and environments as potential health settings. These citations are derived from the Ottawa Charter, which stated:

> *Health is created and lived by people within the settings of their everyday life; where they learn, work, play and love.*

It is evident, therefore, that health promotion can and should take place where people congregate and meet when carrying out the activities of daily living. The notion that health cannot be understood in isolation from social conditions (Naidoo and Wills, 1998) is also implicit within the Charter. Therefore, wherever people eat, relax and study this could potentially result in a harmful effect on their health.

Cusack et al. (1997) point out that the approaches highlighted in the Charter may help address factors that are within the control of not only the individual, but also those who form society, such as those in religion, education and media. The nurse can adapt and use the structure described within the Charter to address the health-care needs of the patient and the community, thereby promoting health.

When the nurse begins to consider interventions aimed at promoting health, he/she needs to be aware of the strategies and processes outlined in the Charter. These processes – advocating, mediating and enabling – will help to empower the individual and the community to determine their own health promotion activities. They can help place the individual and the community at the centre of any decision-making activities related to their health-care needs. In order to achieve complete physical, mental and social wellbeing, the individual or the community group must be able to identify and achieve ambitions, to satisfy needs and to change or manage within the environment.

The Charter (WHO, 1986) identifies three basic strategies for health promotion:

- advocacy
- enabling
- mediation

These three strategies create the essential conditions for health, enabling all people to achieve their full potential and mediating between the different interests in society (WHO, 1998).

## ADVOCACY

Good health is a major resource for social, economic and personal development and also an important dimension of quality of life. Political, economic, social, cultural, environmental, behavioural and biological factors can impact positively or negatively on health. Health promotion aims to make these conditions favourable, through advocacy for health.

## ENABLING

Health promotion focuses on achieving equity in health. Health promotion action aims to lessen the differences in current health status and ensure the availability of equal opportunities and resources to enable all people to achieve their full health potential. This includes a secure foundation in a supportive environment, access to information, life skills and opportunities to make healthy choices. People cannot achieve their fullest health potential unless they are able to control those things that determine their health.

## MEDIATION

The prerequisites and prospects for health cannot be ensured by the health sector alone. Health promotion demands coordinated action by all concerned, including governments, health and other social and economic sectors, non-government and voluntary organisations, local authorities, industry and the media.

The three strategies above are supported by five priority action areas. The five priority areas associated with the Charter are (see Figure 5.2):

- Developing personal skills.
- Creating supportive environments.

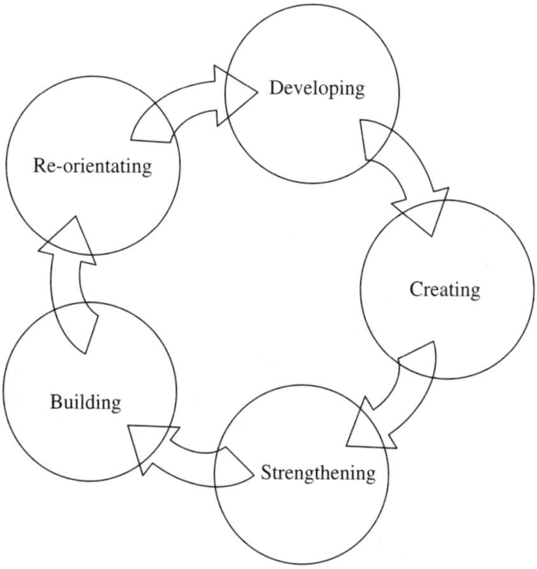


**Figure 5.2** The inter-related five priority action areas
*Source*: WHO, 1986.

- Strengthening community action.
- Building healthy public policy.
- Reorientating services in the interest of health.

## DEVELOPING PERSONAL SKILLS

Personal and social development is supported through health promotion by the provision of information, education and enhancing life skills. The choices available to people to take more control over their health and their environments are improved, and they are able to select preferences that are beneficial to health. Personal development enables people to adopt a life-long learning approach, by preparing themselves for all its stages, and to manage and cope with chronic illness and injuries. Opportunities arise for this to occur in schools, homes, at workplaces and in community settings through actions involving educational, professional, commercial and the nonstatutory sectors.

## CREATING SUPPORTIVE ENVIRONMENTS

The basis for a socio-ecological approach to health is noted in the inextricable links that there are between people and their environments. Health promotion encourages people to take care of each other, the community and the natural and built environments. To achieve this involves creating living and working conditions that are:

- safe
- stimulating
- satisfying
- enjoyable

An assessment of the health impacts of technology, work, energy production and urbanisation is needed. This will include the protection of natural and built environments, along with the conservation of our natural resources. Changing patterns of life, work and leisure have a significant impact on health. Work and leisure can and should be a source of health for people. How society organises work can help create a healthy society. Health promotion generates living and working conditions that are safe, stimulating, satisfying and enjoyable.

## STRENGTHENING COMMUNITY ACTION

Community action that is associated with the formulation and setting of priorities, the making of decisions, planning strategies and implementing them to attain improved health can happen through health promotion. However, for this to occur the empowerment of communities, their ownership and the control of their own activities and destinies are required. This will draw on existing human and material resources within the communities, with the aims of:

- enhancing self-help
- enhancing social support
- encouraging public participation and direction in health matters

Access to information, various learning opportunities and funding support are crucial if this is to occur in a meaningful manner.

## BUILDING HEALTHY PUBLIC POLICY

Health is the responsibility of policy makers in all areas, for example those in the workplace, the health-care sector and schools. Policy makers must be conscious of the consequences of their decisions and responsibilities for health. Health promotion policy aims to join and bring together legislation, the economy (including taxation for example) and also changes that occur at an organisational level to meet aims and objectives. This will only become a reality if joint action is taken to guarantee safer and healthier goods and services, healthier public services and cleaner, more enjoyable environments.

Health promotion therefore goes beyond health care. It places health on the agenda of policy makers in all sectors and at all levels, directing them to be aware of the health consequences of their decisions and to accept their responsibilities for health.

REORIENTATING HEALTH SERVICES

The health sector has had a tendency to focus on the provision of clinical and curative services. This must be challenged and there must be a concerted effort to move beyond this. The focus should be sensitive to and respecting of cultural needs; supportive of the needs of individuals and communities; and generating an awareness of the need to enhance relationships between the health sector and broader social, political, economic and physical environment sectors.

It is essential that a change in the attitude and the organisation of health services takes place, refocusing them on the holistic needs of the individual as a whole person. If this is to occur it will require specific attention in the health research literature with changes in professional education and training – an inter-disciplinary approach is advocated. Health-care professionals must work together towards a health-care system that plays a part in the pursuit of health.

The Ottawa Charter (WHO, 1986) has the potential, as a useful framework, to assist nurses to provide health promotion activity. The Charter goes beyond the individual in the public health debate and can overcome the problem of victim blaming. It enables and empowers individuals and communities (Yeo, 1993).

The fundamental principles associated with the Charter can be used successfully in many settings and environments and with various client groups, for example those with learning disabilities and/or mental health problems (WHO, 2000; National Health Service Education for Scotland, 2005). Loeb et al. (1998) point out that the mental health of individuals is influenced by many things, including public policy and the environment in which the individual finds him/herself.

The vision outlined in the Ottawa Charter was reaffirmed by the Jakarta Declaration (WHO, 1997). The Jakarta Declaration identifies five further priorities that will lead health promotion in the twenty-first century:

- Promote social responsibility for health.
- Increase investments for health development.
- Consolidate and expand partnerships for health.
- Increase community capacity and empower the individual.
- Secure an infrastructure for health promotion.

## PRODUCING AND PROVIDING PATIENT INFORMATION

This section of the chapter provides you with information regarding the production of patient information to enhance health promotion. The quality of information presented to patients can have an impact on the experience they have with health-care providers (Department of Health, 2003). The importance of improving information that is given to patients has been cited in some key government publications, for example *The NHS Plan* (Department of Health, 2000), Kennedy Report into the Bristol Royal Infirmary (2001) and *Good Practice in Consent* (Department of Health, 2001b).

Often those who want to lead a healthy life will require information (Sarafino, 2006). They may need to know:

- What to do.
- When to do it.
- Where to do it.
- How to do it.

Patient information refers to information that is produced and provided in any medium for the benefit of patients. Information that is produced can relate to information on specific diseases, for example diabetes mellitus, it can be associated with health services such as going into hospital or related to health promotion activities, for example smoking cessation (Duman, 2003).

Crane and Patel (2005) suggest that there are three things that need to be considered when writing information (from a medical perspective):

- What does the patient want to know?
- What messages does the medical profession want to get across?
- What is the most appropriate way to give the information?

Many nurses who provide and produce health information do so in a written form, through pamphlets, leaflets, posters or single sheets of paper. Written materials are often used to support one-to-one interactions with patients. Only 50 per cent of information can be recalled five minutes after a consultation with a patient, and patients' recall after a consultation has been demonstrated to be poor (Parkin and Skinner, 2003). Using literature to help patients participate in their own care can therefore be a useful resource.

Hospitals, charities and support groups produce their own literature related to a wide and varied range of topics (Crane and Patel, 2005). Providing patients with written information means they can take it away and absorb the contents at their own pace and in their own place.

The content of the information must be of a high quality if patients are to use it to enhance their health. Bennet and Bridger (1992) have noted that sometimes the standard is inadequate or the material is poorly presented. Just as it is important to ensure that you employ effective verbal communication with patients, it is important to ensure that written communication skills (remember these are nonverbal communication skills) are also effective. Attention to the information provided is important as it can instil confidence in patients, remind them of what is happening or what is going to happen, and allow them to make informed decisions. The Wanless Report recommends that improved health information be developed to help individuals engage with their own health care in an informed way (HM Treasury, 2002).

The Department of Health (2003) outlines five principles that it considers to underpin good patient communication:

- Improve health.
- Provide the best care.
- Act professionally.
- Work efficiently.
- Treat everybody equally.

Any written information provided to patients has the potential to hold up these values and the following should also be considered. Communication should be:

- Clear – so it can be understood.
- Straightforward – using fewer words and keeping to the necessary information.
- Modern – using everyday language and current images.
- Accessible – available to as many people as possible, avoiding jargon, up to date.
- Honest – based on current evidence.
- Respectful – sensitive to cultural needs and people, avoiding stereotypes.

Duman (2003) provides a process map to help develop patient information resources (see Figure 5.3).

The reasons for the provision of information are varied (see Table 5.2).

Prior to beginning the process of developing patient information, there are some key questions that must be answered. It is important to determine why the information needs to be produced. There may be corporate or departmental policies that need to be adhered to and these will include issues such as house style. These defined styles ensure that the information produced is consistent with the organisation's (and in some instances national) core values, for example there may be a thesaurus covering the use of preferred terms. Any information produced could render the organisation liable in law for the consequences of that information, therefore advice must be obtained on legal liability.

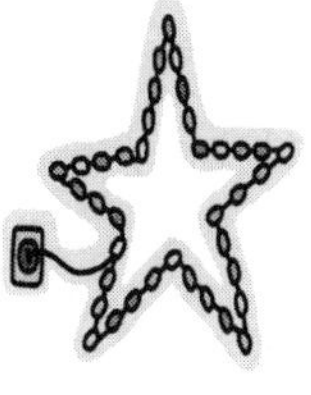

Imagine you had to go into hospital for a surgical procedure or for some form of treatment. Make a list of the information you would like to receive to

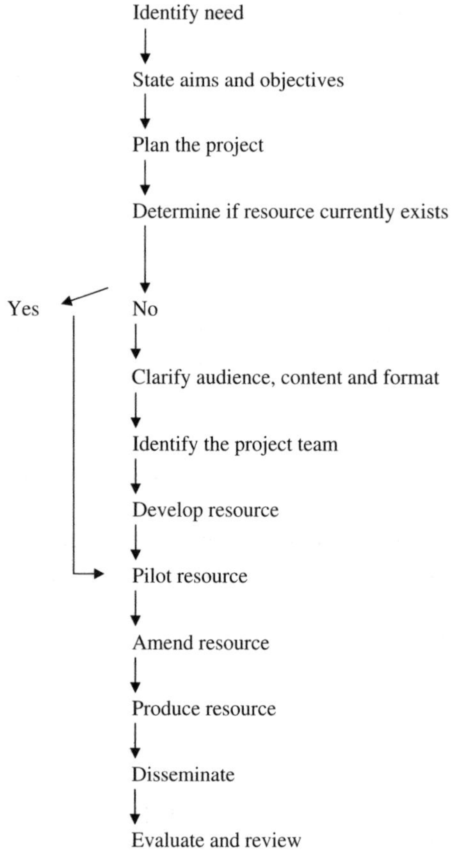


**Figure 5.3** The process map for developing patient information resources
*Source*: Duman, 2003.

**Table 5.2** Some reasons for providing patients with information

- To understand what is wrong.
- To gain a realistic idea of prognosis.
- To make the most of consultations.
- To understand the process and likely outcomes of possible tests and treatments.
- To assist in self-care.
- To provide reassurance and help to cope.
- To help others understand.
- To legitimise help seeking and concerns.
- To identify further information and self-help groups.
- To identify the best health-care providers.

*Source*: Crane and Patel, 2005; Department of Health, 2003; Coulter et al., 1998.

ensure that you are about to make the right decision for the treatment that is planned for you.

Your list might include some of the points highlighted below.

If information is being provided that offers the patient advice regarding any procedure that requires him/her to give explicit informed consent, then this information must adhere to and comply with the requirements provided by the Department of Health regarding consent (Department of Health, 2001b). The following are required as a minimum:

- The aim of the procedure and the intended benefits.
- What the procedure will involve.
- What kind of anaesthesia is likely to be used.
- Serious or frequently occurring risks if they exist for that procedure and the risks of doing nothing if applicable.
- Any additional procedures that are likely to be necessary.
- Any alternative treatments that may be available if appropriate.
- How long the patient may be in hospital.
- What the patient will experience before, during and after the procedure, for example details of the procedure, common side effects and pain relief if appropriate.

Table 5.3 provides questions that need to be considered during the planning stage.

It is vital that the target audience is clearly stated. For example, it may be patients who are at risk of contracting chlamydia (a sexually transmitted infection), however one leaflet or resource may not be appropriate for all potential groups, for example:

- women
- men
- men who have sex with men
- women who have sex with women
- adolescents

**Table 5.3** Issues to be considered during the planning stage

- Who is the package for (e.g. the target audience)?
- How can an assurance be made that the information provided is relevant to the audience?
- How do you envisage it will be used?
- What medium would be suited to the target audience?
- What measures will be taken to ensure that the information produced will be easily understood?
- Does it fit with the organisation's corporate image (e.g. its general aims and information policy)?

*Source*: Adapted from Duman, 2003.

The approach (i.e. the format) used should always be responsive to the target group, taking into account their needs and wishes. It is therefore important to have some insight into the target audience, taking some time to determine their particular characteristics. You should always listen to members of the target audience and their carers, aiming to ascertain how they want the information provided.

Producing and providing patient information can be a complex task. The nurse needs to ensure that the medium used is appropriate for the target audience, the content of the material is factually correct and that it conforms to the organisation's aims and objectives (corporate image). It is advisable at a draft production stage to show the material to at least one expert in the field (patient and/or health-care professional) to determine the accuracy of its content (Crane and Patel, 2005). Once feedback has been received, it will be necessary to show the information to a group of patients to gain their feedback, after which adjustments and alterations may be needed.

It must be remembered that patient information in the form of leaflets or pamphlets, despite increasing in popularity, is no substitute for spoken communication with the nurse. The written supplementary information provided can be used to expand and reinforce what has been said during a discussion or consultation, but never to replace the need for a face-to-face explanation of issues or concerns.

Crane and Patel (2005) provide some simple advice that may help to enhance the understanding of the information that you may provide. The following may help to ensure that you produce patient literature that will help the patient:

- Break down the information into small chunks – a question-and-answer format may help.
- Begin by stating what information you plan to offer, provide it and summarise it – say what you are going to say, say it and say it again.
- Choose the words that you intend to use carefully.
- Technical terms can be used (Abergavenny, 2003), however you must ensure that you have correctly assessed the needs of the audience.
- Use personal terms such as 'you' (as opposed to patient) and 'we' (as opposed to nurses).
- Take time to consider how much information is needed. Be aware, for example, that not all patients want to know their prognosis, particularly where the condition is serious (Schattner, 2002).

In Table 5.4 you will find a checklist that provides an outline of issues that should be taken into account when producing a leaflet or booklet. The checklist is not a complete list and it may be that not all of the items will be relevant. It should be used as a guide only.

**Table 5.4** Items that should be considered by the nurse when devising leaflets and booklets for operations, treatments and investigations

- ☐ What is the leaflet about and who is it for?
- ☐ What is the procedure?
- ☐ Why are they having the procedure? (Give the benefits and alternatives where appropriate)
- ☐ What preparation do they need or not need?
- ☐ Do they need a general anaesthetic, sedation or local anaesthetic?
- ☐ What happens when they arrive at the hospital/clinic/surgery, who will meet them?
- ☐ Will they be asked to sign a consent form or is verbal consent needed?
- ☐ What does the procedure involve? How long does it last? What does it feel like?
- ☐ What happens after the procedure – pain control, nursing checks, e.g. observations, stitches?
- ☐ How long will they be at the hospital/clinic/surgery?
- ☐ Do they need someone with them or any special equipment when they get home?
- ☐ What care do they need at home?
- ☐ What follow-up care is needed? Do they need to visit their doctor?
- ☐ What can go wrong, what signs to look out for and what to do if something goes wrong?
- ☐ When can they start their normal activities again, for example driving, sport, sex or work?
- ☐ Who can they contact if they have any more questions?
- ☐ Tell people where they can find more information, for example support groups and websites.

*Source*: Adapted from Department of Health, 2003.

When the information has been produced and is being used by the patient (or patient group) it must be evaluated to ensure that it is still current and relevant. Changes within health care and health provision are occurring at an exponential rate, new facts are uncovered, new treatments devised and erstwhile approaches to treatment or care may be discarded, therefore it is vital that evaluation and review take place. Duman (2003) suggests that evaluation and review take place about one year after the information's inception and at the maximum two years.

## CONCLUSIONS

The role of the nurse is challenging and one aspect of this complex role is to promote the interests of patients. This will include helping them to gain access to health and social care information and to support their choices related to their health-care needs.

Health promotion cannot be seen as a purely technical activity, it requires a variety of effective communication skills. The nurse must develop and hone his/her skills associated with health promotion. The current health agenda with its focus on health promotion means that the nurse will have to develop and build on a wide range of skills to provide pro-active health promotion with the ultimate aim of enhancing patient care.

The nurse should approach health promotion with an acceptance of the existing knowledge and beliefs of the patient. It should be remembered that some patients may only be able to adopt a healthier lifestyle if certain conditions are present and some of the conditions may be outside the immediate control of the patient and the nurse.

When opportunities arise to promote the patient's health the nurse should act accordingly (Whittam, 2003) in order to:

- Prevent disease and reduce mortality rates.
- Reduce risks associated with disease.
- Promote healthier lifestyles.

The nurse must consider the social factors that contribute to health and ill health as opposed to locating the cause in the individual. Health promotion activity does not occur in a vacuum. The health of a person, poor or good, is not always their own fault. Behaviours and the choices individuals make about their health are not always as a result of a lack of knowledge; other factors may be at play such as fear and denial.

This chapter has provided definitions of some key terms that are used within the health promotion arena. It must be noted, however, that definitions by their very nature can be restrictive and at best can only provide a summary of complex ideas and activities. In spite of these restrictions and limitations, definitions can assist when trying to comprehend the fundamental ideas and concepts associated with health promotion activities. It is important to define key terms that are associated with health promotion, if health promotion is going to be effective,

There are several models of health promotion that exist to help the nurse, patient and the community achieve 'health'. The use of these models and the various available frameworks (e.g. the Ottawa Charter and the Jakarta Declaration) provide guidance as well as situating health promotion within the wider social and political domain.

The provision and production of health promotion materials need much consideration if the patient is to receive high-quality advice. This chapter has provided information to help readers understand some important issues that must be considered if they are planning on producing health promotion materials for use with the public.

Finally, the formulation of new public health strategies and the need to orientate health services must be a priority for the government and the nursing profession in order to ensure that health promotion remains high on the political and social agenda.

## REFERENCES


Abergavenny, R.D. (2003) 'Patients prefer "medical labels" to lay language, study finds'. *British Medical Journal.* Vol 11, p 181.

Acheson, D. (1988) *Public Health in England.* Department of Health. London.

Becker, M.H. (1974) *The Health Belief Model and Personal Health Behaviour.* Slack. New Jersey.

Beattie, A. (1991) 'Knowledge and control in health promotion: A test case for social policy and theory' in Gabe, J., Calnan, M., and Bury, M. (eds) *The Sociology of the Health Service.* Routledge. London. pp 162–202.

Bennet, J. and Bridger, P. (1992) 'Communicating with patients'. *British Medical Journal.* Vol 305, p 1294.

Bridle, G., Riemsma, R.F., Patthenden, J., Sowden, A.J., Mather, L., Watt, I. and Walker, A. (2005) 'Systematic review of the effectiveness of health behavior interactions based on the transtheoretical model'. *Psychology and Health.* Vol 20, No 3, pp 283–301.

Colquhoun, D. and Kellehear, A. (1996) (eds) *Health Research in Practice: Personal Concerns and Public Issues.* Chapman Hall. London.

Coulter, A., Entwistle, V. and Gilbert, D. (1998) *Informing Patients: An Assessment of the Quality of Patient Information Materials.* King's Fund. London.

Crane, R. and Patel, B. (2005) 'Producing patient literature'. *Student British Medical Journal.* Vol 13, p 200.

Cusack, L., Smith, M. and Byrnes, T. (1997) 'Innovations in community heath nursing: Examples from practice'. *International Journal of Nursing Practice.* Vol 3, pp 133–136.

Department of Health (1992) *The Health of the Nation.* Department of Health. London.

Department of Health (1999a) *Making a Difference: Strengthening the Nursing, Midwifery and Health Visiting Contribution to Health and Social Care.* Department of Health. London.

Department of Health (1999b) *Saving Lives: Our Healthier Nation.* Department of Health. London.

Department of Health (2000) *The NHS Plan: A Plan for Investment, A Plan for Reform.* Department of Health. London.

Department of Health (2001a) *Shifting the Balance of Power.* Department of Health. London.

Department of Health (2001b) *Good Practice in Consent Implementation Guide.* Department of Health. London.

Department of Health (2003) *Toolkit for Producing Patient Information.* Department of Health. London.

Department of Health (2005a) *Choosing Health: Making Healthier Choices Easier.* Department of Health. London.

Department of Health (2005b) *Delivering Choosing Health: Making Healthier Choices Easier.* Department of Health. London.

Duman, M. (2003) *Producing Patient Information: How to Research, Develop and Produce Effective Information Resources.* King's Fund. London.

Dunkley, J. (2000) *Heath Promotion in Midwifery Practice: A Resource for Health Professionals.* Bailliere Tindall. Edinburgh.

Ewles, L. and Simnett, I. (2003) (5th edn) *Promoting Health: A Practical Guide.* Bailliere Tindall. Edinburgh.

Forster, D., Pannell, D. and Edwards, M. (1999) 'Health promotion' in Edwards, M. (ed.) *The Informed Practice Nurse.* Ch 4 pp 100–138.

Hampson, G. (2000) (4th edn) *Practice Nurse Handbook.* Blackwell. Oxford.

Hayes, L. (2005) 'Public health and nurses . . . What is your role'. *Primary Care Journal.* Vol 15, No 5, pp 22–25.

HM Treasury (2002) *Securing Our Future Health: Taking a Long-Term View.* HM Treasury. London.

Illich, I. (1976) *The Limits to Medicine: Medical Nemesis: The Expropriation of Health.* Penguin. Harmondsworth.

Kennedy Report into the Bristol Royal Infirmary (2001) *Learning from Bristol: The Report of the Public Inquiry into Children's Heart Surgery at the Bristol Royal Infirmary 1984–1995.* Her Majesty's Stationery Office. Command 5207.

Lisle, M. (2001) 'Organisational health: A new strategy for promoting health and well-being' in Scriven, A. and Orme, J. (eds) (2nd edn) *Health Promotion: Professional Perspectives.* Palgrave. Basingstoke. Ch 20 pp 222–235.

Loeb, D., Markham, W., Naidoo, J. and Wills, J. (1998) 'Mental health promotion' in Naidoo, J. and Wills, J. (eds) *Practicing Health: Dilemmas and Challenges.* Bailliere Tindall. London. Ch 13 pp 255–276.

Long, A. (2003) 'Public health: The promotion and protection of health' in Basford, L. and Slevin, O. (eds) (2nd edn) *Theory and Practice of Nursing: An Integrated Approach to Caring Practice.* Nelson Thorne. Cheltenham. Ch 32 pp 601–612.

Melling, K., Gleeson, J. and Hunter, K. (2004) 'Developing health promotion practice' in Chilton, S., Melling, K., Drew, D. and Clarridge, A. (eds) *Nursing in the Community: An Essential Guide to Practice.* Arnold. London. Ch 10 pp 95–102.

Montazeri, A., McGhee, S. and McEwan, J. (1998) 'Fear inducing and positive image strategies in health education campaigns'. *Journal of the Institute of Health Promotion and Education.* Vol 36, No 3, pp 68–75.

Naidoo, J. and Wills, J. (1998) (eds) *Practicing Health: Dilemmas and Challenges.* Bailliere Tindall. London.

Naidoo, J. and Wills, J. (2000) (2nd edn) *Health Promotion: Foundations for Practice.* Bailliere Tindall. London.

Naidoo, J. and Wills, J. (2001) 'Health promotion' in Naidoo, J. and Wills, J. (eds) *Health Studies: An Introduction.* Bailliere Tindall. London. Ch 10 pp 274–307.

Naidoo, J. and Wills, J. (2005) (2nd edn) *Public Health and Health Promotion: Developing Practice.* Bailliere Tindall. London.

National Health Service Education for Scotland (2005) *The Right Preparation: The Framework for Learning Disability Education in Scotland.* National Health Service Education for Scotland. Edinburgh.

Nutbeam, D. (2000) 'Health literacy as a public health goal: A challenge for contemporary health education and communication. Strategies in to the 21st century'. *Health Promotion International.* Vol 15, pp 259–267.

Nursing and Midwifery Council (2004) *Code of Professional Conduct: Standards for Conduct, Performance and Ethics.* NMC. London.

Parkin, T. and Skinner, T.C. (2003) 'Discrepancies between patient and professionals recall and perception of an outpatient consultation'. *Diabetic Medicine.* Vol 20, pp 909–914.

Russell, J. (2005) *Introduction to Psychology for Health Carers.* Nelson Thornes. Cheltenham.

Sarafino, E.P. (2006) (5th edn) *Health Psychology: Biopsychosocial Interactions.* Wiley. New Jersey.

Schattner, A. (2002) 'What do patients really want to know?'. *Quality Journal of Medicine.* Vol 95, pp 135–136.

Sigerist, H.E. (1946) *The University at the Crossroads.* Schuman. New York.

Stroebe, W. (2000) *Social Psychology and Health.* Open University. Buckingham.

Tannahill, A. (1985) 'What is health promotion?'. *Health Education Journal.* Vol 44, No 4, pp 167–168.

Tones, K. (2001) 'Health promotion: The empowerment imperative' in Scriven, A. and Orme, J. (eds) (2nd edn) *Health Promotion: Professional Perspectives.* Palgrave. Basingstoke. Ch 1 pp 3–18.

Tones, K. and Green, J. (2004) *Health Promotion: Planning and Strategies.* Sage. London.

Whittam, S. (2005) 'Maintaining a safe environment' in Holland, K., Jenkins, J., Solomon, J. and Whittam, S. (eds) *Applying the Roper, Logan and Tierney Model in Practice.* Churchill Livingstone. Edinburgh. Ch 3 pp 43–87.

World Health Organisation (1948) *Preamble to the Constitution of the World Health Organisation.* International Health Conference. New York.

World Health Organisation (1978) *Report on the International Conference on Primary Health Care, Alma Ata, 6–12th September.* WHO. Geneva.

World Health Organisation (1986) *Ottawa Charter for Health Promotion 1st International Conference on Health Promotion. November 17th–21st.* WHO. Ottawa.

World Health Organisation (1997) *The Jakarta Declaration on Leading Health Promotion into the 21st Century.* WHO. Geneva.

World Health Organisation (1998) *Health Promotion Glossary.* WHO. Geneva.

World Health Organisation (2000) *Women's Mental Health: An Evidence Based Review.* WHO. Geneva.

Wright, C. (2001) 'Community nursing: Crossing boundaries to promote health' in Scriven, A. and Orme, J. (eds) (2nd edn) *Health Promotion: Professional Perspectives.* Palgrave. Basingstoke. Ch 5 pp 51–64.

Yeo, M. (1993) 'Towards an ethic of empowerment for health promotion'. *Health Promotion International.* Vol 8, No 3, pp 225–235.

# 6 Assessment of Needs

The effective assessment of needs is paramount if the subsequent planning, implementation and evaluatory processes are to be successful. This chapter describes in detail how to undertake and document a comprehensive, systematic and accurate nursing assessment. The patient's physical, psychological, social and spiritual needs are considered. Models of nursing are briefly discussed in order to explain that undertaking an assessment of needs in isolation (the gathering of data) will limit care interventions. A guide or framework (a model of care) will help to enhance the patient's experience, and promote holistic nursing care.

Various assessment strategies are described and a range of assessment tools that are used to guide the collection of data for assessing the needs of the patient are also outlined.

## THE NURSING PROCESS

The nursing process is a systematic, patient-centred, goal-oriented approach to caring that provides a framework for nursing practice; it allows the nurse and the patient to work together (Taylor et al., 2005). Slevin (2003) refers to the nursing process as a problem-solving approach to the implementation of nursing, and nursing intervention takes place within the context of the nursing process; while Fryer (2003) describes it as a systematic inquiry into how patients' needs would be assessed, planned, implemented and evaluated.

The nursing process is nursing practice in action. It is a step-by-step approach to the provision of nursing care to patients. The nurse uses various skills to progress through the process in an orderly, systematic manner, with planned actions that are directed or aimed at achieving a particular goal or aim. The aim of the nursing process is to encourage the nurse together with the patient to make decisions and to solve problems in a more holistic manner, as opposed to a task-oriented approach to the delivery of nursing care.

In the UK it is common for theorists and practitioners to describe the nursing process as having four phases or components (Slevin, 2003; see Figure 6.1):

- assessment
- planning
- implementation
- evaluation

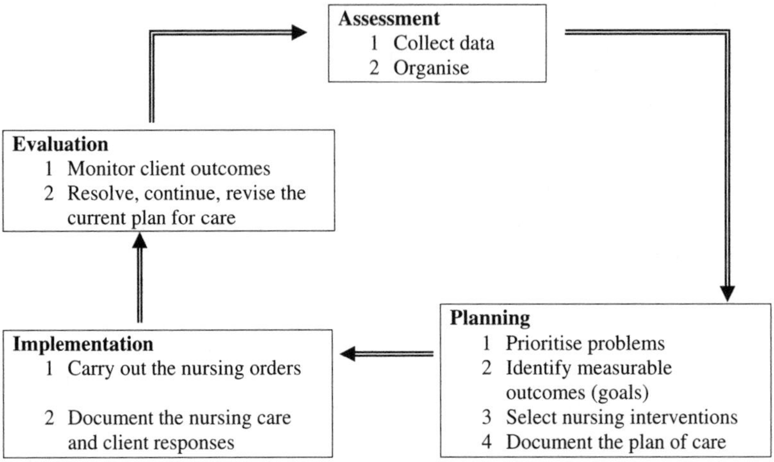


**Figure 6.1** The four-stage nursing process

A five-stage nursing process is gaining popularity in the UK. Previously the five-stage or five-component nursing process was used predominantly in the USA (see Figure 6.2):

- assessment
- nursing diagnosis
- planning
- implementation
- evaluation

The steps of the nursing process are not separate items; they are parts of a whole and are inter-related. This chapter will discuss the five stages. Table 6.1 provides a summary of the five phases/stages of the nursing process.

## WHAT IS ASSESSMENT?

Assessment is the first stage or step in the nursing process and is the systematic and continuous collection of facts or data. There are three key features associated with the assessment phase:

- *Communication* – obtaining a health history.
- *Measurement* – physiological measurements, the use of risk-assessment tools (Bird, 2005).
- *Observation* – observing the patient's nonverbal signs of pain (Feldt, 2000); observing the patient in his/her total environment, especially when in his/her

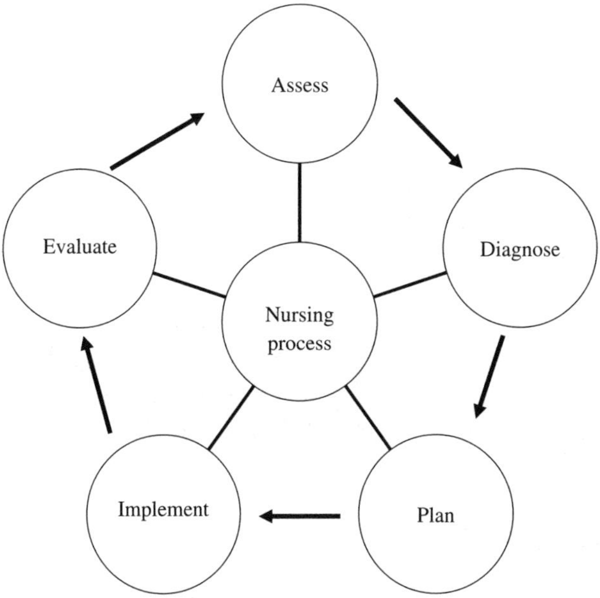


**Figure 6.2** The five-stage nursing process

own home (Rayman, 2004). Observation of the patient takes place each time the nurse and patient have any contact. The nurse observes many things such as the patient's mood, interactions with others, emotional responses, and detecting early signs of health deterioration, e.g. pallor, sweating and cyanosis.

Nicol et al. (2003) suggest that the assessment is crucial to the whole nursing process. When the data has been collected and analysed this will allow the nurse with the patient (if appropriate) to identify problems and strengths of the patient. Assessment can take place anywhere, for example in the hospital, in the patient's home or in the workplace.

Heath (2000) suggests that assessment is regarded as the data-collection phase that allows the nurse to make judgements about the patient's health, situation, needs and wishes. Assessment also helps to establish priorities and allows the planning of care. Assessment does not focus solely on the physical aspects of care, it also takes into account the patient's complete social and mental wellbeing.

The purpose of assessment, according to Rayman (2004), is to establish a database about the following:

- physical wellbeing
- emotional wellbeing

**Table 6.1** An overview of the five stages of the nursing process

| Stage/step of the nursing process | Description | Reason | Actions |
|---|---|---|---|
| **Assessing** | Collection, validation and communication of patient data | Make judgements about the patient's health status, the ability of the patient to manage his/her own health care and determine the need for nursing | Establish a database by:<br>• Obtaining a nursing history<br>• Conducting a physical and if needed psychological assessment<br>• Review of the patient's nursing and medical notes<br>• Seek secondary data from other health-care professionals, the patient's carer(s)<br>Continually update the database<br>Validate the data<br>Communicate data/findings (document findings) |
| **Diagnosing** | Analysis of patient data to determine patient's strengths and health problems that nursing interventions can prevent or resolve | Develop and prioritise a list of nursing diagnoses | Interpret and analyse patient data<br>Ascertain patient strengths and health problems<br>Devise and validate nursing diagnoses<br>Develop and document a list of nursing diagnoses that have been prioritised |

| | | | |
|---|---|---|---|
| **Planning** | Identify measurable outcomes and set goals that can prevent, relieve or resolve the problems identified. Select and describe appropriate nursing interventions. Document the plan of proposed care | To develop an individualised care plan that can be evaluated. To produce evidence that demonstrates an individual assessment of needs has taken place | Determine priorities<br>Document proposed outcomes and put into place an evaluatory strategy<br>Decide on appropriate nursing interventions<br>Communicate proposed plan of care |
| **Implementation** | The 'doing' stage. The plan of care is implemented at this stage | Assist and support the patient to achieve the stated goals, to enhance health, prevent disease, illness and deterioration in condition, provide comfort and maintain dignity | Carry out/implement the planned care<br>Continue to gather data and modify the plan of care in response to the patient's condition<br>Document actions and omissions |
| **Evaluation** | Monitoring and measuring of patient outcomes and effects of nursing interventions, with reference to interventions that may have helped or exacerbated the patient's condition<br>Consider revision of the plan of care if needed | To continue with plan of care, modify nursing activities or terminate interventions | Refer to original database to determine if there has been a change in the patient's condition as a result of the planned and implemented nursing interventions<br>Measure how well the plan of care has benefited the patient's condition<br>Determine if there are certain interventions that have adversely effected the patient's condition<br>Modify care plan if appropriate<br>Document findings |

*Source*: Taylor et al., 2005, Timby, 2005; Kozier et al., 2004; Beretta, 2003.

- intellectual functioning
- social relationships
- spiritual condition

It is important to note that data is not collected as a one-off activity. Data collection occurs continuously – it is a continuous process. Ongoing assessment will alert the nurse to any changes in the patient's health as well as any changes in response to nursing intervention; a patient's condition can change quickly.

Kozier et al. (2004) note that the activities associated with the assessment phase of the nursing process will include:

- Making a reliable observation.
- Being able to distinguish relevant from irrelevant data.
- Being able to distinguish important data from unimportant data.
- Validating, organising and categorising the data according to a framework.
- Making judgements.

Establishing a database means that the nurse has to gather information and this is usually done by interviewing the patient (or his/her carer, family or significant other). This allows the nurse to obtain a nursing history. Epstein et al. (1997) suggest that it is the history that guides the nurse though a series of questions designed to build a profile of the patient and his/her problems. The history-taking event ends with the nurse having a deeper understanding of the patient and the ability to go on and make a diagnosis.

The way the nurse can go about obtaining a patient history is described below. More data can be collected by examining the patient if needed. Further information can be gleaned from the patient's nursing/medical notes and other health-care professionals, for example a physiotherapist or occupational therapist. A database may contain the information detailed in Table 6.2.

## OBTAINING A PATIENT HISTORY

Chapter 4 outlined the skills the nurse needs to possess in order to communicate effectively with the patient. This aspect of this chapter builds on those nursing skills and provides insight into how best to obtain a patient history.

The accuracy of the information that the nurse collects or gathers from a patient during a consultation (clinical interview) has the potential to influence the diagnosis and subsequent treatment of the patient. Obtaining a patient history in a competent manner is crucial to the patient encounter and patient outcome (Matthews, 1998).

The patient and the nurse are partners in care. The clinical interview, according to Peate (2005), is at the heart of the nurse–patient relationship and this confirms the bond between the two parties, in order to begin to provide care for the patient. The patient needs the help of the nurse, who in turn needs

**Table 6.2** Some components of a patient history database

**Demographic data**
- The patient's name (include here the name he/she wishes to be known by)
- Address
- Age
- Sex
- Marital status
- Occupation
- Religious preferences (if any)

**Reason for admission/chief complaint**
The reason the patient (or his/her guardian) gives for admission should be documented. The response the patient gives to your question should be documented – verbatim and in inverted commas ' ' so that the patient's understanding of his/her condition/complaint can be noted in his/her own words.

**History of present illness**
Ask the patient:
- When did the symptoms start?
- Was the onset of the symptoms sudden or gradual?
- How often does the problem occur?
- Where is the exact location of the distress/problem?
- Describe the character of the complaint, for example the intensity of pain, the nature of the sputum – colour and consistency, give details about any vomit (colour, quantity) or any discharge (colour, quantity and from where).
- Any activity the patient was performing when the problem arose.
- Do any activities aggravate or alleviate the condition, for example coughing or passing urine, lying down?

**Past history**
Ascertain any relevant past history. Ask the patient about:
- Any childhood illness (current or in the past).
- Any immunisations (as a child or/and an adult) and when they were given.
- Any known allergies, e.g. allergies to medicines, foods, other agents such as plasters, and the type of reaction that occurs when exposed to the allergen.
- Any accidents or illnesses (how, when, where).
- Any hospitalisation or time spent in hospital – reasons, any surgical interventions, any complications.
- Medication they may be taking: include here prescribed medications, medications bought over the counter and use of recreational drugs. Note dose, route and frequency.

**Family history of illness**
Spend time with the patient asking about any family history of illness in order to determine if there are any risk factors for certain diseases (e.g. sickle cell anaemia). Ask about the current health of siblings, parents, grandparents, their ages if still alive and, if deceased, the cause of death.

**Lifestyle**
The nurse can use a model of care to help guide this aspect of the assessment process (models of care are discussed later in this chapter). The issues below can help guide the discussion.

**Table 6.2** *Continued*

Ask about personal habits such as the frequency and amount of:
- Tobacco use (type).
- Alcohol consumption (type).

Ask the patient to describe their typical diet:
- Any special dietary needs.
- Number of meals consumed in a day.

Consider asking about leisure activities:
- How much exercise is taken and what type?
- Hobbies or interests.

**Social history**
Social data will help to complete the picture of the patient and will provide information based on the following:
- Family relationships.
- Any particular ethnic/cultural beliefs.
- Occupational history (current and past occupations).
- Economic status (is the patient self-employed for example).
- Whether the patient is receiving any social services to help him/her cope at home, e.g. home help or district nursing services.

**Psychological data**
- Is the patient aware of any stressors that impact negatively on his/her health? What is his/her perception of them?

**Communication data**
Determine how the patient communicates:
- Can the patient verbally respond (e.g. is he/she conscious)?
- What language does the patient prefer to communicate in (is English the patient's first language)?
- Does the patient use eye movements, gestures, touch, posture to interact with others?

*Source*: Adapted from Kozier et al., 2004.

information from the patient in order to offer that help. A professional relationship needs to be developed and maintained between the patient and the nurse in order to provide the most effective care.

It is important for the patient to know from the outset how the data will be managed, what the nurse intends to do with the information gathered, what will be written, where this will be stored and who will be able to access it. Being open about the management of the information the patient wishes to give to the nurse may put the patient's mind at rest that the information collected will be treated confidentially, with respect, kept safe and when disclosure is to be made to a third party this will be done with the patient's consent and will be made in his/her best interests.

The clinical interview can be looked at as having three parts:

- Beginning the interview and introductions.
- Obtaining the history.
- Terminating the interview.

Obtaining a health history from a patient demands a skilled, confident and competent nurse. The more often you undertake a nursing assessment and the gathering of information through the clinical interview, the more proficient you will become (Nusbaum and Hamilton, 2002).

There are no hard-and-fast rules of obtaining a health history; each nurse will have his/her own approach. The nurse should aim to create a comfortable atmosphere with a relaxed, but professional and friendly approach. The way in which the interview is carried out will determine the amount of information the patient may be prepared to reveal and some patients may have to reveal some very intimate and personal issues. If the patient is to reveal intimate, personal and potentially embarrassing information, he/she may find this difficult and hence the nurse must provide a safe environment in which to do this.

Each aspect of the clinical interview is addressed briefly in the following section.

### Meeting, Greeting and Seating

The approach taken will depend on where the interview is taking place. For example, if it is in the patient's own home then the nurse will need to wait to be invited into the patient's home and take his/her cues from the patient or his/her family.

If, however, the information-gathering event takes place in a clinical setting such as a hospital ward, a clinic or a GP surgery, the nurse must stand up as the patient enters the room, greet him/her, face the patient and look at him/her directly – smile. Greet the patient verbally (being aware of the nonverbal greeting you are simultaneously making). Explain to the patient who you are (even though you will have some form of name badge or identity on you) and the reason for the consultation, for example 'to obtain a clear picture of the problem/issue'. Ascertain at this stage how the patient would like you to refer to him/her. Using terms that make assumptions about the patient should be avoided, for example when enquiring about a patient's sexual orientation it is advised that the nurse use the term 'partner' as opposed to 'boyfriend' or 'girlfriend', 'husband' or 'wife'. Ask about the patient's partner instead of asking if he/she is married or not. The response the patient gives may confirm if he/she is married or not.

Deciding to conduct the interview with the patient alone or with his/her partner present needs much thought. It could be that the patient may not be as open or forthcoming with information if the partner is present; however, joint consultations can provide much important detail. The nurse will need to exercise his/her professional judgement in coming to a decision about this issue.

It may be appropriate to shake the patient's hand, but be aware of cultural values: some cultures may not accept a female touching a male and vice versa. Invite the patient to where he/she should sit: indicate this clearly by gesture and verbally. The nurse should then sit down in a nonthreatening manner. Explain that you will be taking some notes during the interview, reaffirming that the information given will be treated in confidence.

Noise and interruptions can be disconcerting and cause distraction; if possible a quiet room should be sought in which to conduct the interview. Seating and the way this has been arranged should be given consideration. If possible, the patient's seat should be placed in such a way as to avoid the use of a desk, which could appear confrontational; arrange the seats so that they are at the side of the desk. Doing this gives the nurse an opportunity to observe the patient's body language – remember, however, that this type of arrangement also allows the patient to observe your body language. The nurse must also consider how he/she is dressed for the interview: a dress code may be apparent in some clinical areas and this will dictate how the nurse should dress. Epstein et al. (1997) suggest that the way the health-care professional is dressed can have implications for the relationship.

When the interview takes place (the timing of the interview) needs to be given consideration: try to avoid meal times or rest periods. Sufficient time must be set aside by the nurse, and if possible inform the patient of how much of his/her time you may need to take to conduct the interview. Depending on the reason for the interview, the time required will vary. Tomlinson (1998) suggests that when carrying out a sexual health interview, for example, between 45 and 60 minutes will be needed.

Make the patient feel as comfortable as possible, encourage him/her to feel safe, relaxed and to talk openly. On some occasions the patient may reveal information that the nurse may find shocking, however it is crucial that a non-judgemental approach be taken. Often nurses make use of several techniques to promote comfort intuitively:

- Greeting the patient.
- Seating arrangements.
- Ensuring privacy (a 'do not disturb' sign, telephones diverted and mobile telephones switched off).

## Obtaining the History

When introductions have been performed and the patient feels comfortable, the nurse needs to ask questions to generate more insight into the patient's needs. It may help the patient if the nurse reiterates and explains the reasons questions are being asked. For example: 'I am asking these questions so that I can assess your needs fully and work out the right care for you, therefore I need to know a bit more detail about your health.'

If the nurse undertakes the history-taking exercise as if he/she is asking questions from a questionnaire or a list that is to be run through with the patient, then this approach is in danger of losing all of its potential worth. Asking a lot of questions will result in the patient providing a lot of answers. There is a danger that the problem the patient has presented with may not have been identified because the nurse did not hear, as he/she has not allowed the patient to give details. The nurse must listen to the patient and if needed allow or give the patient permission to tell his/her story.

Questioning approaches have been briefly discussed in Chapter 4. However, to reiterate:

- Use appropriate opening questions, for example: 'Could you tell me what it was that led to you come here today for help?'
- Use verbal facilitation to encourage his/her patient to tell his/her story in his/her own words, for example encourage the patient to continue talking by saying: 'Please go on and tell me some more about it', 'What happened next?', 'You said just then that you felt a pain.'
- Nonverbal facilitation should also be used, for example head nodding, looking, attentive posture.
- Listen, allow the patient sufficient time to talk and avoid interrupting too quickly with questions or reassurance.
- Encourage the patient to focus by bringing the patient back to the point if he/she talks about unrelated areas.
- Seek clarification of any issues you are unsure about and encourage the patient to do the same.
- Avoid the use of jargon, both the jargon the patient may be using or any that you may be using – seek clarification.
- Avoid bias by the use of leading questions, for example: 'Are you depressed?', 'You couldn't breathe very well?' Try instead to use open-ended questions, such as: 'How was your mood at that time?', 'How was your breathing?'
- Take care to avoid using multiple questions, such as: 'How are you and how has your weight been?'
- Encourage the patient to be precise about the issues, such as dates of onset of key symptoms, problems or events, nature of previous treatments. Cross-check key points, for example: 'Could I just clarify this . . .'
- During the physical examination, use all the above communication skills appropriately, being particularly attentive to the patient's responses to your palpation and percussion. Consider incorporating your auditory, tactile and olfactory senses.
- Above all, respect the patient.

### Terminating the Interview

The ending of the relationship is just as important as the formulation. At the end of the interview ensure that there is time to summarise what the patient has told you. Make it clear to the patient that you would like to sum up the history with him/her to verify the accuracy of your account of his/her problems/issues and to determine if anything important has been missed out. Ask if there is anything he/she would like to add before the interview is concluded. Thank the patient for his/her time.

When a health history is required from children, young people and people with learning disabilities this may present challenges, as the carer or parents may have accompanied the patient and may tend to answer for him/her. Furthermore, the patient may be unwilling to divulge information with a third party present. The use of dolls, puppets and images to demonstrate what is being discussed can help. Wakley et al. (2003) suggest breaking each period of communication/interaction into shorter parts, after each section checking that all parties have understood what is being said. The nurse needs to be aware of his/her limitations and be prepared to refer the patient to a more appropriate health-care professional if he/she is feeling out of his/her depth.

## MEASUREMENTS/RISK-ASSESSMENT TOOLS

The second important feature of the assessment phase is the ability to carry out measurements, for example physiological measurements, or risk assessments using recognised risk-assessment tools such as pain assessment or risk-assessment tools associated with the prevention of pressure ulcers.

### The Skin and the Risk of Pressure Ulcers

The largest and heaviest organ in the body is the skin; this is the primary defence against pathogenic invasion (Doughty, 2004). The skin is a sensory organ and has several physiological functions.

A pressure ulcer or pressure sore can be defined as an area of skin and tissue loss that has been caused by long-standing or extreme soft-tissue pressure. Pressure ulcers often develop because of external pressure that causes an occlusion of blood vessels and endothelial damage to both the arterioles and microcirculation (Courtenay, 2002).

External pressure is a primary causative factor associated with the onset of pressure ulcers, and because of this it follows that some bones that are close to the skin, for example shoulders, hips, heels and the sacrum, are possible sites for ulcer formation. The pressure sent from the surface of the skin to the bones results in compression of the underlying tissue.

When conducting a holistic assessment of the patient. the nurse must take into account certain intrinsic risk factors that may result in the development of a pressure ulcer, for example:

- reduced mobility or immobility
- sensory impairment
- acute illness
- level of consciousness
- extremes of age
- vascular disease
- severe chronic or terminal illness
- previous history of pressure-sore damage
- malnutrition and dehydration

Extrinsic factors also exist that may cause or predispose a patient to tissue damage, and where possible these should be removed or diminished to prevent injury. For example:

- pressure
- shearing
- friction

If the nurse is to prevent or minimise the effects of pressure ulcers, then one important aspect of nursing practice will be to identify those patients who may be at risk of developing them and the nurse does this by conducting an in-depth, holistic assessment of the patient. A pressure ulcer (sore) risk calculator is needed to provide an objective assessment of risk. Risk-assessment tools, however (e.g. the Waterlow scale, 1985), should only be used as an aide mémoire and can never replace clinical judgement (NICE, 2001). Figure 6.3 describes the Waterlow scale.

There are many risk-assessment tools available to help the nurse make objective (as opposed to subjective) judgements and each clinical area will choose the tool that best suits the patient's needs. The timing of the assessment of risk should be based on each individual patient, but this should be within six hours of the start of admission and assessment must be ongoing. The importance of ongoing assessment has already been discussed in this chapter. The NMC (2002) states that all aspects of care must be documented; this is also true of the outcome of assessment and reassessment of a patient who may be at risk of developing pressure ulcers.

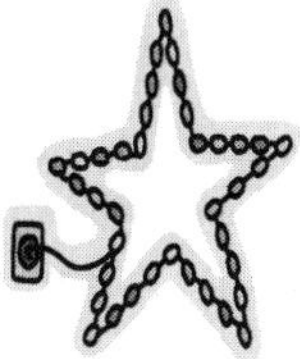

Can you list and describe any other types of risk-assessment tool you may have seen in use? The following are tools that are often used in clinical settings:

| **Build/weight for height** | **Visual skin type** | **Continence** | **Mobility** | **Sex Age** | **Appetite** |
|---|---|---|---|---|---|
| Average **0**<br>Above average **2**<br>Below average **3** | Healthy **0**<br>Tissue paper **1**<br>Dry **1**<br>Oedematous **1**<br>Clammy **1**<br>Discolour **2**<br>Broken/spot **3** | Complete **0**<br>Occasionally incontinent **1**<br>Catheter/incontinent of faeces **2**<br>Doubly incontinent **3** | Fully mobile **0**<br>Restricted/difficult **1**<br>Restless/fidgety **2**<br>Apathetic **3**<br>Inert/traction **4** | Male **1**<br>Female **2**<br>14–49 **1**<br>50–64 **2**<br>65–75 **3**<br>75–80 **4**<br>81+ **5** | Average **0**<br>Poor **1**<br>Anorectic **2** |

| **Special risk factors:** | **Assessment value** |
|---|---|
| (1) Poor nutrition e.g. terminal cachexia **8**<br>(2) Sensory depravation e.g. diabetes, paraplegia, CVA **5**<br>(3) High dose antiinflammatory or steroid use **3**<br>(4) Smoking 10+ per day **1**<br>(5) Orthopaedic surgery/fracture below waist **3** | At risk = **10**<br>High risk = **15**<br>Very high risk = **20** |

**Directions for use:**

1 Assess the patient, circling the number in each category in which the patient fits.
2 Add up all the numbers, including 'special risk factors'.
3 If the total places the patient within the 'at risk', 'high risk' areas, turn the card over and read the suggested preventative aids listed on the back.
4 Record the circled numbers in the patient's documentation, giving the total and the date.
5 Assess each patient as per protocol.

**Figure 6.3** The Waterlow scale.
*Source*: Waterlow, 1985.

- The Glasgow coma scale (this tool measures levels of consciousness).
- Pain-assessment scales (there are many of these tools in use and there are specific ones related to specific patient groups, e.g. children).
- The rule of nines, which helps the nurse to assess the extent of a burn (see Figure 6.4).
- The Lund and Browder chart (Lund and Browder, 1944), used predominantly in assessing the extent of a burn in a baby but can be used in children and adults.

## MAKING A NURSING DIAGNOSIS

Step two of the nursing process requires the nurse to make a nursing diagnosis. Having gathered the information, performed a risk assessment and undertaken a physical examination, the nurse then identifies the health-related problem. Analysis of the data gathered is now needed to determine if the findings are normal or abnormal (Timby, 2005). The nurse must now consider carefully the data that has been collected and he/she begins to interpret, analyse and synthesise it (Taylor et al., 2005).

The diagnosis can be cited as 'actual' or 'potential'. For example, the patient may have been assessed by the nurse and as a result of his/her condition there

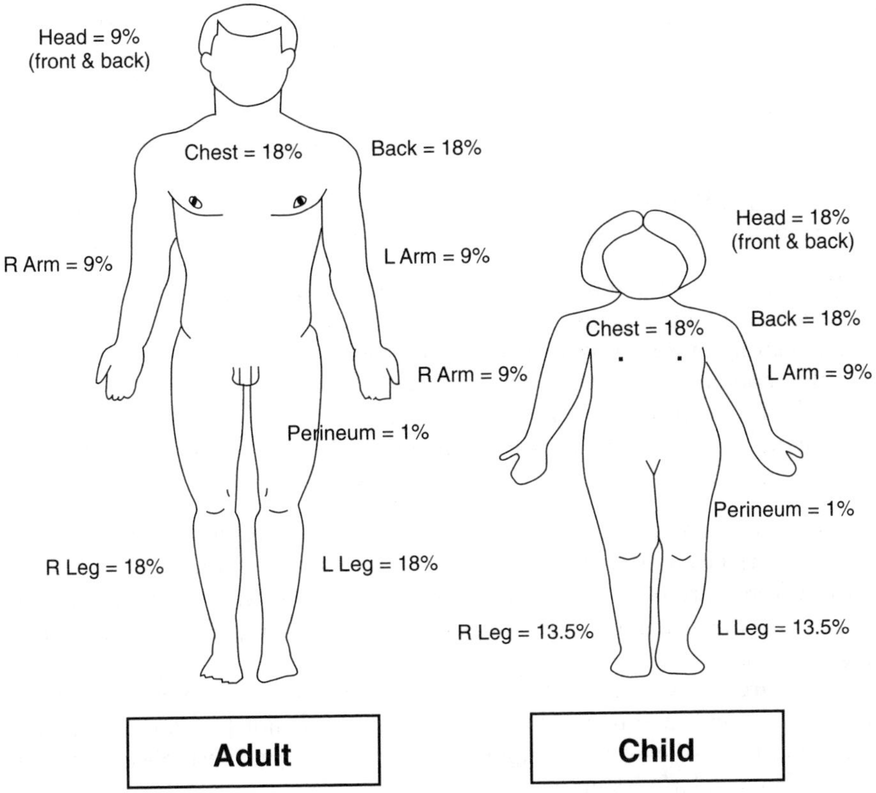


**Figure 6.4** The rule of nines assessment tools for both an adult and a child

may be problems associated with sleep and the problems can be actual or potentially occurring. A list will have been formulated by the nurse and statements will have been compiled that reflect the problems identified (Kozier et al., 2004).

Alfaro-LeFevre (2002) states that the diagnosis stage of the nursing process is a pivotal point in the process, as the accuracy and relevancy of the whole nursing care plan will depend on the nurse's ability to be able to identify both the problems and their cause. The creation of a care plan that pro-actively promotes health and prevents problems before they begin will depend on the nurse's ability to recognise risks.

## PLANNING

The nurse works with the patient and family (if appropriate) in order to establish priorities, identify the expected patient outcomes, choose interventions to help alleviate or prevent problems and communicate the plan of care – the planning stage. The identification of measurable goals or outcomes is given much thought at this stage. Once the plan of care is decided on and documented, the nurse with the patient and family must ensure that the goals stated are revised as and when appropriate. The nurse should ask the question: 'How can the patient's needs be met?'

Sibson (2005) suggests that consideration must be given to what nursing care will be undertaken to prevent or manage problems. This will include:

- Preventing identified problems from becoming actual problems.
- Solving actual problems.
- Alleviating those problems that cannot be solved and assisting the individual to cope positively with these problems.
- Preventing recurrence of a treated problem.
- Helping a person to be as pain free and comfortable as possible when death is inevitable.

Some problems the patient presents with will require immediate attention and they are given highest priority. For example, a patient who is liable to self-harm will require help and nursing interventions that will prevent harm. It is imperative that the nurse determines which problems require the most immediate attention.

There are many ways to determine priorities and one way is to use (as a guide) Maslow's hierarchy of needs. This model is not the only model and different areas of care may employ different methods to establish priorities. Table 6.3 considers this hierarchy.

The plan of care that will be formulated once the goals have been set can be seen as a prescription for care. The goal statements and the interventions required to meet the patient's needs must be documented. The components of a measurable goal should comprise the following, using the mnemonic **STAMP**:

**S**pecific – the goal must be specific with details and avoid being vague.
**T**ime element – time limits should be applied. The time limits will depend on the goal set, e.g. whether it is a long-term goal or a short-term goal. The target date or time for achievement should be specified when possible.
**A**chievable – and the goal must be realistic for the patient and the situation he/she finds him/herself in.
**M**easurable – the proposed intervention should be measurable.
**P**atient centred – 'The patient will . . .'

The following is an example of a goal statement that contains all of the components stated above. It is a goal statement for a patient who is asthmatic:

*Mrs Jones will be able to perform, using a peak flow meter, a peak flow rate of 400 ml 20 minutes after having had a prescribed bronchodilator nebuliser.*

**Table 6.3** An adaptation of Maslow's hierarchy of needs

| | 
|---|
| **Self-actualisation**<br>Realising full potential, 'becoming everything one is capable of becoming'. |
| **Cognitive needs**<br>Knowledge and understanding, curiosity, exploration, needs for meaning and predictability. |
| **Esteem needs**<br>The esteem and respect of others and self-esteem and self-respect. A sense of competence. A sense of worth. |
| **Love and belongingness**<br>Receiving and giving love, affection, trust and acceptance. Affiliating, being part of a group (family, friends, work). Relationships with others. |
| **Safety needs**<br>Protection from potentially dangerous objects or situations, e.g. the elements, physical illness. The threat is both physical and psychological (e.g. 'fear of the unknown'). Importance of routine and familiarity. Protection from danger or threat. |
| **Physiological needs**<br>Food, drink, oxygen, temperature regulation, elimination, rest, activity, sex. These are the basic requirements. |

*Source*: Adapted from Maslow, 1954.

This goal is specific **(S)**, it is also precise and detailed, it allows Mrs Jones and all who care for her to understand what this goal is trying to achieve in relation to her prescribed medication (the nebuliser). There is a clear time **(T)** element attached to the goal statement – 20 minutes after the nebuliser has been given. It is achievable **(A)** and realistic and Mrs Jones should be able to perform a peak flow of 400 ml as the nurse has assessed her condition. It is measurable **(M)** and the measure is the 400 ml after 20 minutes she is expected to be able to produce after the drug (a bronchodilator has been given to her). The goal is patient **(P)** centred, it is for Mrs Jones as it has been stated that she is the person for whom the goal has been devised.

Producing measurable outcomes can be difficult. The following are some verbs that can help you write measurable outcomes:

- identify
- define
- explain
- apply
- demonstrate
- select

The following are verbs that are to be avoided when composing measurable outcomes as they are too general and difficult to measure (Taylor et al., 2005). Compare them with the observable and measurable verbs in the list above:

- know
- understand
- become aware
- learn

It takes time to write competent goal statements. You must remember practice makes perfect. Using the **STAMP** mnemonic may help you to take into account all the important components.

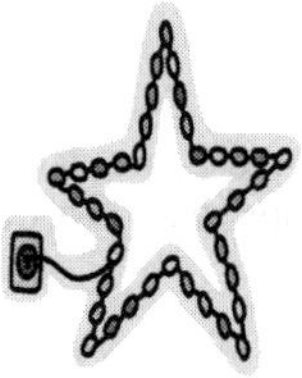

In the following goal statement, can you determine the STAMP components for this patient?

*By the end of the week (8/9/07) Mrs Mehta will be able to walk the length of the ward with the aid of one other person twice daily.*

'By the end of the week' gives (T), 'Mrs Mehta' gives (P), and (A) and (M) are contained in the goal of walking the ward with another person's help twice daily. You will have to decide if it is specific and a good test for this is if you had to nurse Mrs Mehta, would you be able to determine the aim of the goal statement?

How might the following statement be rewritten in order for it to become specific and clear?

*Encourage fluids.*

This statement is not specific, it is ambiguous and is in danger of being interpreted differently by different people, and as a result the care provided may be inconsistent and inadequate. You might have considered adding the patient's name and being more specific about the type of fluid, how often the patient is to have the fluid and when. A revised statement might look like this:

*Provide Lily with 100 ml of oral fluid of her choice every hour while she is awake.*

According to Gega (2004), the language used when writing a problem statement should be:

- user friendly
- nonjudgemental
- personalised

Gega (2004) also provides some helpful points to test if the language used conforms with the criteria above. The nurse can ask him/herself the following:

- Would this make sense to my patient?
- If this were me, would I mind someone else saying this about me?
- Would I be happy for my patient to read this?
- Does this describe my patient's personal experiences of the problem?

## IMPLEMENTATION

The penultimate stage of the nursing process is the implementation stage, often referred to as the 'doing' stage. The implementation stage will only be as good as the activity undertaken in the planning stage; here the quality of the goal statements and the ability to communicate them are vital. If the goal statement is written in a nonsensical manner, for instance it is not measurable or achievable, then the care that is subsequently provided is in danger of harming the patient. During the planning stage the nurse will have to have documented the proposed nursing interventions for others to read and adhere to.

Reference to the care plan will advise the nurse what nursing interventions are to be performed, how the proposed nursing interventions are to be performed, when they are to be performed and by whom – the what, how, when and who. As with all other aspects of the nursing process the nurse continues to gather and collect data, amending and reviewing care as this new data is gathered, informing the plan of care in an ongoing manner. All care provided (or any that has been omitted) must be documented in line with local policy and in keeping with the tenets associated with the NMC's guidelines (2002).

McClosky and Bulechek (2000) define a nursing intervention as any treatment that a nurse performs to enhance patient outcomes. These nursing interventions can include both direct and indirect nurse-initiated care.

The nurse must remember to act in partnership with the family (if appropriate) when implementing care. Always take time to explain to the patient what you are doing and why, and explain this to the patient in a language that he/she understands. Prior to implementing the proposed nursing actions you must always reassess the patient to determine that the proposed action is still required and appropriate.

## EVALUATION

The final stage allows the patient and the nurse to work together to measure and decide if the proposed outcomes that were detailed in the nursing care plan have been achieved. Evaluation does not occur as a one-off activity, it is ongoing and occurs throughout the patient's stay or during his/her contact with the nurse. While this stage is considered as the last step it is not, in reality it is an ongoing activity. The evaluation stage is discussed in more detail in Chapter 10.

## NURSING MODELS

Nurses can use nursing models in a variety of settings to help guide practice and, in particular, the assessment stage of the nursing process. Wright (1990) provides a definition of a nursing model. He states that nursing models include a collection of ideas, knowledge and values about nursing and they enable nurses to make explicit the manner in which they work with patients as individuals or groups. A common theme emerges when attempting to define nursing models: they attempt to express the reality of nursing and have the potential to enable nurses to work towards common goals (Ramsay, 1998).

Conceptual models of nursing attempt to articulate reality, but they can only do this by providing the nurse with a descriptive representation of the beliefs concerning nursing. Fawcett (1995) postulates that central to any nursing model are the following:

- The meaning of nursing.
- The individuals receiving nursing care.
- The meaning of health.

Several models of care exist that will help nurses provide the patient with consistency and continuity. The choice of model will depend on the patient and the philosophy of care used in the care area. Examples of models are:

- Orem's Self-Care model (1995).
- Roper, Logan and Tierney's model (1996).
- Casey's Partnership Nursing model (1988).
- Peplau's model (1988).

One of the most popular and most widely used models in the UK is the Roper, Logan and Tierney model based on a model of living (Roper et al., 1996). Briefly, this model helps guide the nurse, especially during the assessment stage of the nursing process, by encouraging the nurse to consider the following five components or concepts:

- Twelve activities of living.
- The lifespan.
- The dependence/independence continuum.
- The five factors that influence the activities of living.
- Individuality in living.

Figure 6.5 provides a diagrammatic overview of the model of living.

When the nurse uses Roper et al.'s model he/she concentrates on the activities of living, basing the assessment on the patient's usual abilities/routine. When the nurse ascertains what the patient usually does in relation to the activities of living, a comparison can then be made based on what the patient is like now. The activities are not assessed in isolation, the nurse must also consider what effect the five influencing factors may have on the patient's

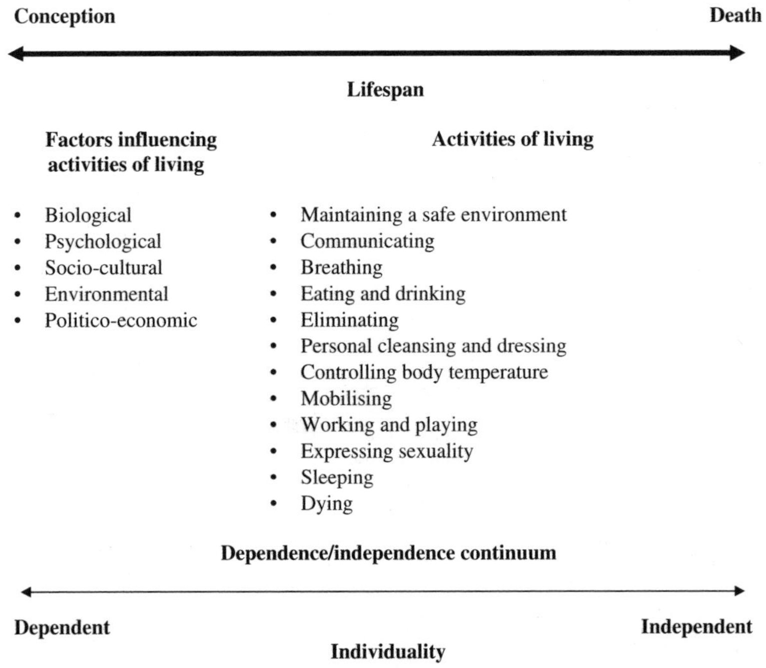


**Figure 6.5** A diagrammatic representation of the model of living
*Source*: Adapted from Roper et al., 1996; Holland, 2003.

abilities to carry out the activities of living, where he/she is in relation to lifespan and the degree of dependence/independence. When carrying out the assessment the nurse must at all times consider the patient as a unique individual, thereby supporting the notion of a holistic, individual approach to nursing care.

Orem's model is American in origin and is based on the concept of self-care. Orem uses universal self-care requisites on which to base a nursing assessment (see Table 6.4).

When using Orem's model the aim of assessment is to determine the patient's ability to self-care (Beretta, 2003). Having identified a shortfall in self-care, the nurse then needs to consider self-care limitations and self-care deficits that have become apparent as a result of the assessment. The nurse's role is to help the patient with the identified deficits.

Casey's Partnership model is used in the paediatric setting. Figure 6.6 provides a diagrammatic representation of the model.

The aim of the model is to explain and encourage parental participation in care. Family-centred care in relation to this model considers the needs of the child within the context of the family unit; the family members are seen as the primary carers. The wellbeing of the child is central, however there is a

**Table 6.4** Orem's self-care model and the universal self-care requisites

- Maintenance of sufficient intake of air.
- Maintenance of sufficient intake of water.
- Maintenance of sufficient intake of food.
- Provision of care associated with elimination of processes and excrements.
- Maintenance of a balance between solitude and social integration.
- Prevention of hazards to life, human functioning and human wellbeing.
- Promotion of human functioning and development within social groups in accordance with human potential, known human limitations and the human desire to be normal.

*Source*: Orem, 1995.

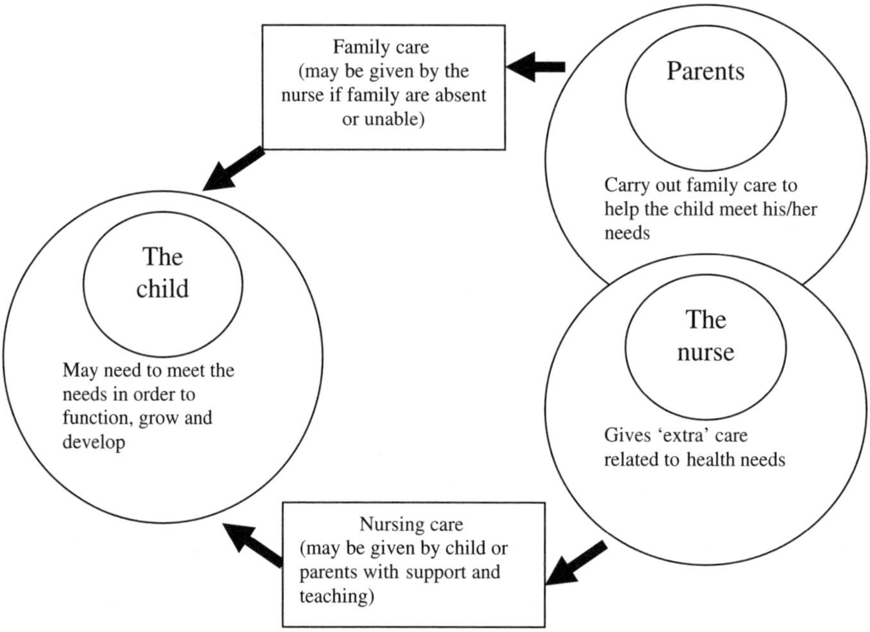


**Figure 6.6** A diagrammatic representation of Casey's Partnership model
*Source*: Casey, 1988.

recognition that care, if it is to be effective, will depend on negotiation and partnership between the nurse and the primary carers. Samwell (2000) suggests that each party has an equal part in the relationship.

## CONCLUSIONS

The concept of the nursing process has been used for many years in both the US and UK. It is a systemic, patient-centred, goal-oriented approach to nursing care, providing the nurse with a framework on which to deliver nursing care. The nursing process is (when appropriate) carried out with the patient.

A five-stage nursing process is gaining popularity in the UK:

- assessment
- nursing diagnosis
- planning
- implementation
- evaluation

The first stage of the nursing process is pivotal; this stage involves the continuous collection of data or facts and the nurse uses various strategies to achieve this. For example, he/she communicates, measures and observes. During this stage judgements are made about the patient's health status. The diagnostic stage demands that the nurse analyses the data in order to determine the patient's strengths and health problems that can be prevented or resolved. Measurable outcomes and goals are set during the planning stage. The purposes of these goals are to prevent, relieve or resolve the problems identified during the diagnostic phase. The outcome of planning is to produce individualised care plans that can be evaluated to determine if care interventions have been successful. Implementation is associated with doing: the nurse implements the care planned. The patient is assisted and supported in an attempt to achieve the stage goals, to enhance health and to prevent disease. Evaluation of the care provided is the final stage of the process. After monitoring and measuring the effects of nursing interventions the nurse, in conjunction with the patient, modifies the care plan if needed.

There are several models of care available to the nurse that can help guide practice. They attempt to express the reality of nursing and encourage nurses to work towards common goals. Nursing models are conceptual representations of reality and there are three central components associated with them: the value of nursing, the individuals receiving nursing care and the meaning of health. They are frameworks that help the nurse to make a comprehensive assessment of the 'whole' being. The model chosen cannot be used in isolation: the nurse must also use a systematic approach to care. The nursing process is aimed at providing high-quality, responsive nursing care.

## REFERENCES

Alfaro-LeFevre, R. (2002) (5th edn) *Applying the Nursing Process.* Lippincott. Philadelphia.

Beretta, R. (2003) 'Assessment: The foundations of good practice' in Hinchliff, S., Norman, S. and Schober, J. (eds) (4th edn) *Nursing Practice and Health Care.* Arnold. London. Ch 6 pp 121–146.

Bird, J. (2005) 'Assessing pain in older people'. *Nursing Standard.* Vol 19, No 19, pp 45–52.

Casey, A. (1988) 'A partnership with child and family'. *Senior Nurse*. Vol 8, No 4, pp 8–9.

Courtenay, M. (2002) 'Movement and mobility' in Hogston, R. and Simpson, P.M. (eds) (2nd edn) *Foundations of Nursing Practice: Making the Difference.* Palgrave. London. Ch 8 pp 262–285.

Doughty, D.B. (2004) 'Skin integrity and wound healing' in Daniels, R. (ed.) *Nursing Fundamentals: Caring and Clinical Decision Making.* Thompson. New York. Ch 36 pp 1049–1086.

Epstein, O., Perkin, G.D., de Bono, D.P. and Cookson, J. (1997) (2nd edn) *Clinical Examination.* Mosby. London.

Fawcett, J. (1995) (3rd edn) *Analysis and Evaluation of Conceptual Models of Nursing.* Davies. Philadelphia.

Feldt, K. (2000) 'The checklist for non verbal pain indicators'. *Pain Management Nursing.* Vol 1, No 1, pp 13–21.

Fryer, N. (2003) 'Principles of professional practice' in Hinchliff, S., Norman, S. and Schober, J. (eds) (4th edn) *Nursing Practice and Health Care.* Arnold. London. Ch 2 pp 27–47.

Gega, L. (2004) 'Problems, goals and care planning' in Norman, I. and Ryrie, I. (eds) *The Art and Science of Mental Health Nursing: A Textbook of Principles and Practice.* Open University Press. Milton Keynes. Ch 23 pp 665–678.

Heath, H. (2000) 'The nurse's role in assessing an older person'. *Elderly Care.* Vol 12, No 1, pp 3–24.

Holland, K. (2003) 'An introduction to the Roper–Logan–Tierney model for nursing, based on activities of living' in Holland, K., Jenkins, J., Solomon, J. and Whittam, S. (eds) *Roper, Logan and Tierney Model in Practice.* Churchill Livingstone. London. Ch 1 pp 3–22.

Kozier, B., Erb, G., Berman, A. and Snyder, S. (2004) (7th edn) *Fundamentals of Nursing: Concepts, Process and Practice.* Pearson. New Jersey.

Lund, C.C. and Browder, N.C. (1944) 'Estimation of areas of burns'. *Surgery, Gynecology and Obstetrics.* Vol 79, No 3, pp 352–358.

McCloskey, J.C. and Bulechek, G.M. (2000) (3rd edn) *Nursing Interventions Classification (NIC).* Mosby. St Louis.

Maslow, A. (1954) *Motivation and Personality.* New York. Harper and Row.

Matthews, P. (1998) 'Sexual history taking in primary care' in Carter, Y., Moss, C. and Weyman, A. (eds) *Royal College of General Practitioners Handbook of Sexual Health in Primary Care.* Royal College of General Practitioners and Family Planning Association. London. Ch 2 pp 17–50.

National Institute for Health and Clinical Excellence (2001) *Pressure Ulcer Risk Assessment and Prevention.* NICE. London.

Nicol, M., Brooker, C. and Meyer, J. (2003) 'Adult nursing: Setting the scene' in Brooker, C. and Nicol, M. (eds) *Nursing Adults: The Practice of Caring.* Mosby. Edinburgh. Ch 1 pp 3–21.

Nursing and Midwifery Council (2002) *Guidelines for Records and Records Keeping.* NMC. London.

Nusbaum, M.R.H. and Hamilton, C.D. (2002) 'The proactive sexual health history'. *American Family Physician.* Vol 66, No 9, pp 1705–1712.

Orem, D. (1995) (5th edn) *Nursing: Concepts of Practice.* Mosby. St Louis.

Peate, I. (2005) *Manual of Sexually Transmitted Infections.* Whurr. London.

Peplau, H. (1988) *Interpersonal Relationships in Nursing.* Putman. New York.

Ramsay, J. (1998) 'The development and process of children's nursing' in Moules, T. and Ramsay, J. (eds) *The Textbook of Children's Nursing.* Stanley Thornes. Cheltenham. Module 7, Part 3, pp 579–648.

Rayman, S.M. (2004) 'Assessment' in Daniel, R. (ed.) *Nursing Fundamentals: Caring and Clinical Decision Making.* Delmar. New Jersey. Ch 11 pp 196–218.

Roper, N., Logan, W.W. and Tierney. A.J. (1996) (4th edn) *The Elements of Nursing: A Model Based on a Model of Living.* Churchill Livingstone. Edinburgh.

Samwell, B. (2000) 'Nursing the family and supporting the nurse: exploring the nurse–patient relationship in community children's nursing' in Muir, J. and Sidey, A. (eds) *The Textbook of Community Children's Nursing.* Harcourt. London.

Sibson, L.E. (2005) 'The nursing process' in Peate, I. (ed.) *Compendium of Clinical Skills for Student Nurses.* Whurr. London. Ch 2 pp 19–36.

Slevin, O. (2003) 'Problem solving frameworks: the nursing process approach' in Basford, L. and Slevin, O. (eds) (2nd edn) *Theory and Practice of Nursing: An Integrated Approach to Caring Practice.* Nelson Thornes. Cheltenham. Ch 24 pp 447–469.

Taylor, C., Lillis, C. and LeMone, P. (2005) (5th edn) *Fundamentals of Nursing: The Art and Science of Nursing Care.* Lippincott. Philadelphia.

Timby, B.K. (2005) (8th edn) *Fundamental Nursing Skills and Concepts.* Lippincott. Philadelphia.

Tomlinson, J. (1998) 'Taking a sexual health history'. *British Medical Journal.* Vol 317, pp 1573–1576.

Wakley, G., Cunnion, M. and Chambers, R. (2003) *Improving Sexual Health Advice.* Radcliffe. Oxford.

Waterlow, J. (1985) 'A risk assessment card.' *Nursing Times.* Vol 81, No 49, pp 51–55.

Wright, S. (1990) (2nd edn) *Building and Using a Model of Nursing.* Arnold. London.

# 7 Partnerships

While Chapter 6 focused on the assessment aspect of a systematic approach to nursing care, Chapter 7 will consider the ability to formulate and document a plan of nursing care with emphasis on the active involvement of the patient, the family and carers, if appropriate. The key functions of the nursing care plan are discussed and various templates are described, for example written and computerised care planning.

The important issue of record management and the obligations bestowed on authorities concerning the retention of nursing and medical records are discussed. Examples of what are considered 'records' are provided.

The use of integrated care pathways, also known as care pathways or treatment protocols, is detailed. Integrated care pathways can be used for various conditions. It is suggested that integrated care pathways are not cast in tablets of stone, they should and can be reviewed to suit the changing needs of the patient.

The importance of developing and sustaining partnerships in care with the patient, patient organisations and other health and social-care agencies is addressed. The aims of partnership and collaborative working are outlined. The concept of expert patients is described and discussed.

## RECORDS AND THEIR MANAGEMENT

Nurses and other health-care professionals use many different types of records in their day-to-day management of patient care, in both the hospital and the community setting. Often documentation used for record keeping is produced locally, for example a stool chart. The records have usually been designed to meet the individual needs of specific patients or groups of patients in specific settings.

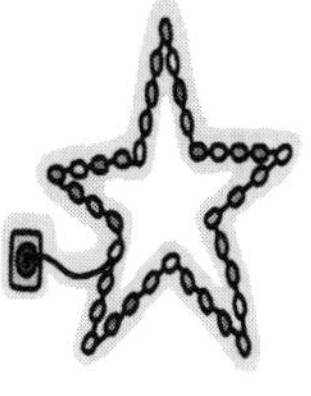

Make a list of patient records that you may have used in a clinical setting or that you think may be used in a clinical setting.

Compare your list to the one provided in the list below:

- observation charts, e.g. for the nurse to record temperature, pulse, respiration
- blood pressure charts
- turning charts
- feeding charts
- peak flow charts
- prescription charts
- percentile graphs
- seizure charts

All NHS records are public records under the terms of the Public Records Act 1958, which sets out responsibilities for everyone who works with such records. In March 1999 the Department of Health issued a Health Service Circular (HSC) and the key purposes of this circular were to improve the management of NHS records in health authorities and NHS Trusts. Table 7.1 outlines the key purposes of the circular.

There are legal requirements surrounding retention periods for patients' records. The legal requirements for retention periods for records differ with the nature of the records (see Table 7.2). The following are some examples of patient records:

- Patient health records (electronic or paper based).
- GP records, including records of private patients seen on NHS premises.
- Accident and emergency, theatre, births, deaths and all other registers.
- Administrative records (including for example notes associated with complaint handling).
- X-ray and imaging reports.
- Photographs, slides and other images.
- Microfiche or film.
- Audio and visual tapes, cassettes, CD-ROM.
- Computer databases, output and disks and all other electronic records.
- Material intended for short-term or transitory use, including notes and spare copies of documents.

**Table 7.1** The key purposes of the HSC 1999/053

| |
|---|
| • Sets out the legal obligations for all NHS bodies to keep proper records. |
| • Explains the actions needed from chief executives and other managers to fulfil these obligations. |
| • Provides good guidance and good practice. |
| • Explains the requirements to select records for permanent preservation. |
| • Suggested minimum periods for retention of NHS records. |

*Source*: HSC, 1999.

**Table 7.2** Information about the retention and disposal of some records

| Record | Retention period |
|---|---|
| Birth registers (i.e. register of births kept by the hospital) | Local decisions should be made with regards to permanent preservation of these records, in consultation with relevant health professionals and places of deposit |
| Death registers (i.e. register of deaths kept by the hospital) | |
| Discharge books (i.e. register of those discharged by the hospital) | |
| Operating theatre records | |
| Pharmacy records | |
| Ward registers | |
| **Retention periods listed below are intended as minimum periods related to clinical needs. It is not necessary to keep every piece of paper generated in connection with patients. Trusts should determine with the relevant professional groups what should be a permanent part of the patient record and what should be regarded as transient and what should be discarded as their value ceases** | |
| Hospital patient case records | |
| Children and young people | Until the patient's $25^{th}$ birthday, or $26^{th}$ if the young person was 17 years at conclusion of treatment, or 8 years after the patient's death, if death occurred after the $18^{th}$ birthday |
| Maternity (all obstetric and midwifery records including those episodes of maternity care that end in still birth or where the child later dies) | 25 years |
| Mentally disordered persons (as defined under the Mental Health Act 1983) | 20 years after no further treatment is necessary or 8 years after the death of the patient if the patient died whilst still receiving treatment |
| Deceased patients | Issues surrounding the retention and destruction of records once a patient has died have been devolved to local authorities and decisions are made at a local level. Generally, records are not destroyed but kept in storage and reduced to microfiche or transferred on to systems that allow for electronic storage |

*Source*: HSC 1999/053.

Patient records, as can be seen, are kept and maintained for a number of purposes. They can be the channel for communication between the health-care team, and if used effectively they can prevent fragmentation, repetition and delays in patient care. For example, the care plan, when reviewed, can be used in the audit process (see Chapter 12 for more discussion of audit) and quality assurance. The institution (for example the general practice setting) may review records to determine if care standards are being achieved. Information can be gleaned from the record(s) to help with research activity, and information gained can be helpful in the treatment of other patients. The care plan and other patient records can be helpful when used as educational tools, for example for use with students of health care.

## CARE PLANNING

The planning of nursing care has been discussed in detail in Chapter 6. However, the nurse needs to be able to construct a nursing care plan in order to ensure that the care that has been planned is carried out in a safe and effective manner, and that the goals that have been set are achieved.

### THE FUNCTIONS OF A NURSING CARE PLAN

A nursing care plan, patient care plan or a plan of nursing care is, according to Taylor et al. (2005), a written guide that directs the efforts of the nursing team as nurses work with patients to achieve their health goals. It allows the documentation and dissemination of clinical nursing information. Nursing care plans (just like any other nursing documentation) can be called on and used in a court of law. It could be suggested, therefore, that nursing care plans are legal documents.

The patient can be actively encouraged to participate in his/her care (if appropriate). This leads to the patient making an informed choice and can result in empowerment. Development of a nursing care plan will aim to help the patient achieve optimal health, habilitation and rehabilitation that are based on assessment and the use of contemporary nursing knowledge.

Figures 7.1, 7.2 and 7.3 are templates that can be used to document care using the nursing process. Not all care plans will follow the same format in these figures. Templates and formats vary from care setting to care setting, according to the needs of the patient and the care area.

| Date | Patient problem | Aim/goal | Nursing intervention | Evaluation | Name and signature |
|---|---|---|---|---|---|
| | | | | | |

**Figure 7.1** An example of a template for a nursing care plan

| Problem/area need | Goals/objectives | Action | Rationale | Review |
|---|---|---|---|---|
| | | | | |

**Figure 7.2** An example of a template for a nursing care plan
*Source*: Adapted from Gega, 2004.

| Nursing diagnosis | Goal (short term) | Goal (long term) | Nursing interventions | Evaluation |
|---|---|---|---|---|
| Pain as a result of a fractured tibia | Mr Jones to state that he is comfortable with pain rating score of below 2 within 15 minutes after the administration of prescribed analgesia | For Mr Jones to state that he is in control of his pain within 24 hours | • Provide prescribed analgesia and monitor effects<br>• Nurse on a bed that is equipped with pressure relief devices<br>• Ensure a two-hourly change of position with help from two nurses<br>• Provide distraction therapies, i.e. radio, television | Mr Jones states he is comfortable and has a pain rating score of below 2 |

**Figure 7.3** An example of a nursing care plan
*Source*: Hogston, 2002.

In some clinical areas the format or template used may be one where all members of the multidisciplinary team write and contribute to care plans, for example:

- social workers
- physiotherapists
- speech and language therapists
- chiropodists
- doctors

In other areas the plan of care may be computer generated. There are advantages and disadvantages associated with computer-generated care plans.

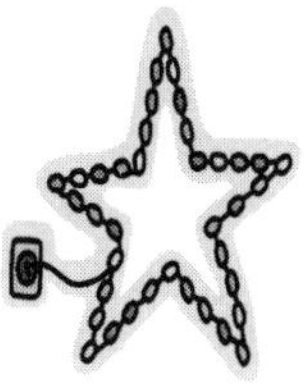

Make a list of the advantages and disadvantages that you think may be associated with computerised care plans.

Check your list against the one provided in Table 7.3.

**Table 7.3** Some advantages and disadvantages of computerised care plans

| Advantages | Disadvantages |
|---|---|
| • Can reduce duplication, e.g. the collection of demographic data.<br>• Can help to improve the quality of record keeping.<br>• Can be accessed by all members of team.<br>• Can be accessed remotely.<br>• Printouts can be easily produced and data reproduced speedily.<br>• May generate a wider knowledge base.<br>• Computers can process data much faster than humans.<br>• Have the potential to reduce time spent on handwriting care plans and can be easier to read.<br>• Recording data can be faster.<br>• Can improve accuracy (e.g. drug calculations) therefore human error can be reduced.<br>• Current methods used to record data can lead to breaches in confidentiality and security with data. | • Can reduce autonomy (patient and nurse).<br>• May lead to a loss of individualisation of care.<br>• Have the potential to become an 'administrative' data-inputting task.<br>• Loss of nursing expertise.<br>• Access to a wider audience because of remote access can lead to breaches in confidentiality and security with data.<br>• Assume that all nurses have the skills required to use computerised care plans.<br>• High costs for hardware and software.<br>• Investment needed in staff development.<br>• Possible IT equipment breakdown.<br>• System may be expensive. |

*Source*: Adapted from Strachen, 1994; Harris, 1990.

## OTHER FORMATS FOR DOCUMENTING CARE ISSUES

Other documents are used when providing care, and they will differ according to the care setting. For example:

- *Communication sheets* – these allow the nurse and other members of the multidisciplinary team to communicate with each other regarding specific aspects of care. They may also be called progress notes.
- *Graphic records* – these documents allow the nurse to chart and record clinical data such as:
  - blood pressure
  - pulse
  - respiratory rate
  - temperature
  - neurological status (e.g. Glasgow coma scale)
  - weight
  - bowel movements
- *Fluid balance charts* (see Figure 7.4) – sometimes called input and output charts. All routes of fluid intake and output are documented in these charts, for example:

  - intravenous fluids
  - any fluids via a gastrostomy tube
  - nasogastric tube
  - vomitus
  - diarrhoea
  - urine
  - sweat
- *Drug charts.*

Ward: *Acorn* Date: *27/2/07*

Surname: *Cohen* Hospital Number: *3AN02785*

Forename: *Gillian*

Date of Birth: *4/1/25*

**Insensible loss is estimated to be per day 750 ml in the apy rexial patient. This should be calculated into the daily fluid balance as loss.**

| Fluid intake | | | | Fluid output | | | | |
|---|---|---|---|---|---|---|---|---|
| **Time** | **Oral** | **Intravenous** | **Other (specify)** | **Urine** | **Vomit** | **Other (specify)** | | |
| **01.00** | | | | | | | | |
| **02.00** | | | | | | | | |
| **03.00** | | | | | | | | |
| **04.00** | | | | | | | | |
| **05.00** | | | | | | | | |
| **06.00** | | | | | | | | |
| **07.00** | | | | | | | | |
| **08.00** | | | | | | | | |
| **09.00** | | | | | | | | |
| **10.00** | | | | | | | | |
| **11.00** | | | | | | | | |
| **12.00** | | | | | | | | |
| **13.00** | | | | | | | | |
| **14.00** | | | | | | | | |
| **15.00** | | | | | | | | |
| **16.00** | | | | | | | | |
| **17.00** | | | | | | | | |
| **18.00** | | | | | | | | |
| **19.00** | | | | | | | | |
| **20.00** | | | | | | | | |
| **21.00** | | | | | | | | |
| **22.00** | | | | | | | | |
| **23.00** | | | | | | | | |
| **24.00** | | | | | | | | |
| **Total** | | | | | | | | |

**Figure 7.4** A fluid balance chart

Local policy and procedure must be adhered to when providing care in the patient's home. In many situations the documentation (including the care plan and other documents used in care provision) is left with the patient and/or his/her family. It may be that some Trusts provide the nurse with a handheld computer device (or laptop) to plan and document care interventions.

## GUIDELINES FOR DOCUMENTING CARE INTERVENTIONS

This aspect of the chapter must be read in conjunction with the standards produced by the NMC (2002) concerning documentation and record keeping, as well as any further guidance issued at a local level.

Any information entered should be a complete and accurate representation of events that have occurred; the data should be concise and factual. Data should be recorded in chronological order and any changes in the patient should be noted or deleted as appropriate. Document the care given as soon as possible and as closely as possible to the time care was carried out. Timing of entries made in any documents must be governed by the patient's condition, for example the patient's condition will dictate the frequency of observations.

Words that are vague should be avoided, such as:

- good
- average
- fine
- normal

These words may have different meanings to different people and as a result can lead to confusion regarding the care provided. Generalisations such as 'slept well' should be avoided as they provide little insight into what has occurred.

All entries must have the nurse's signature and, if appropriate, the nurse's name in full, the date and the time of entry. The 24-hour clock must be used to avoid any mistakes, for example 2.30 pm becomes 14.30 hours. You must always be cognisant that the entry you are making now may be used later by others for various reasons. Only the approved documentation should be used to document and record care.

### ABBREVIATIONS

The use of abbreviations abounds in nursing. When student nurses begin their nurse education they are often overwhelmed with the use of nursing and medical jargon and the abbreviations that are used in nursing care plans and other health and social-care records. The language used at handover in the nursing and medical notes in the early stages is often unfamiliar, and can even be intimidating. As time passes the student begins to learn the new language and he/she absorbs this into everyday life as a nurse.

The language used is often context specific within the different fields of health care. The haphazard use of abbreviations can put the patient and the patient's carer at risk. Abbreviations may start as time savers, but in the long run they may take up more time.

As already discussed, the NMC (2002) has stipulated that abbreviations should not be used in patient records. If local policy allows the use of abbreviations then you should make yourself familiar with the abbreviations that are acceptable in the clinical area where you work, use them as little as possible and print them clearly so as to reduce confusion. Use only the abbreviations on the approved list, which are there to enhance communication between the nurse and others. Prior to using an abbreviation, stop and think about it: ask yourself if it is in the best interest of the patient. A short list of commonly used abbreviations is included at the end of this text.

## CLINICAL/WARD HANDOVERS

One other way of disseminating information about patients is the clinical handover. The purpose of the handover is to transfer essential information necessary for safe, holistic patient care. The role of the handover is to prevent any break in the provision of care. It is where the transfer of professional responsibility and accountability occurs for some, or all, aspects of care for a patient, or group of patients, to another nurse.

Handover often takes place at the beginning or end of each shift. However, there may be other times when handover is needed, for example on transfer to another unit (from the cardiac care unit, for instance) or ward, or on discharge to the care of another health-care professional, for example from the hospital nurse to the community nurse. However, the process of handover varies from ward to ward and hospital to hospital. Some wards have no handover at all. In a hospital ward the work is a continuous process; despite this there are changeovers of nurses and other health-care workers as one turn of duty ends and another commences.

Handover of care can be one of the most unsafe and dangerous procedures that the nurse carries out. If handover of care is not carried out correctly, it can be a major contributory factor in subsequent error and harm to the patient (British Medical Association (BMA), 2004). It is important that during handover the nurse avoids jargon and explains any abbreviations being used (Hoban, 2003).

Each clinical area will develop its own policy regarding handover. This will require a coordinated approach, including other members of the multidisciplinary team. Those hospitals who have been involved in a night-team approach to care (see National Patient Safety Agency (NPSA), 2005) will require a process that will involve the whole team being brought together, to

**Table 7.4** Issues to be considered when planning handover events

| | |
|---|---|
| Who | Should be involved |
| When | Should it take place |
| Where | Should it occur |
| How | Should it happen |
| What | Needs to be handed over |

*Source*: BMA, 2004.

receive and disseminate information from all parts of the hospital, with the aim of coordinating care during the out-of-hours period. Often in a hospital handover takes place at the patient bedside and/or in the nurses/unit office or at the nurse's station.

The handover is another opportunity to engage in partnership with the patient and his/her family. The patient and family should be encouraged to take part in handover (if appropriate) so that they can be a part of the decision-making process regarding their care. The patient will not feel as if he/she is being talked about or being talked over: he/she can be an active participant as opposed to a passive bystander. This approach can also be extended to the GP surgery and in the home setting.

According to the BMA (2004) a competent and confident handover will:

- Protect patient safety.
- Reduce discontinuity of care.
- Decrease repetition.
- Increase service satisfaction.
- Provide educational opportunities (for patients and staff).

Table 7.4 may help when considering handover.

The handover has to be conducted succinctly but thoroughly in order to make sure that all vital information has been provided. This is to ensure that safe and effective care is available, in partnership with the patient and his/her family (if appropriate). Table 7.5 provides some dos and don'ts concerning handover. The principles provided can be adapted to meet both community and hospital settings.

## INTEGRATED CARE PATHWAYS

In many areas of health and social care, an integrated care pathway approach is being increasingly used as the favoured methodology to apply packages of care in a coordinated and integrated way. Clinical governance initiatives introduced by the government (Department of Health, 1998) aim to ensure that care provided is of high quality and has effective outcomes (Solomon, 2003).

**Table 7.5** Some dos and don'ts that may be useful during handover in either the community or hospital setting

| Dos | Don'ts |
|---|---|
| • Provide only essential information.<br>• Identify the patient's nursing problems and if known the cause of them.<br>• Describe objective measurements or observations about the patient and his/her response to care interventions.<br>• Evaluate care provision and other interventions.<br>• State any recent changes in the patient's condition.<br>• Share significant information about the family members if this relates to the patient's problems.<br>• Review discharge plan if this is appropriate for the patient.<br>• Inform staff of any significant change in care provision, e.g. if turning regimes have changed.<br>• Ensure you are clear to other staff about patient and nursing priorities.<br>• Involve the patient and his/her family if appropriate. | • Don't neglect the patient and family during handover.<br>• Don't review all routine aspects of care, e.g. medication (unless significant).<br>• Don't review all biographical data.<br>• Never use subjective/derogatory comments about the patient or his/her family.<br>• Don't describe interventions or results of investigations as 'good' or 'satisfactory', be more specific and state values if available.<br>• Don't engage in idle chat that is irrelevant to patient care.<br>• Don't use jargon or abbreviations that may confuse or intimidate the patient or other members of the team. |

*Source*: Adapted from Hoban, 2003; BMA, 2004; Heath, 1995.

Integrated care pathways are also known as care pathways, treatment protocols, clinical pathways, critical pathways and nursing care pathways. The aim of a care pathway is to improve and enhance the continuity and coordination of care that occur across different disciplines and sectors within the health service. The care pathway forms the single clinical record of care for all health professionals involved in the care and treatment of the patient (Johnson, 1997).

Care pathways or treatment protocols are used for various conditions:

- Orthopaedic conditions, e.g. hip and knee replacements, fractured neck or femur.
- Asthma management for inpatients.
- Stroke rehabilitation.
- Cardiac cases, e.g. heart failure.
- Respiratory conditions, e.g. bronchiolitis, pneumonia.

Middleton et al. (2003) define an integrated care pathway as a multidisciplinary outline of anticipated care. They go on and add that the anticipated care is placed within a time frame, with the key aim of helping the patient with a specific condition or set of symptoms move progressively through a clinical experience to positive outcomes (see Figure 7.4). Throughout the patient care journey (or the clinical experience, as suggested by Middleton et al., 2003), the patient will encounter many and various health professionals in a range of settings. Effective channels of communication between these professionals are therefore a prerequisite for successful continuity of care (Cringles, 2002).

Campbell et al. (1998) suggest that integrated care pathways are in essence care plans that detail the important steps in the care of patients with a specific clinical problem; they describe the expected progress of the patient. The integrated care pathway should be designed by the multidisciplinary team of the local disciplines involved (Integrated Care Pathway Users Scotland, 2005). All those involved in the patient's care would be expected to contribute to the pathway.

The integrated care pathway is often kept at the patient's bedside, which allows the patient to read and refer to it. In some instances (this may be in response to patient choice or local policy) the pathway may be kept centrally, for example at the nurses' station. Professional discretion will be needed regarding pathways that contain sensitive information, such as a difficult or provisional diagnosis. Some integrated pathways have a section available for the patient to write his/her comments (see Figure 7.5).

It must always be remembered that integrated care pathways are not cast in stone and should be used as a guideline to make sure that the most appropriate care is given. The pathway should not be followed blindly and at all times clinical judgement should be used by the nurse. Variations from the pathway can and do occur, often as a result of clinical autonomy in response to a change in the patient's condition. There is much more to the delivery of high-quality care than just following guidelines and procedures. The unique biology of the patient associated with his/her special circumstances guides care and treatment. Integrated care pathways should be reviewed on a regular basis in the light of new practices or new evidence emerging.

| | | | | | |
|---|---|---|---|---|---|
| **Name** | | | | | |
| **Named nurse** | | | | | |
| **Reason for admission** | | | | | |
| **Anticipated length of stay (delete as appropriate)** | **1, 2, 3, 4, 5, 6, 7 days** | | | | |
| **Intervention** | **Pre-admission (outpatients/pre-admission clinic)** | **Day of admission Day 0** | **Day 1** | **Day 2** | **Variance/patient's comments** |
| **Clinical assessment** | | | | | |
| **Treatment** | | | | | |
| **Medication** | | | | | |
| **Discharge plan** | | | | | |
| **Investigations/tests** | | | | | |
| **Activities** | | | | | |
| **Outcome** | | | | | |
| **Health education/promotion** | | | | | |

**Figure 7.5** An example of a clinical pathway matrix

In some instances care pathways can be seen as algorithms. Algorithms are developed and used to provide a map of logical and sequential steps towards effective case management. They offer, in a flow-chart format, an outline of the decisions to be made and the care to be provided for a given patient or patient group for a specific condition in a step-by-step sequence. Figure 7.6 provides a pathway to care for a person with schizophrenia. Care pathways provide clinical guidelines and are based on the best available evidence (evidence-based practice is addressed in Chapter 8).

## DEVELOPING AND SUSTAINING PARTNERSHIPS

Carnwell and Carson (2005) state that the need to work in 'partnership', in 'collaboration', to take on 'joined-up thinking' and to deliver services that are 'seamless' constitute terminology that is policy driven. Often, however, what is discussed in theory (e.g. what partnership is) and what is happening in practice (e.g. what partnerships do) can drift apart.

It has already been stated that no one professional group can work in isolation in order to achieve improvements in the health of the public (see for example Chapter 5 and health education, Chapter 13 and inter-professional working and learning, and also the above discussion concerning integrated care pathways). Partnerships are needed. Figure 7.7 demonstrates who some of the key stakeholders may be who work in partnership with and for the patient. Together this partnership can become a powerful model for enhancing health improvements for the nation – at work, from an individual perspective or at a family level.

Collaboration as opposed to competition is central to the government's health agenda (Department of Health, 2001a). One aspect of this collaboration is partnership. National policy is moving towards more integrated public services. Partnership working between various agencies with the patient at the centre brings substantial benefits. In 2004 the Department of Health (Department of Health, 2004a) published its plans to describe the way in which the NHS needed to change in order to become a truly patient-led service. The NHS needs to offer more choice to patients, provide more information for them to make choices, make available more personalised care, and encourage real empowerment of people for them to be able to improve their health. The relationship the NHS currently has with the users of the service – the patients – needs to be addressed. A move is required to provide an NHS that no longer does things to and for the patient, one that is patient led, where the service provided works with patients to support them with their health needs (Department of Health, 2005a).

One of the key aims is to move from a centrally directed system to a patient-led system. The Department of Health (2003) suggests that the combined knowledge and expertise of the partners have the potential to create synergy and offer new opportunities and innovations for service delivery. A bottom-up

**Figure 7.6** A pathway of care for a person with schizophrenia

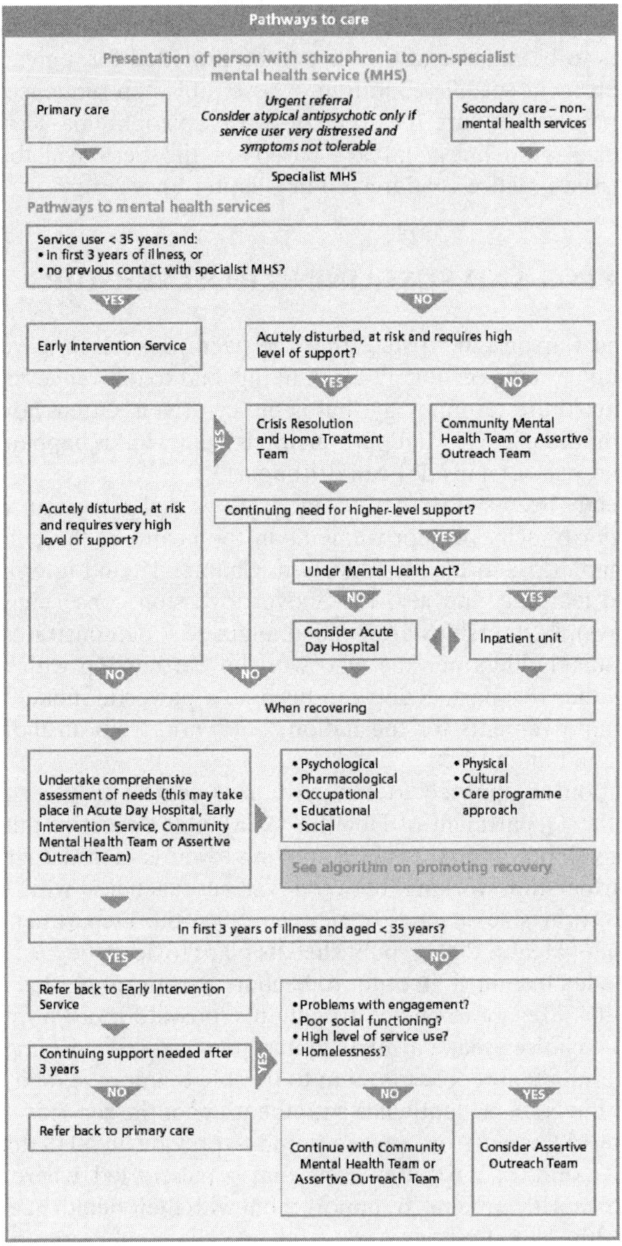


*Source*: National Institute for Health and Clinical Excellence (2002). This is Crown Copyright material which is reproduced with the permission of the Controller of HMSO and the Queen's Printer for Scotland.

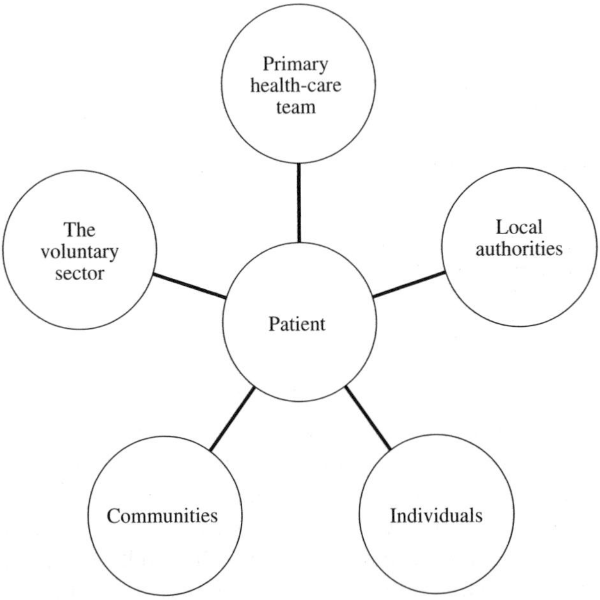


**Figure 7.7** Some of the key stakeholders who work in partnership with and for the patient

approach is suggested (Department of Health, 2005a) that will encourage local innovation and creativity, responding to the needs and wishes of the patient.

While working in partnership is strongly advocated, it is time consuming. When attempting to develop and sustain these relationships, the professionals involved must be prepared to work together and have clear aims. Clarity of purpose is vital, as well as a willingness to work together in a flexible and creative manner, deploying skills that can be best used to serve the needs of the patient. Everyone must remember that they are accountable for their own practice in the form of their code of professional conduct, as well as their accountability to their employing authority and to the partnership itself (Holland, 2003). Members of the partnership must be willing to own the activities they undertake and share responsibilities.

There are challenges to be faced when working in partnership. Ethical and moral issues can arise when working in partnership and these issues are complex (Allison, 2005). The tensions arise primarily as a result of attempting to balance competing responsibilities within various agencies. Conflict can occur as a result of attempting to find the best way to meet the needs of the patient within inter-professional communities (Department of Health, 2001b). Some of the potential challenges associated with partnership working have been highlighted in Table 7.6.

**Table 7.6** Some of the challenges associated with partnership working

| |
|---|
| • Separate legislative frameworks that inform partnership working.<br>• Culture clashes, ideological differences and rivalry between organisations.<br>• Difficulty maintaining continuity of care when there are multiple agencies involved.<br>• Difficulties in establishing accountability arrangements when multiple organisations are involved.<br>• Lack of clarity and role confusion.<br>• A potential for some of the larger agencies to dominate and not fully appreciate and respect the work of smaller agencies. |

*Source*: Adapted from NHS Executive, 2000; Department of Health, 2000; Drugs Prevention Advisory Service, 1999; Carnwell and Buchanan, 2005.

Partnerships do not work in a vacuum. Because of constraints, policy, regulation and priorities, employing authorities and government bodies can have a significant effect on the success (or failure) of the aims of the partnership. A change of culture within the NHS is needed in order to be responsive to patient-led care provision (Department of Health, 2005a). A patient-led NHS needs to address the barriers that impede progress. Not all previous practice has had a negative effect on patient-led care, and indeed many positive practices in the past will allow the NHS to move forward in order to reach its goals. The NHS has a rich legacy in the way it operates, it has an absolute commitment to quality and the patients it serves. However, it is very hierarchical, with professional divides, inflexible processes and bureaucratic systems (Department of Health, 2005a). See Figure 7.8.

There are several ongoing strategies (local and national) that are promoting partnership working, for example:

- Building on the Best, which is improving choice for patients in health care.
- The move to improve the management of chronic disease – empowering and supporting patients to manage their own conditions.
- The expert patient programme – the aim is to help to build equal, informed partnerships between patients and health and social-care professionals (see below).
- The government's strategy to put in place a more formal relationship between the statutory and the voluntary and community sectors – working closely with the voluntary and community sectors to deliver the expert patient training course, making the concept of expert patient become reality.
- The various national service frameworks (NSFs), for example the NSF for Long-Term Conditions (Department of Health, 2005b).

Partnership working can be achieved, and it can help to facilitate health-care professionals and the patient working together in collaboration. Agencies involved in partnership working can deliver a more effective service (Carnwell and Buchanan, 2005).

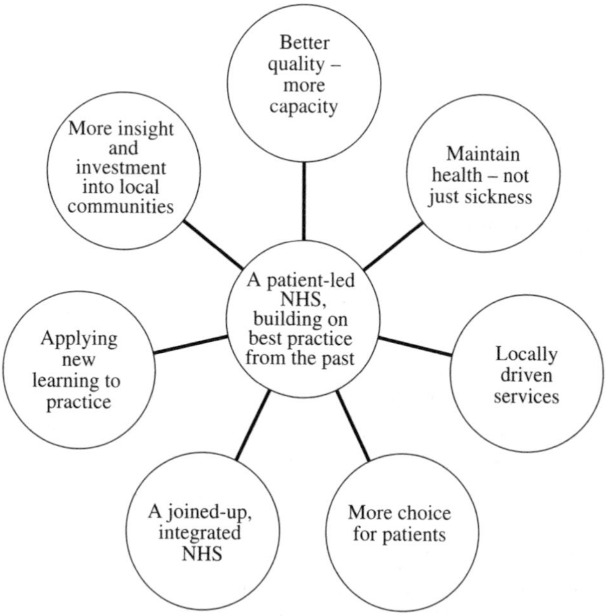


**Figure 7.8** Some aspects of service provision that will move towards providing a patient-led NHS
*Source*: Adapted from Department of Health, 2005a.

Working in partnership is not easy, and indeed it will not be a panacea for all ills that befall service provision. However, providing a service in a more fluid and dynamic manner can enable the various health and social-care agencies to respond speedily and effectively to changes that occur within communities and with individuals.

## THE EXPERT PATIENT

One example of working in partnership with the patient is the development of the concept of the expert patient (Department of Health, 2001a). The idea was alluded to in an earlier government publication, *Saving Lives* (Department of Health, 1999), and then reaffirmed in the *NHS Plan* (Department of Health, 2000).

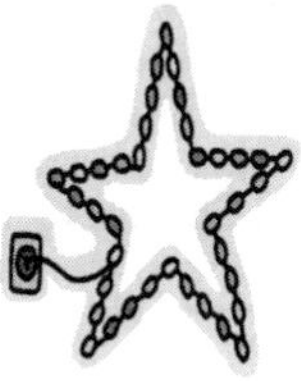

What conditions do you think may be classed as long term/chronic?

You might have considered the following:

- cardiac disease
- stroke
- cancer
- arthritis
- enduring mental health illnesses
- diabetes mellitus
- asthma
- epilepsy

One of the key components of the expert patient initiative (Department of Health, 2001a) is that patients (particularly those with long-term chronic conditions) should be seen as more than passive recipients of care. According to the Department of Health (2004b), it is estimated that 60 per cent of adults in England report a chronic health problem. The extent of the problem is demonstrated in Table 7.7.

Holman and Lorig (2000) point out that chronic disease has become the principal medical problem and that the patient must become a co-partner in the process of dealing with it. Emphasis is being placed on the relationship between the NHS and the people it provides a service to – one in which nurses and other health professionals and patients are true partners together, seeking the best solutions to each patient's problem.

In the UK approximately 25 per cent of those people with a long-standing problem have three or more problems. This results in more complex care provision for this group of the population (Department of Health, 2004b). This is outlined in Figure 7.9.

Patients should become key decision makers in the treatment process (Department of Health, 2001a) and this can become a reality if patients are empowered (through the provision of information and other resources) to

**Table 7.7** Chronic conditions and their impact

| Condition | Impact |
|---|---|
| Diabetes mellitus | The number of diabetics is currently estimated at 1.3 m people, with another million who may be undiagnosed |
| Chronic obstructive pulmonary disease (COPD) | Affects in the region of 600 000 people |
| Asthma | Affects approximately 3.7 m adults and 1.5 m children |
| Epilepsy | There are approximately 400 000 sufferers |
| Mental ill health | Affects up to 1 in 6 of the population, including 1 in 10 children |

*Source*: Department of Health, 2004b.

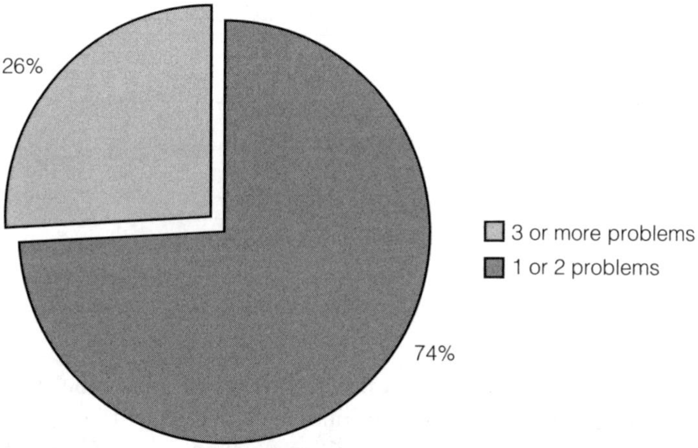


**Figure 7.9** Proportion of people with a chronic disease with three or more problems
*Source*: Department of Health, 2004b.

take on some of the responsibility for their conditions and its management. When working in partnership with their health and social-care providers, patients can assume greater control over their lives. However, in order to achieve this, patients need to be supported. Self-management programmes can be designed to provide this support and to reduce the severity of symptoms and improve confidence, along with an improvement in self-efficacy and resourcefulness. The NHS will need to work in partnership not only with the patient, but with other government departments and agencies (for example the Department for Work and Pensions) and patient organisations.

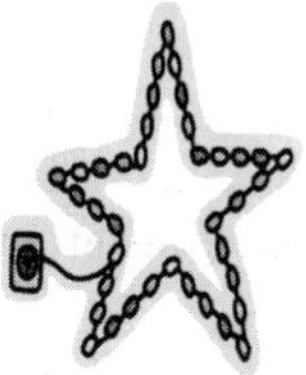

In Table 7.8 complete the conditions that you think are associated with the patient organisations listed. For example, the Terence Higgins Trust is a patient organisation concerned with helping people with HIV/AIDS.

Self-management programmes led by people who themselves live with a chronic condition are seen as a positive way of achieving government objectives detailed in the expert patient initiative (Department of Health, 2001a). A programme has been developed that will lead to more lay self-managed interventions, with the aim to provide people with long-term illnesses with the

**Table 7.8** Patient organisations

| Organisation | Patient group |
|---|---|
| Terence Higgins Trust | People with or affected by HIV/AIDS |
| Ovacome | |
| Laryngectomee Trust | |
| Marc's Line | |
| Rethink | |
| ABC | |
| Sense | |
| PEACH | |

confidence to manage their condition better. It is envisaged that by 2007 the programmes (for key chronic conditions) will be mainstreamed within all NHS areas (Long-term Medical Conditions Alliance (LMCA), 2001). Ten prerequisites for the successful implementation and provision of lay-led self-management programmes have been identified (see Table 7.9).

Successful lay-led self-managed programmes will result in (Department of Health, 2001a):

- Many more patients with chronic diseases improving, remaining stable or deteriorating more slowly.
- Many more patients being able to manage more effectively certain aspects of their condition, for example pain.
- Patients with chronic diseases who become expert being likely to be less severely incapacitated by fatigue, sleep disturbance and low levels of energy.
- Most patients with a chronic disease having the skills to cope with the emotional consequences of their disease.
- Many people with chronic disease gaining and retaining employment.
- Many more patients with chronic diseases successfully using health-promoting strategies.
- Most patients with chronic diseases becoming more effective in accessing appropriate health and social-care services.
- People with chronic diseases making greater use of adult education and employment training programmes.
- Many more patients with chronic diseases becoming more informed about their condition and their medication, feeling empowered in their relationship with health-care professionals, and having a more positive sense of self-esteem.
- People with chronic diseases spending fewer days a year as hospital inpatients or attending outpatient clinics.
- People with chronic diseases contributing their skills and insights for the further improvement of services.
- People with chronic disease working as counsellors, information workers and advocates for others.

**Table 7.9** The prerequisites for the successful implementation and provision of lay-led self-management programmes

- Understanding and support are required for self-management initiatives within organisations at all levels.
- Raising awareness among health professionals and community workers in local areas will increase the long-term sustainability of the programme and help to build effective partnerships.
- Central coordination is a vital resource and the key to facilitating the most effective use of available resources.
- A well-planned and resourced recruitment process for volunteer tutors is a worthwhile long-term investment. They are the key resource and ensuring that they are able to have a long-term commitment to the programme is essential.
- Tutors must be recruited from a range of social backgrounds, so that the courses appeal to a broad spectrum of people from diverse social and cultural groups.
- A sound quality assurance framework for supporting and monitoring the volunteer tutors is essential.
- Organisations running self-management programmes need to resource a dedicated member of staff or volunteer who can support the tutors by taking on administrative tasks. These tasks are essential to running successful courses.
- There is a need for high-quality materials to market courses to target audiences in the locality.
- Joint working across agencies creates high levels of reciprocity, cost-effectiveness and outreach and is most effective within formalised agreements.
- Central coordination facilitates cross-sector working and a greater understanding of differing agendas.

*Source*: Adapted from Cooper, 2001.

**Table 7.10** Some of the initial findings from the first expert patient programme pilot study

- 45% said they felt more confident that they would not let common symptoms (pain, tiredness, depression and breathlessness) interfere with their lives.
- 38% felt that such symptoms were less severe 4–6 months after completing the course.
- 33% felt better prepared for consultations with health professionals.
- 7% reductions in GP consultations.
- 10% reductions in outpatient visits.
- 16% reductions in A&E attendances.
- 9% reductions in physiotherapy use.
- Over 94% of those who took part felt supported and satisfied with the course.

*Source*: Hawley, 2005.

The first expert patient programme pilot study was internally evaluated. Over 1000 participants undertaking the expert patient's programme provided data for the evaluatory study. The data demonstrated that the programme is achieving its aims (Hawley, 2005); see Table 7.10.

Chronic disease management is an important issue and failing to manage these diseases effectively means that patients may suffer unnecessary complications of their illness and can even be dying prematurely (Department of

**Table 7.11** Types of self-care support with examples

| Support/care | Information and knowledge | Training and networking | Facilities and equipment |
|---|---|---|---|
| Prevention/ promotion | Interactive online courses, information on health TV | Lifestyle courses, personal training | Gyms, personal portals |
| Diagnosis | Home health-care literature | Training in self-diagnosis | Home pregnancy test, blood and urine tests |
| Decision on action to take | Telephone helpline, interactive video on treatment discussions | Decision support, patient peer groups, internet discussion groups | Personal portals, decision algorithm |
| Treatment/ medication | First aid manuals, software tools for mental health self-help | First aid courses, self-help courses | First aid kit: over-the-counter medicines, home dialysis, public access defibrillators |
| Monitoring and evaluation | Self-maintained medical records | Supermarket 'MOTs' | Home or public access BP monitors, blood glucose testing kits |

*Source*: Department of Health, 2004b.

Health, 2004b). By enhancing partnerships in care with patients and patient groups, these premature deaths and unnecessary complications can be reduced. However, partnerships in care do not merely mean the provision of information for the patient. There are various other steps that can be taken that can help provide a genuine partnership in care. Table 7.11 demonstrates how much more is needed to provide self-care support.

The examples shown in Table 7.11 will become a reality over time as there will be a rise in the information variable (and type of information), as well as the ability of the population to build on and use IT to support self-care. More home monitoring systems will become available and there will, it is envisaged, be a greater desire for some patients to be the focus of control (Department of Health, 2004b).

## CONCLUSIONS

Involving patients in their care has many advantages for both the patient and the health service provider. Patient and family involvement can demonstrate that you have provided patients with information in order for them to make informed decisions about their care. It also demonstrates that you have provided patients with an understanding of the intended nursing actions. The nursing care plan can be one way of doing this. The concept of the expert patient and the ability to work in true collaboration *with* the patient *for* the patient has potential that is only just being taken into consideration by health and social-care agencies.

The nursing care plan cannot be underestimated as a communication tool and the nurse needs to give careful consideration to its construction. Think about the language when you write a care plan. Avoid using terms that reflect the diagnosis only, also include what the patient's experiences are – how he/she feels, what his/her needs are. Steer clear of using vague, general and ambiguous statements; instead use terms that can be measured and evaluated. Never use value judgements in describing the patient or the patient's behaviours. When appropriate, the patient and his/her family should always be a part of care-planning activities. The patient should also be actively encouraged to take part in handover sessions, which can occur at the bedside in the hospital or in the patient's own home. This chapter has outlined the importance of a carefully considered handover and implications for patient care.

The retention and management of patient records (and what constitutes patient records) are guided by government directives and local policy. If used effectively, the records and documents can prevent fragmentation of care, reduce repetition and prevent delays in care. Care plans, for example, can be used as a part of quality control or in the audit process.

Integrated care pathways can be used in various clinical settings for a variety of conditions. The key aim is to provide a coordinated approach to patient care across health and social-care disciplines. Integrated care plans provide guidance but can never substitute for professional judgement.

In order to provide a service where the patient is at the centre and he/she is part of the decision-making process, the nurse must develop and sustain partnership with various key stakeholders in the nursing and social-care domains. The use of the expert patient has been discussed: this concept is relatively new in the UK and is currently undergoing evaluation. It is envisaged that the patient will become a key decision maker in the treatment process through empowerment. The patient will take on some responsibility for his/her condition and its subsequent management. The NHS will have to work in partnership with the patient and also other government departments (e.g. the Department of Transport) and patient organisations.

## REFERENCES

Allison, A. (2005) 'Ethical issues of working in partnership' in Carnwell, R. and Buchanan, J. (eds) *Effective Practice in Health and Social Care: A Partnership Approach.* Open University. Buckingham. Ch 3 pp 37–50.

British Medical Association (2004) *Safe Handover: Safe Patients. Guidance on Clinical Handover for Clinicians and Managers*. BMA. London.

Campbell, H., Hotchkiss, R., Bradshaw, N. and Porteous, M. (1998) 'Integrated care pathways'. *British Medical Journal.* Vol 316, No 7125, pp 133–137.

Carnwell, R. and Buchanan, J. (2005) 'Learning from partnerships: Themes and issues' in Carnwell, R. and Buchanan, J. (eds) *Effective Practice in Health and Social Care: A Partnership Approach*. Open University. Buckingham. Ch 1 pp 261–270.

Carnwell, R. and Carson, A. (2005) 'Understanding partnerships and collaboration' in Carnwell, R. and Buchanan, J. (eds) *Effective Practice in Health and Social Care: A Partnership Approach*. Open University. Buckingham. Ch 1 pp 3–20.

Cooper, J. (2001) *Partnerships for Successful Self-Management: The Report of the Living with Long-Term Illness (Lill) Project*. LMCA. London.

Cringles, M.C. (2002) 'Developing an integrated care pathway to manage cancer pain across primary, secondary and tertiary care'. *International Journal of Palliative Care.* Vol 8, No 5, pp 247–255.

Department of Health (1998) *A First Class Service: Quality in the New NHS.* The Stationery Office. London.

Department of Health (1999) *Saving Lives: Our Healthier Nation*. The Stationery Office. London.

Department of Health (2000) *The NHS Plan: A Plan for Investment, A Plan for Reform*. The Stationery Office. London.

Department of Health (2001a) *The Expert Patient: A New Approach to Chronic Disease Management for the 21st Century*. Department of Health. London.

Department of Health (2001b) *Valuing People: A New Strategy for Learning Disability for the 21st Century*. Department of Health. London.

Department of Health (2002) *Keys to Partnership: Working Together to Make a Difference to People's Lives*. Department of Health. London.

Department of Health (2003) *The NHS Improvement Plan: Putting People at the Heart of Public Services*. Department of Health. London.

Department of Health (2004a) *Making Partnership Work for Patients, Carers and Service Users*. Department of Health. London.

Department of Health (2004b) *Chronic Disease Management: A Compendium of Information*. Department of Health. London.

Department of Health (2005a) *Creating a Patient-led NHS: Delivering the NHS Improvement Plan*. Department of Health. London.

Department of Health (2005b) *The National Service Framework for Long Term Conditions*. Department of Health. London.

Drugs Prevention Advisory Service (1999) *Doing Justice to Treatment.* DPAS. London.

Gega, L. (2004) 'Problems. goals and care planning' in Norman, I. and Ryrie, I. (eds) *The Art and Science of Mental Health Nursing: A Textbook of Principles and Practice*. Open University Press. Milton Keynes. Ch 23 pp 665–678.

Harris, B.L. (1990) 'Becoming deprofessionalized: One aspect of the staff nurse's perspective on computer-mediated nursing care plans'. *Advances in Nursing Science*. Vol 13, No 2, pp 63–74.

Hawley, K. (2005) Report on the EPP Parent Pilot Course: January 2004–January 2005. NHS. London.

Health Services Commission (1999) *For the Record – Managing Records in NHS Trusts and Health Authorities*. HSC 1999/053. London.

Heath, H.B.M. (1995) *Foundations in Nursing Theory and Practice*. Mosby. London.

Hoban, V. (2003) 'How to . . . handle handover'. *Nursing Times*. Vol 99, pp 54–55.

Hogston, R. (2002) 'Managing nursing care' in Hogston, R. and Simpson, P.M. (eds) (2nd edn) *Foundations of Nursing Practice: Making the Difference*. Palgrave. Basingstoke. Ch 1 pp 1–25.

Holland, K. (2003) 'Nursing and the context of care' in Holland, K., Jenkins, J., Solomon, J. and Whittam, S. (eds) *Roper, Logan and Tierney Model in Practice*. Churchill Livingstone. Edinburgh. Ch 2 pp 23–39.

Holman, H. and Lorig, K. (2000) 'Patients as partners in managing chronic disease'. *British Medical Journal.* Vol 320, pp 526–527.

Integrated Care Pathway Users Scotland (2005) *Introducing Care Pathways.* NHS ICP Users Scotland. Edinburgh.

Johnson, S. (1997) *Pathways of Care*. Blackwell. Oxford.

Long-term Medical Conditions Alliance (2001) *Supporting Expert Patients*. LMCA. London.

Middleton, S. and Roberts, A. (2000) (eds) *Integrated Care Pathways: A Practical Approach to Implementation.* Butterworth-Heinemann. Oxford.

Middleton, S., Barnett, J. and Reeves, D. (2003) 'What is an integrated care pathway?'. www.evidence-based-medicine.co.uk. Vol 3, No 3, pp 1–8. Last accessed 11.08.2005.

NHS Executive (2000) *Working in Partnerships: Developing a Whole Systems Approach: Good Practice Guide*. NHS Executive. London.

National Institute for Health and Clinical Excellence (2002) *Clinical Guideline 1: Schizophrenia*. NICE. London.

National Patient Safety Agency (2005) *Hospital at Night: Patient Safety Risk Assessment Guide*. NPSA. London.

Nursing and Midwifery Council (2002) *Guidelines for Records and Records Keeping*. NMC. London.

Solomon, J. (2003) 'Eating and drinking' in Holland, K., Jenkins, J., Solomon, J. and Whittam, S. (eds) *Roper, Logan and Tierney Model in Practice*. Churchill Livingstone. Edinburgh. Ch 6 pp 163–198.

Strachen, H. (1994) 'There are benefits from computerising the nursing care plan!'. *Journal of the British Computer Society Nursing Specialist Group*. Vol 6, No 1, p 8.

Taylor, C., Lillis, C. and LeMone, P. (2005) (5th edn) *Fundamentals of Nursing: The Art and Science of Nursing Care*. Lippincott. Philadelphia.

**le 8.1** Components of foreground questions – PICO

| ient or tient's blem/ ndition | Intervention | Comparative intervention [(optional) Is there an alternative treatment to compare with the intervention?] | Outcome |
|---|---|---|---|
| tients h mild pertension | does anti-hypertensive medication when compared with | exercise and diet | make a difference in the reduction of hypertension? |
| emature bies with kle cell ait | what are the current treatments | | in the management of high temperature and infection? |
| en roviding re for atients ith type 2 iabetes | does standard care when compared with | primary/community care | make a difference to patient outcomes and reduction in cost? |

to consult your knowledge manager or information consultant ing resources centre. They may direct you to specialist journals abases such as Medical Literature On-line (Medline) and Cumu- to Nursing and Allied Health Literature (CINAHL). You may earch the World Wide Web for information about your topic. s of information are:

wed journals, which include research-based articles within cation range. The research-based articles should provide enough out the methodology so that informed judgements can be made study's validity and the clinical relevance of the findings.
nt publications, which include funded research reports, discussion nference proceedings, government policies and enquiry results.
ions and professional bodies often provide free information and urces of evidence.
nd abstracts to theses.
e collections on past students' work, specific dictionaries and aedias.

# 8 Evidence-based Practice

**Dr MAXINE OFFREDY**

Safe and effective nursing care is based on the best available evidence. This chapter encourages the reader to apply knowledge and skills indicative of safe and effective nursing practice. The key aspect of the chapter relates to the student's ability to use research and best evidence findings that underpin safe and effective nursing practice. The stimulus for evidence-based practice has its origins in evidence-based medicine, but its components are relevant to the practice of all health-care professionals. Patients in the acute and community settings are cared for by multiprofessional teams and nursing interventions can affect patient morbidity and mortality. A proficient practitioner must be able to demonstrate the ability to meet the needs of patients associated with a range of interventions that support and optimise health and wellbeing.

The commencement of the evidence-based movement is attributed to the physician and epidemiologist Archie Cochrane, who drew attention to the dearth of evidence about the effects of health care. He suggested that there should be efforts to summarise the results of research (specifically summaries arising from randomised clinical trials) available to decision makers (Cochrane, 1979). However, the term 'evidence-based medicine' was coined at McMaster University medical school as a way of describing problem-based learning (Bennett et al., 1987). Sackett et al. (1996) define evidence-based medicine as:

> *the conscientious, explicit and judicious use of current best evidence about the care of individual patients. The practice of evidence-based healthcare means integrating individual clinical expertise with the best available external, clinical evidence from systematic research.*

This strategy has been applied to the broader practice of health care, including nursing. Thus, evidence-based practice is a concept that is used to capture the essence of evidence-based medicine. The primary aim of evidence-based practice is defined as the 'identification and application of the most efficacious intervention to maximise the quality and quantity of life for individual patients' (Sackett et al., 1997). The demand for high-quality care has come from a number of sources, including government, patients and their carers, the public and the nursing profession. This demand is accompanied by organisational change within health-care provision and the need to ensure that limited resources are used to provide health care that is based on the best available evidence (Department of Health, 1998). The chapter commences by explaining the stages of evidence-based practice.

## STAGES OF EVIDENCE-BASED PRACTICE

Evidence-based practice has five stages, namely:

- A clear question is developed arising from the patient's problem.
- The questions are used to search the literature for evidence relating to the problem.
- The evidence is appraised critically for its validity and usefulness.
- The best available current evidence, together with clinical expertise and the patient's perspectives, is used to provide care.
- The patient outcomes are evaluated through a process of audit and peer assessment, including self-evaluation of the research process.

An explanation of each stage and their subdivisions follows.

## A CLEAR QUESTION IS DEVELOPED ARISING FROM THE PATIENT'S PROBLEM

This stage consists of two aspects: types of questions and finding the answers to your questions. When nursing a patient it is not unusual for you to consider why the patient is being cared for in that way, or whether there is an alternative way to provide that care. How would you find out the answer to your concern or problem? One of the points that you need to be clear about is the question that you want to ask. This may not be as easy as it sounds, because if you do not ask the right type of question, you will not get the correct answer to your concern or problem.

### TYPES OF QUESTIONS

You will need to decide on the type of information you require and thus the question that needs to be asked. There are two types of questions: background questions and foreground questions.

#### Background Questions

These questions allow you to find out more about the patient/problem or condition under scrutiny. It is a question about who, what, when, where, why and how, and is related to a problem. For example: what causes vomiting? Note that there are no inclusion or exclusion criteria and this type of search would



produce a large amount of info
your focused question/s. Backg
the condition and may help to f

#### Foreground Questions

Unlike background questions, fo
tion about managing the patient
Foreground questions can be rela

- *Diagnosis* – selecting the most
the results of a particular test.
- *Treatment* – what is the most ef
problem?
- *Harm or aetiology* – what are th
and how can these be minimised
- *Prognosis* – what is the likely co
patients?
- *Service redesign* – is it cost effecti
2 diabetes from secondary to prin

Sackett et al. (1997) devised a fran
ground questions: **P**atient or **P**roblem
and **O**utcome. The initials give rise to
may be a comparative intervention,
provides an example of how PICO m
tion, the next step is to locate the answ
section.

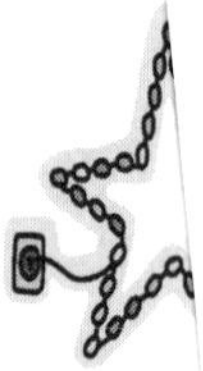

Consider a patient in your care. Ident
current treatment or care; that is, the int
to formulate a foreground question. You
out this chapter.

### FINDING THE ANSWERS TO YOUR

A number of resources may be at your di
nurse specialist or a nurse consultant, if th



Tab

| | |
|---|---|
| Component of the clinical question | Pa pa pr co |
| Example | In pa wi hy |
| Example | In p ba si tr |
| Example | Wh p c p v c |

may also like
at your learn
as well as dat
lative Index
also like to
Other sourc

- Peer-revie
their publ
details ab
about the
- Governm
papers, c
- Organisa
further s
- Indexes
- Referenc
encyclop

- Conference proceedings.
- Pharmaceutical company information.
- Discussion and networking groups.
- Newspapers.

You may be overwhelmed with information, depending on how much research has been done in the area you are searching. If this is the case, you will need to narrow your search to obtain a manageable amount of articles. The second stage of evidence-based practice, searching the literature, provides information about undertaking this procedure, which is discussed below.

## THE QUESTIONS ARE USED TO SEARCH THE LITERATURE FOR EVIDENCE RELATING TO THE PROBLEM

Now that you have formulated your question, the next step is to search the literature for evidence. This raises three important questions: What do we mean by evidence? In particular, what do we mean by best evidence? How can we search the literature for evidence? Having answered these three questions, a decision has to be made on the worth of the material found. A discussion on each of these follows.

### WHAT IS THE MEANING OF EVIDENCE?

Polit and Beck (2004) say that there is no consensus about what is meant by evidence for evidence-based practice (EBP), but there is general agreement that the results from 'robust' or 'best' research studies are of importance. A dictionary definition of evidence (Collins, 1986) includes:

- ground for belief or disbelief
- data on which to base proof or to establish truth or falsehood
- serve to indicate, attest

The common thread running through the above is that evidence needs to be observed and be subjected to scrutiny.

Cochrane's (1979) emphasis on quantitative research, specifically randomised control trials, gave rise to a view that quantitative research evidence was more valued than other forms of research evidence. However, qualitative and quantitative research are equally necessary in the generation of research-based nursing knowledge to inform nursing practice. For example, if we wish to find out the experiences of a specific group of people living with long-term conditions, a qualitative design may be best suited for this study. On the other hand, if we want to measure the effectiveness of one treatment over another, a quantitative design would be suitable. The evidence-based medicine movement has shifted to include clinically relevant research evidence by all health-care practitioners, whether it is of a quantitative or qualitative nature (Sackett et al., 2000). Higgs and Jones (2000) extend the view of what constitutes evidence by proposing that 'evidence is knowledge derived from a variety of sources that has been subjected to testing and has been found to be credible'. Thus 'evidence' may encompass knowledge broader than research-based information. We now turn to discussing the meaning of best evidence.

## WHAT IS THE MEANING OF BEST EVIDENCE?

Current best evidence includes clinical practice guidelines, which are usually nationally developed by expert researchers and which have undergone research trials. The National Institute for Health and Clinical Excellence (NICE, formerly The National Institute for Clinical Excellence, also formerly known as NICE) and National Service Frameworks (NSFs) are examples of authoritative national guidance developed to achieve consistent clinical standards across the NHS (Department of Health, 1998).

Clinical guidelines are recommendations by NICE on the relevant treatment and care of people with specific diseases and conditions within the NHS. The guidelines assist health professionals in their work, but they do not replace their knowledge and skills.

The aim of good clinical guidelines is to improve the quality of health care. They can change the way health care is delivered and improve people's chances of getting as well as possible. Well-constructed and up-to-date clinical guidelines have the added advantages of:

- Providing recommendations for the treatment and care of people by health professionals.
- Being used to develop standards to assess the clinical practice of individual health professionals.
- Being used in education and training sessions of health professionals.
- Assisting patients and carers to make informed decisions, thus improving communication between the patient, carer and health professional (Department of Health, 1998).

The clinical guidelines used in nursing should be updated by nurses and other health-care professionals as new empirical evidence becomes available. It is important to bear in mind that not all research is of best quality and practices may be described as research based even when the research process is questionable. Some published research can be of poor quality and result in conflicting evidence. When this is used as a basis for a change in practice, it may mean that patients may not receive the optimum care. Cullum et al. (1997) point to the paucity of evaluative research undertaken to distinguish between effective and noneffective nursing practices. Careful searching for evidence is therefore important.

## HOW TO SEARCH FOR EVIDENCE: STEPS IN LITERATURE SEARCH

This section provides a guide to the principles of searching the research literature. It is outside the remit of the section to give extensive and detailed information about the art of searching. However, the information given in Figure 8.1 provides good guidance on searching the literature. Conducting a literature search can be a lengthy and complex process, but the time taken is well worth the investment. You will need to be organised and systematic in your approach, as it is important to keep detailed records of the searches made and the information found.

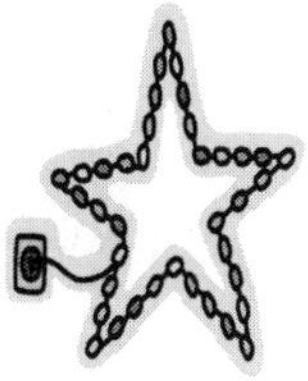

You may wish to use your formulated question to follow the example used in Table 8.2, discussed below. Try to follow the procedures with your own question.

Take the first example in Table 8.1, which is replicated as Table 8.2. Using the PICO example, you will need to set parameters by reviewing the literature in relation to some main themes pertinent to your topic. For example, you will need to have clear in your mind a definition of mild hypertension. You may wish to use the British Hypertensive Society's guidelines or any other suitable definition. You may also want to specify which type of hypertensive medication you would like to find evidence about. These need to be noted. You may also want to note alternative spellings, synonyms and acronyms for use in your search. As you proceed with your search, you may wish to be more specific by having inclusion and exclusion criteria.

### Inclusion Criteria

Inclusion criteria are characteristics that are essential to the problem under scrutiny. They are sometimes referred to as eligibility criteria; in other words, the sample population must possess the named characteristics. Examples of inclusion or eligibility criteria include:

- appropriate age groups
- language, for example English
- location or geography
- time period, for example between 1995 and 2000
- evidence-based medicine

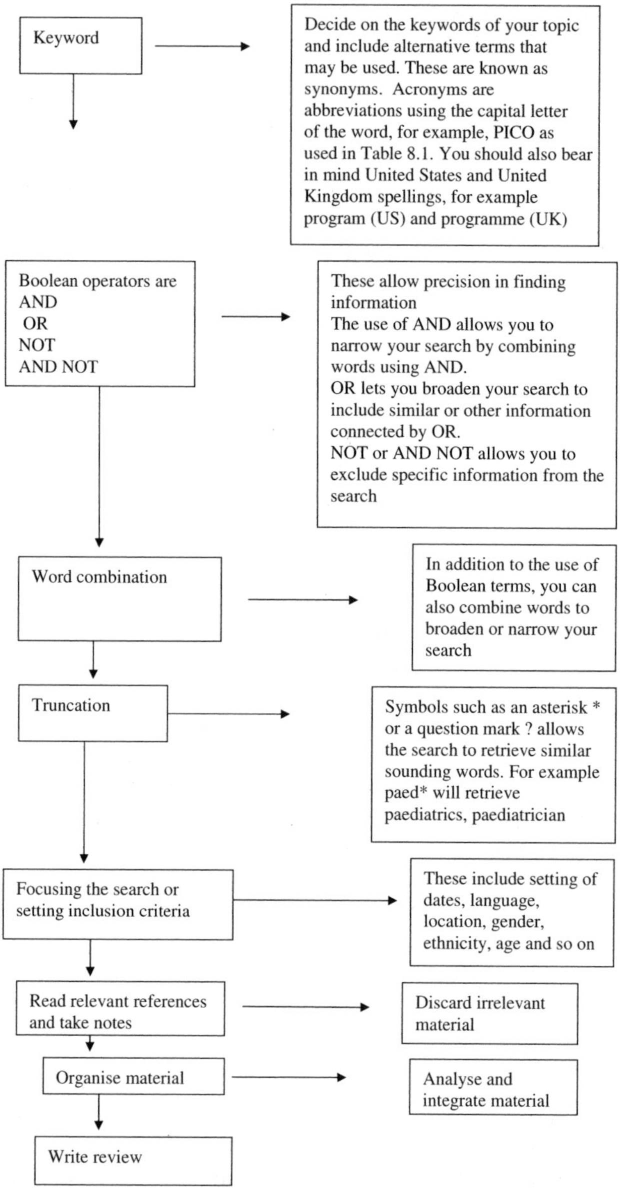


**Figure 8.1** Steps in the literature search
*Source*: Adapted from Hart, 1998; Burns and Grove, 2003; Polit and Beck, 2004.

**Table 8.2** Illustration of PICO's use in identifying components of a question

| Component of the clinical question | Patient or problem | Intervention | Comparative intervention [(optional) Is there an alternative treatment to compare with the intervention?] | Outcome |
|---|---|---|---|---|
| Example | In patients with mild hypertension | does anti-hypertensive medication when compared with | exercise and diet | make a difference in the reduction of hypertension? |

The inclusion criterion of evidence-based medicine will mean that the results of the search will be limited to articles reviewed in databases such as Health Technology Assessment (HTA), Cochrane Database of Systematic Reviews (CDSR) and Databases of Abstracts of Reviews of Effectiveness (DARE). DARE complements the CDSR by providing a selection of quality-assessed reviews in those subjects where there is currently no Cochrane review (Acton, 2001; Greenhalgh, 1997).

### Exclusion Criteria

Exclusion criteria are characteristics that you specifically do not wish to include in your search, such as Caucasians with diabetes if the problem pertains to Afro-Caribbean males with diabetes. The inclusion and exclusion criteria are important characteristics of a research study as they have implications for both the interpretation and the generalisability of the findings (Polit and Beck, 2004).

Having obtained the literature, you will need to decide on the worth of the material found. This can be done by assessing the information by using a hierarchy of evidence or by appraising the literature using the research process. Discussion of both these follows next.

## THE EVIDENCE IS APPRAISED CRITICALLY FOR ITS VALIDITY AND USEFULNESS

### HIERARCHY OF EVIDENCE

An aid commonly used to assess the worth of the material found, and which is used in clinical decision making, is the hierarchy of evidence (Table 8.3).

**Table 8.3** An example of the hierarchy of evidence

| Rank: | Methodology | Description |
|---|---|---|
| 1 | **Systematic reviews and meta-analyses** | **Systematic review**: review of a body of data that uses explicit methods to locate primary studies, and explicit criteria to assess their quality.<br>**Meta-analysis**: A statistical analysis that combines or integrates the results of several independent clinical trials considered by the analyst to be 'combinable', usually to the level of reanalysing the original data, also sometimes called *pooling, quantitative synthesis*.<br>Both are sometimes called 'overviews'. |
| 2 | **Randomised controlled trials** (finer distinctions may be drawn within this group based on statistical parameters like the confidence intervals) | Individuals are randomly allocated to a control group and a group which receives a specific intervention. Otherwise the two groups are identical for any significant variables. They are followed up for specific end points. |
| 3 | **Cohort studies** | Groups of people are selected on the basis of their exposure to a particular agent and followed up for specific outcomes. |
| 4 | **Case-control studies** | 'Cases' with the condition are matched with 'controls' without, and a retrospective analysis used to look for differences between the two groups. |
| 5 | **Cross-sectional surveys** | Survey or interview of a sample of the population of interest at one point in time. |
| 6 | **Case reports** | A report based on a single patient or subject; sometimes collected together into a short series. |
| 7 | **Expert opinion** | A consensus of experience from the good and the great. |
| 8 | **Anecdotal** | Something your friend told you after a meeting. |

*Source*: http:www.shef.ac.uk/scharr/ir/units/systrev/hierarchy.htm.

Hierarchies of evidence were first used by the Canadian Task Force on the Periodic Health Examination in 1979, and have subsequently been developed and used in assessing the effectiveness of research studies (Canadian Task Force on the Periodic Health Examination, 1979; Sackett, 1986; Cook et al., 1995; Guyatt et al., 1995; Petticrew and Roberts, 2003). They allow research-based evidence to be graded according to their design, are ranked in order of decreasing internal validity (National Health Service Centre for Reviews and Dissemination, 1996), and indicate the confidence decision and policy makers can have in their findings. However, the hierarchy of evidence remains a source of debate, as the use of the term is contentious when applied to health promotion and public health (Petticrew and Roberts, 2003).

Although there is an undeniable necessity for quantitative research, this approach is not suitable for many issues encountered in nursing practice. Patients' views about health care are not always quantifiable, for example their experiences of living with a long-term condition; the effects of treatment; or their choice of treatment. These need to be considered when delivering health care and the concept of a hierarchy of evidence is often problematic when appraising the evidence for social or public health interventions. These issues cannot be addressed appropriately in a quantitative study; a qualitative approach is more suitable, as this way of conducting research focuses on the meanings and understandings of people's experiences (Burns and Grove, 2003). Another way of deciding on the worth of the material found is by appraising the evidence guided by a systematic process. A number of factors are important in the execution of this process and these are considered below.

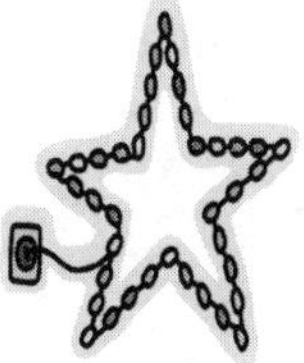

Using a research paper found from your literature search of your question/topic, attempt to review as much of the paper by using the process outlined below in appraising the evidence.

## DECIDING THE WORTH OF THE MATERIAL FOUND

### Appraising the Evidence

Reviewing the literature requires developing a complex set of skills acquired through practice. A comprehensive review of the literature is important (Gray, 2004) because it:

- Provides an up-to-date understanding of the subject and its significance to practice.
- Identifies the methods used in the research.
- Helps in the formulation of research topics, questions and direction.
- Provides a basis on which the subsequent research findings can be compared.

There are a number of ways in which evidence may be appraised. Burns and Grove (2003), Grbich (1999) and Polit and Beck (2004) suggest that a research appraisal can be divided into several sections. Using the subdivisions and considering the points suggested below will assist with this activity.

**The Structure of the Report**

- Is the organisation of the report logical?
- Does the report follow the sequence of steps of the process of research:
  - introduction
  - identification of the research problem
  - planning
  - data collection
  - data analysis
  - discussion
  - conclusions
  - recommendation

The way in which a report is organised may vary from one researcher to the next. However, in all cases the organisation should be logical. It should begin with a clear identification of what is to be studied and how, and should end with a summary or conclusion recommending further study or application. You should bear in mind that different journals may require a different layout, but the key issue is logical progression.

**The Abstract**

- Does the abstract, in a concise paragraph, clearly describe:
  - what was studied
  - how it was studied
  - how the sample was selected
  - how the data were analysed
  - the main findings of the research

The abstract provides a summary of the question and the most important findings of the study. It outlines how these differ from those of previous studies, and gives some indication of the methodology undertaken. It is usually up to 200–300 words long (depending on the guidelines for specific journals and the thesis formats of the relevant university). The abstract serves to provide the reader with a quick overview of what the research has done and found.

**The Introduction**

The introduction serves to explain 'why' and 'how' the research problem came to be defined in this particular way. It reviews critically previous relevant literature, pointing out any limitations in findings, methodology or theoretical interpretation. It also provides a pathway to the methodology section by clarifying the need for research to be undertaken in the chosen topic, especially with the methodological orientation or techniques chosen by the researcher.

### The Problem Statement/Purpose of the Research

You should consider whether:

- The general problem has been introduced promptly.
- The problem has been substantiated with adequate background and the need for the study.
- The general problem has been narrowed down to a specific research problem or to a problem with sub-problems as appropriate.
- The hypotheses directly answer the research problems.

### The Literature Review and Theoretical Rationale for the Study

- You should aim to consider whether this section is relevant, clearly written, well organised and up to date and whether the reliability of the methods and data collection are addressed (your reasons should be substantiated).
- Was there a sufficient review of the literature and theoretical rationale to assure you that the author had considered a broad spectrum of the possibilities for investigating the problem?
- Is it clear how the study will extend previous findings?

A thesis requires an extensive literature review, while in a journal article the author will usually cite the *major* pieces of work that are particularly relevant.

### Methodology

The methodology section must fully inform readers of the step-by-step processes undertaken in conducting the study. You should consider the appropriateness of the research methods chosen, including:

- sampling approach
- data-collection methods
- validity and reliability of observations or measurements

Consideration of the following sub-headings and questions will help in providing this information.

*The Population and Sample*

- Is the study population specific enough so that it is clear to what population the findings may be generalised?
- Is the sample representative of the population defined?
- Would it be possible to replicate the study population?
- Is the method of sample selection appropriate?
- Was any bias introduced by this method?
- Is the sample size appropriate and how is it substantiated?

*Instrumentation*

- Are the data-collection methods appropriate to the study?
- Do they obtain the data that the researcher seeks?
- Is the author specific regarding the validity and reliability of the instruments used?

*Procedure for Data Collection*

- Were steps taken to control extraneous variables?
- Were collection methods replicable?

*Ethical Considerations*

- The rights of subjects.
- The impact of ethical problems on the merit of the study and the wellbeing of the subjects.
- Steps to protect subjects.
- Indications of violations of ethical principles and suggestions as to how these could have been avoided.
- Inclusion in the report of any ethical considerations.
- Presentation of evidence that indicates that the rights of the study's subjects have been protected.

*The Pilot Study*

- Was a pilot study undertaken?
- Were any changes made following the pilot study?

**Analysis of Data**

- Were the analyses reported clearly and related to each hypothesis?
- Is it clear what statistical methods were used and what values were obtained?
- Is there a statement of whether or not the data support the hypotheses?
- Is a complete discussion of the data given?
- Has a thorough examination of each hypothesis, including the use of appropriate statistical analysis and the decision to accept or reject the hypothesis, been included?
- Has explanation been given on how missing data were handled?
- Have experts been used to assist in the analysis of the data?

**Discussion**

- Is the discussion critically presented?
- Can the findings be generalised?

**Conclusions and Limitations**

- Has the author related the findings to the theoretical position of the study?
- Did the researcher identify methodological problems?
- Does the author over-generalise?
- Are the implications of the findings for practice identified?
- Are there suggestions for further research?

**References and Bibliography**

- Are references cited relevant to the study?
- Do the reference list and bibliography reflect:
  - the review of the literature
  - search for and/or development of valid and reliable instruments/methodology

Hart (1998) warns that when reading a review or undertaking a review, you should be aware of your own value judgements and try to avoid personalised destructive criticisms. The fourth stage of evidence-based practice, putting evidence into practice, will now be explained.

## THE BEST AVAILABLE CURRENT EVIDENCE, TOGETHER WITH CLINICAL EXPERTISE AND THE PATIENT'S PERSPECTIVES, IS USED TO PROVIDE CARE

The discussion in this section encompasses three aspects: the factors that need to be taken into account when putting evidence into practice; factors affecting the implementation of evidence-based practice; and ways of promoting evidence-based practice. The discussion commences with factors that need to be taken into account.

### FACTORS TO BE TAKEN INTO ACCOUNT WHEN PUTTING EVIDENCE INTO PRACTICE

Getting research into practice is a complex and time-consuming task and involves behaviour change on the part of the individuals, teams and organisations involved (Royle and Blythe, 1998). Making decisions about care is an iterative process that involves consideration of the potential benefits and harm of treatment and needs of the individual (Wulff and Gøtzsche, 2000). These factors can create uncertainty about how and whether research evidence can be put into practice. At a time when cost pressures are evident in health-care delivery and there is a need for holistic evidence-based care, evidence of clinical governance as well as quality improvement targets, nurses must be aware of the key factors that should be taken into account when putting evidence into practice. These include:

- The need to take into account that there are different types of evidence and that not all research studies provide robust evidence.
- The different sources of evidence, for example patient comfort; alteration in life style; evidence from specialist nurses and national guidelines.
- The type of setting, which is key to implementing change. Teaching/learning organisations and those that take part in research, whether at a local or national level, are more likely to be open to introduce evidence-based practice than institutions where nurses are seldom provided with the opportunities for updating their knowledge and skills. Decision making in the former institutions is bottom up rather than top down, as health-care professionals feel valued and are supported to find new ways of working. Leadership has a key role to play in the change process.
- Understanding of cultures, values and beliefs to overcome potential barriers to change.
- The need for nurses to be articulate about the research evidence. Knowledge about the different paradigms is important, because those whom the nurses may be trying to convince for funding to support change may prefer the quantitative approach to research. That is, their preference is for information in a numerical form, collected and analysed in a systematic, objective and measurable way with definite conclusions. This approach to obtaining data is not always conducive to nursing. The qualitative approach, which tries to understand and explain the phenomena under study and is generally seen as less scientific, is often more appropriate to many of the issues central to nursing, and less receptive to policy makers and decision makers (Sackett et al., 2000; Rycroft-Malone et al., 2004; Melnyk et al., 2004).

Overall, nurses need the ability to take into account not just the evidence but the evidence of case-based knowledge in clinical practice, patient preferences and factors and the particular clinical scenario before deciding on appropriate management (Jennings and Loan, 2001; Rycroft-Malone et al., 2004). This involves assessing the evidence for the appropriate problem; considering the appropriateness of both anecdotal evidence and direct clinical experience in relation to the clinical problem; as well as incorporating the patient's views and deciding whether the patient under discussion is similar to patients addressed by the research or guidelines. Consideration should be given to the issue that similar decision scenarios may not be identical since they may be conducted in different clinical settings and target different patient subgroups. It is also important to note whether or not there is an additional patient problem, as this might influence safety and effectiveness. Further, it should be noted that patients' beliefs about the value of treatment, their assessment of personal risk and their reluctance to change treatment might also influence their treatment preferences (Wulff and Gøtzsche, 2000). In addition, other factors that may affect the implementation of evidence-based practices include individual and organisational factors. These are discussed next.

## FACTORS AFFECTING THE IMPLEMENTATION OF EVIDENCE-BASED PRACTICE

The barriers to evidence-based practice have been documented in studies by Kajermo et al. (1998), Retsas (2000), Jennings and Loan (2001) and McKenna et al. (2004) and can be grouped under two subheadings.

### Individual Factors

- Lack of interest in research.
- Lack of confidence in reading and understanding the research process.
- Lack of training in research issues and consequently lack of skills required for critical analysis, particularly when there is a plethora of evidence, some of which may be conflicting.
- Anticipated outcomes of using research.

### Organisational Factors

- Cost pressures at work resulting in lack of, or limited, funding for research courses.
- Insufficient time within work commitments.
- Lack of patient compliance.
- Inadequate library and computer facilities.
- Inaccessibility of research findings.
- Lack of support from peers, managers and other health-care professionals.

McKenna et al. (2004) opine that identifying barriers to implementing evidence-based practice is only one step to changing practice. Studies by Haines and Donald (1998) and Rycroft-Malone et al. (2002) have identified ways that could assist in promoting the uptake of research findings; these are itemised below.

## WAYS OF PROMOTING THE UPTAKE OF RESEARCH FINDINGS

- Determine that there is an appreciable gap between research findings and practice.
- Define the appropriate message (for example the information to be used).
- Identify champions to promote the message of change.
- Decide which processes need to be altered.
- Involve the key players (for example those people who will implement change or who are in a position to influence change, such as managers).
- Identify the barriers to change and decide how to overcome them.
- Decide on specific interventions to promote change (for example the use of guidelines or educational programmes).
- Identify levers for change; that is, existing mechanisms that can be used to promote change.

- Determine whether practice has changed in the way desired; use a clinical audit to monitor change.

Implementing evidence-based practice has become a priority in the NHS (Department of Health, 1998), where health-care professionals are urged to use up-to-date research evidence in order to give patients the best possible care. Winch et al. (2002) proffer the view that incorporating evidence-based practice principles into nursing requires more than shifting nurses from an oral to a reading tradition. It requires nurses at all levels to embrace practices and attitudes such as interest, professional pride, positiveness, willingness to undertake change and a commitment to life-long learning (Thompson et al., 1999).

Findings from Melnyk et al.'s (2004) study support the view that knowledge and beliefs about evidence-based practice are important indicators for change in behaviours. However, it is important for nurses to believe that evidence-based practice will result in better patient outcomes in order for changes in practice to occur. Of equal importance was the presence of a mentor who facilitated use of databases, such as the Cochrane Database of Systematic Reviews. Knowledge of learning and searching databases tend to support the use of evidence-based practice as well as support from experts in the field, research departments, library resources and administrators. Melnyk et al.'s (2004) study supports the findings of an earlier work by Nagy et al. (2001), who identified six factors that represent the conditions nurses view as necessary for the development of evidence-based practice. These are:

- a supportive organisation
- nurses' belief in the value of research-based evidence for improvement in patient care
- searching, reading and evaluating research studies
- clinically relevant research
- knowledge of research language and statistics
- protected work time for activities related to evidence-based practice

The final stage in evidence-based process is evaluation. This is discussed next.

## THE PATIENT OUTCOMES ARE EVALUATED THROUGH A PROCESS OF AUDIT AND PEER ASSESSMENT, INCLUDING SELF-EVALUATION OF THE RESEARCH PROCESS

This final stage of evidence-based practice will provide a brief discussion on clinical audit, peer and self-evaluation as a means of evaluating the outcomes as a result of implementing a change in practice. The research process was discussed earlier. The discussion begins with clinical audit.

## CLINICAL AUDIT

Clinical audit is a clinically-led initiative that seeks to improve the quality and outcome of patient care through structured peer review, whereby clinicians examine their practices and results against agreed explicit standards and modify their practice where indicated (NHS Executive, 1996). The key feature of clinical audit is that it provides a framework to enable improvements in health-care delivery to be made to ensure that what should be done is being done. Clinical audit has six stages (Clinical Governance Support Team, 2005):

- Identify the problem or issue.
- Set criteria and standards.
- Observe practice and collect data.
- Compare performance with criteria and standards.
- Implement change.
- Sustain change.

As with the research process, clinical audit follows a systematic process to identify best practice, which is measured against set criteria. Action is taken to improve care based on the data collected and monitoring procedures are implemented to sustain improvement. Clinical audit is discussed in detail in Chapter 12.

## PEER ASSESSMENT AND SELF-EVALUATION

Peer assessment and self-evaluation (sometimes referred to as self-assessment) constitute a process in which individual practitioners comment on and judge their colleagues' or their own work. It can be used both in formative and summative assesments. It provides the opportunity for the individual to make independent judgements of their own and of others' work. Practitioners take responsibility for monitoring and making judgements about how the process of implementation has been undertaken, thereby determining their level of knowledge and skills (Kaufmann et al., 2000).

The processes of peer assessment and self-evaluation require a high degree of professional ethics and objectivity (Weaver and Cotrell, 1986). There are four main advantages of this type of evaluation (Kaufman et al., 2000; Weaver and Cotrell, 1986):

- Helping students to become more autonomous, responsible and involved in practices around them.
- Encouraging students to analyse work done by others critically, rather than simply seeing a mark.
- Assisting in clarifying the assessment criteria.
- Giving students a wider range of feedback.

The disadvantages are (Kaufman et al., 2000; Weaver and Cotrell, 1986):

- Students may lack the ability to evaluate each other.
- Students may not take the process seriously, allowing friendships and entertainment value to influence their marking.
- Students may not like peer marking because of the possibility of being discriminated against, being misunderstood.

The final aspect of the evaluation is the undertaking of the research process. This is outlined above.

## SOME CRITICISMS OF EVIDENCE-BASED PRACTICE

Evidence-based practice has its critics. Over three decades ago Freidson (1970) pointed out that clinical experience derived from personal observation, reflection and judgement is required to translate scientific results into treatment of individual patients. Building on this view, authors such as Naylor (1995) and Armstrong (2002) point out that evidence-based practice reduces professional autonomy by encouraging rigid and prescriptive practices that fail to take into account the complexities of clinical situations. Armstrong (2002) argues that evidence-based practice is in opposition to a patient-centred model of care. Applied programmes in public health are too complex and context driven to be adequately described by evidence-based practice strategies. Woolf et al. (1999) also voiced reservations about evidence-based guidelines by suggesting that however well intentioned, evidence-based guidelines and policies could cause unintended harm to patients.

Arising from these views is the issue of whether Randomised Control Trials (RCTs) should be considered the gold standard for evidence-based practice and the appropriateness of hierarchies that promote meta-analyses as the best available evidence (Kitson, 1997; Rolfe, 1999; Petticrew and Roberts, 2003). RCTs inform about which treatment is better, but not for whom it is better; RCTs give an oversimplified and artificial environment that might bear little resemblance to day-to-day reality (Petticrew and Roberts, 2003). Thus the ideal of Sackett et al.'s (1997) view of integrating individual clinical experience with the best external evidence might only be realised by health professionals with a wealth of clinical experience and research knowledge. It should also be taken into account that when patients are given an active role in their treatment decisions that may result in a less successful outcome regarding uptake of optimal treatment, particular skills are required of the clinician to maintain a balanced view to convey to the patient why a particular course of action is recommended.

## CONCLUSIONS

The discussion presented in this chapter offers guidance to help the reader to apply knowledge and skills in obtaining and using the literature to underpin practice. Central to evidence-based practice are the patient, the environment and individuals within that arena in which change is to occur. Evidence is not a static concept; practitioners must make every effort to keep abreast of the latest research data pertaining to their area, bearing in mind that they are accountable for their practice. From the point of view of the organisation, protected time must be set aside for nurses to engage in evidence-based nursing activities. Well-resourced facilities and effective managerial support for evidence-based practice will be seen as a positive step for other members of the health-care professions to regard evidence-based practice as a way of thinking and practising.

## REFERENCES


Acton, G.J. (2001) 'Meta-analysis: A tool for evidence-based practice'. *AACN Clinical Issues: Advanced Practice in Acute and Critical Care.* Vol 12, No 4, pp 539–545.

Armstrong, D. (2002) 'Clinical autonomy, individual and collective: The problem of changing doctors' behaviour'. *Social Science of Medicine.* Vol 55, No 10, p 1771.

Bennett, K.J., Sackett, D.L., Haynes, R.B., Neufeld, V.R., Tugwell, P. and Roberts, R. (1987) 'A controlled trial of teaching critical appraisal of the clinical literature to medical students'. *Journal of the American Medical Association.* Vol 257, pp 2451–2454.

Burns, N. and Grove, S.K. (2003) (3rd end) *Understanding Nursing Research.* Saunders. Philadelphia.

Canadian Task Force on the Periodic Health Examination (1979) 'The periodic health examination'. *Canadian Medical Association Journal.* Vol 121, pp 1193–1254.

Clinical Governance Support Team (2005) *A Practical Handbook for Clinical Audit.* Clinical Governance Support Team. London.

Cochrane, A.L. (1979) *A Critical Review, with Particular Reference to the Medical Profession. Medicines for the Year 2000.* Office of Health Economics. London.

*Collins Paperback English Dictionary* (1986) Collins. London.

Cook, D.J., Guyatt, G.H., Laupacis, A., Sackett, D.L. and Goldberg, R.J. (1995) 'Clinical recommendations using level of evidence for antithrombotic agents'. *Chest.* Vol 108, pp 227s–230s.

Cullum, N., diCenso, A. and Ciliska, D. (1997) 'Evidence-based nursing: An introduction'. *Nursing Standard.* Vol 11, No 28, pp 30–33.

Department of Health (1998) *A First Class Service: Quality in the New NHS.* Department of Health. London.

Freidson, E. (1970) *Profession of Medicine: A Study of the Sociology of Applied Knowledge.* Dodd, Mead. New York.

Gray, D.E. (2004) *Doing Research in the Real World.* Sage. London.

Grbich, C. (1999) *Qualitative Research in Health.* Sage. London.

Greenhalgh, T. (1997) 'Papers that summarise other papers (systematic reviews and meta-analyses)'. *British Medical Journal.* Vol 315, pp 672–675.

Guyatt, G.H., Sackett, D.L., Sinclair, J.C., Hayward, R., Cook, D.J. and Cook, R.J. (1995) 'Users guide to the medical literature: 1X. A method for grading healthcare recommendations'. *Journal of the American Medical Association.* Vol 274, pp 1800–1804.

Haines, A. and Donald, A. (1998) 'Steps in promoting the uptake of research findings'. *British Medical Journal.* Vol 317, pp 72–75.

Hart, C. (1998) *Doing a Literature Review: Releasing the Social Science Research Imagination.* Sage. London.

Higgs, J. and Jones, M. (2000) 'Will evidence-based practice take the reasoning out of practice?' in Higgs, J. and Jones, M. (eds) (2nd edn) *Clinical Reasoning in Health Professionals.* Butterworth Heinemann. Oxford. pp 307–315.

Jennings, B. and Loan, L. (2001) 'Misconceptions among nurses about evidence-based practice'. *Journal of Nursing Scholarship.* Vol 33, No 2, pp 121–127.

Kajermo, K.N., Nordstrom, G., Krusebrant, A. and Bjorvell, H. (1998) 'Barriers to and facilitators of research utilisation as perceived by a group of registered nurses in Sweden'. *Journal of Advanced Nursing.* Vol 27, pp 798–807.

Kaufman, D.B., Felder, R.M. and Fuller, H. (2000) 'Accounting for individual effort in cooperating learning teams'. *Journal of Engineering Education.* Vol 89, No 2, pp 133–140.

Kitson, A. (1997) 'Using evidence to demonstrate the value of nursing'. *Nursing Standard.* Vol 11, No 28, pp 34–39.

McKenna, H., Ashton, S. and Keeney, S. (2004) 'Barriers to evidence-based practice in primary care'. *Journal of Advanced Nursing.* Vol 45, No 2, pp 178–189.

McKibbon, K.A. and Marks, S. (2001) 'Posing clinical questions: Framing the question for scientific enquiry'. *AACN Clinical Issues: Advanced Practice in Acute and Critical Care.* Vol 12, No 4, pp 477–481.

Melnyk, B.M., Fineout-Overholt, E., Feinstein, N.F., Li, H., Small, L., Wilcox, L. and Kraus, R. (2004) 'Nurses' perceived knowledge, beliefs, skills, and needs regarding evidence-based practice: Implications for accelerating the paradigm shift'. *World Views on Evidence-Based Nursing.* Vol 1, No 3, pp 185–193.

Nagy, S., Lumby, J., McKinley, S. and MacFarlane, C. (2001) 'Nurses' beliefs about the conditions that hinder or support evidence-based practice'. *International Journal of Nursing Practice.* Vol 7, pp 314–321.

National Health Service Centre for Reviews and Dissemination (1996) *Undertaking Systematic Reviews of Research on Effectiveness. CRD Guidelines for Those Carrying Out or Commissioning Reviews.* University of York. York.

Naylor, C.D. (1995) 'Grey zones of clinical practice: Some limits to evidence based medicine'. *Lancet.* Vol 345, pp 840–842.

NHS Executive (1996) *Promoting Clinical Effectiveness. A Framework for Action in and through the NHS.* NHS Executive. London.

Petticrew, M. and Roberts, H. (2003) 'Evidence, hierarchies and typologies: Horses for courses'. *Journal of Epidemiology and Community Health.* Vol 57, pp 527–529. http:///jech.bmjjournals.com/cgi/content/ful/57/7/527.

Polit, D.F. and Beck, C.T. (2004) *Nursing Research: Principles and Practice.* Lippincott Williams and Wilkins. Philadelphia.

Retsas, A. (2000). 'Barriers to using research evidence in nursing practice'. *Journal of Advanced Nursing.* Vol 31, No 3, pp 599–606.

Rolfe, G. (1999) 'Insufficient evidence: The problem of evidence-based nursing today'. *Nurse Education Today.* Vol 19, No 6, pp 433–442.

Royle, J. and Blythe, J. (1998) 'Promoting research utilisation in nursing: The role of the individual, organisation, and environment'. *Evidence-based Nursing.* Vol 1, pp 71–72.

Rycroft-Malone, J., Harvey, J., Kitson, A., McCormack, B., Seers, K. and Titchen, A. (2002) 'Putting evidence into practice: Ingredients for change'. *Nursing Standard.* Vol 16, No 37, pp 38–43.

Rycroft-Malone, J., Seers, K., Titchen, A., Harvey, G., Kitson, A. and McCormack, B. (2004) 'What counts as evidence in evidence-based practice?'. *Journal of Advanced Nursing.* Vol 47, No 1, pp 81–90.

Sackett, D.L. (1986) 'Rules of evidence and clinical recommendations on the use of antithrombotic agents'. *Chest.* Vol 89, pp 2s–3s.

Sackett, D.L., Richardson, W.S., Rosenberg, W. and Haynes, R.B. (1997) *Evidence-based Medicine: How to Practise and Teach EBM.* Churchill Livingstone. Edinburgh.

Sackett, D.L., Richardson, W.S., Rosenberg, W. and Haynes, R.B. (2000) (2nd edn) *Evidence-based Medicine: How to Practise and Teach EBM.* Churchill Livingstone. Edinburgh.

Sackett, D.L., Rosenberg, W., Gray, J.A., Haynes, R.B. and Richardson, W.S. (1996) 'Evidence-based medicine: What it is and what it isn't'. *British Medical Journal.* Vol 312, pp 71–72.

Thompson, P.E., Bell, P. and Prevost, S. (1999) 'Overcoming barriers to research based practice'. *Medsurg Nursing: The Journal of Adult Health.* Vol 8, No 1, pp 59–63.

Weaver, W. and Cotrell, H.W. (1986) 'Peer evaluation: A case study'. *Innovative Higher Education.* Vol 11, pp 25–39.

Winch, S., Creedy, D. and Chaboyer, W. (2002) 'Governing nursing conduct: The rise of evidence-based practice'. *Nursing Inquiry.* Vol 9, No 3, pp 156–161.

Woolf, S.H., Grol, R., Hutchinson, A., Eccles, M. and Grimshaw, J. (1999) 'Potential benefits, limitations, and harms of clinical guidelines'. *British Medical Journal.* Vol 318, pp 527–530.

Wulff, H.R. and Gøtzsche, P.C. (2000) (3rd edn) *Rational Diagnosis and Treatment. Evidence-based Clinical Decision Making.* Blackwell Science. Oxford.

# 9 Sociocultural Issues

This chapter considers the social, cultural, legal, political and economic influences associated with the provision of nursing care in relation to antidiscriminatory practice. Consideration is given to the sociocultural factors that impinge on the patient's ability to enjoy good health and wellbeing. It is noted in this chapter that there are some groups in society who could be said to be marginalised or oppressed and the sociocultural issues that may lead to this marginalisation are outlined. Three particular groups are used to illustrate the issues that members of a marginalised society may face.

In Chapter 3 diversity and culture were discussed in relation to several factors, for example practices associated with specific religions and religious beliefs. Some key terms were defined in that chapter and the reader is encouraged to revisit the definitions of those key terms while using this chapter. It has already been stated that what is considered the norm in one culture may not be case in another culture (Holland, 2003).

Nurses practise nursing within a social, political and economic context. Professional and patient autonomy is a key feature of the nurse's role. The nurse must consider how culture, economic conditions and overall lifestyle can impinge on an individual's health. Developing skills to understand how these factors can influence a person's health will help the nurse understand the patient (Taylor et al., 2005).

Demonstrating accountability for nursing care that has been and is being delivered means that the nurse must take into account social, spiritual, cultural, legal, political and economic factors. The nurse must also understand and apply the values that underpin antidiscriminatory working practices.

## SOCIOCULTURAL FACTORS

The term sociocultural, according to Sarafino (2006), means involving or relating to social and cultural issues that embrace ethnic and income variations within and across nations. Consideration of the social determinants of health means that health and social wellbeing is being thought about from a social, economic, environmental and political perspective. Epidemiologists have identified sociocultural differences in health and they have determined that there are specific types of cancer, for example cancers that are more prevalent in certain cultures than others.

Wight and Henderson (2004) consider the sociocultural factors that can influence a young person's sexuality. They have identified the following factors associated with sexual behaviour, but it must be remembered that they are discussing these factors in relation to young people:

- social class
- educational level
- family composition
- ethnicity
- parenting style

The sociocultural factors outlined above have the potential to shape a young person's sexual behaviour from the childhood experiences to which they have been exposed. It is during childhood and adolescence that the process of marginalisation may begin (Lehtinen et al., 1997). Societal and cultural contexts not only influence and give meaning to perceptions of health and illness, but also to other bodily (physical and psychological) changes and symptoms (Heath and McCormack, 2002; Taylor and Muller, 1995). Roper et al. (1996) suggest that sociocultural factors have considerable influence on the person's ability to carry out the activities of living.

## MARGINALISED SOCIETIES

Three particular groups in society who could be said to be marginalised or oppressed will be considered. They may have similar yet different sociocultural issues that can have an effect on their health. A person's social position affects their health, appearance and chances in life. There are many complex reasons why people are marginalised by society, for example they may feel marginalised because of their difference. This chapter will consider the following three groups in an attempt to provide some insight into the issues that may be apparent when caring for these groups of people:

- the homeless
- prisoners
- homosexuals

Prior to considering each group, recall the various components or dimensions that affect all humans (see Figure 9.1). Remember that health integrates all the human dimensions and as a result the nurse must consider each component in order to provide individualised care.

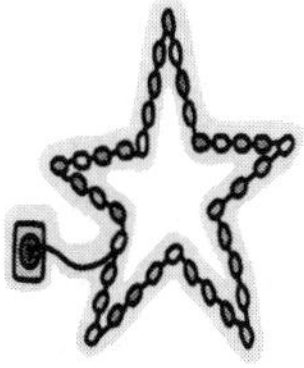

Consider the following situation.

> There are two candidates for a kidney transplant. One is a homeless person and unemployed and has a 95 per cent chance of surviving the operation; the other person is a company manager and has an 85 per cent chance of survival. Who should get the kidney?

This is clearly a difficult case scenario to answer. The example is there to illustrate a point – when decisions are made about many things in life we can take into account the sociocultural and socioeconomic attributes of a person's life. To make a response or to begin to answer the above scenario, you may need to acquaint yourself once again with the ethical frameworks discussed in

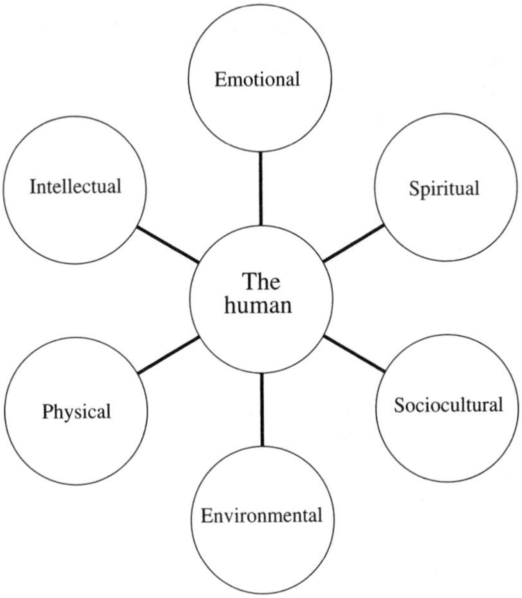


**Figure 9.1** The interdependent components of the human being

Chapter 2. The influencing factors or the criteria used to allocate resources can be medically or socially based. In the decision-making process related to resource allocation, this may hinge on several aspects of the scenario, including the fact that one of the transplant candidates is homeless (a social factor).

If social criteria alone were used to make recommendations for those who required renal transplants, then aspects such as the person's wealth, marital status, psychological stability and religious affiliation may be taken into the equation and then this would be unacceptable. It is easy for us to be disapproving of the idea of using social criteria to make decisions about life and death situations, but often medical criteria merge into social criteria.

The following factors (individually or a collection of them) can be key factors that may lead to marginalisation. Serious deficiencies in any (or all) of the following areas of a person's life may render them susceptible to marginalisation:

- *Accommodation* – the person may live in substandard accommodation that is often unstable or temporary. Renting or owning accommodation depends on income.
- *Income* – often people are on a low income, e.g. those receiving disability allowance or pensions, which is their only source of income. The assets they own may be some clothes and a little furniture.
- *Diet* – many have a poor and inadequate diet. A number may have no proper cooking facilities and they rely on cheap and unhealthy takeaway food.
- *Social support* – social isolation is a major problem and many marginalised people live alone. Many of them have split from their families and no longer have contact with them. Few, if any, have close friends. Most of them have no one to turn to if they are facing particular problems.
- *Health* – the general health of many marginalised communities is poor as a result of their lifestyle. Chronic illness is not uncommon.
- *Disabilities and disorders* – disability or other conditions may preclude them from, or limit their opportunities to participate in, regular community activities. Psychiatric illness, behavioural problems, physical disability and learning disability are common among the marginalised of society. They may also be experiencing some form of substance abuse, for example alcohol and nicotine.
- *Self-esteem* – lack of self-confidence is very common among marginalised people. As a result of continuous putdowns in their lives, they may feel they are of little value and frequently believe that no one is interested in them. Lack of self-esteem is often the hardest thing facing a person who has been marginalised. It is not the lack of material goods such as shelter or food, but being seen as having no worth, being devalued as a person. Feeling as if you are of little worth leads to a loss of dignity as a human. Living a 'dehumanised' existence with few friends and little social contact only exacerbates the situation.

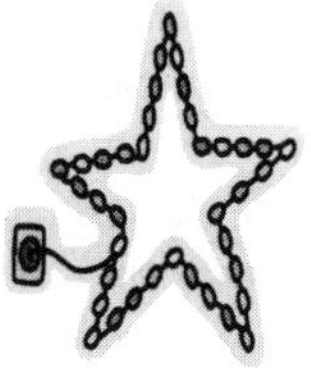

Thinking about the factors above, make a list of people who you think could be seen as marginalised.

Your list must be very long; any one of us may have experienced or may experience any of the factors above. Whole societies can be marginalised. Burton and Kagan (2004) state that marginalisation is a multiconcept, dynamic and fluid idea that can change according to social status; it also has a temporal element attached to it. You might have included the following in your list:

- the elderly
- those with a psychiatric illness
- those who suffer from a stigma (e.g. those with cancer or an infectious disease)
- people who have a physical disability
- people with a learning disability
- addicted people (e.g. addicted to drugs, alcohol, nicotine)
- travellers
- prostitutes
- refugees
- the uneducated
- the poor

Smith (1999) suggests that sometimes medicine fails marginalised people and unfortunately those who care for marginalised groups themselves become marginalised. This is evidenced by low recruitment rates to the psychiatry of learning disability; it is not seen as a 'high-status' speciality.

Marginalisation is complex, it is a multifaceted process produced by restricted activity or capacity. Marginalisation leads to exclusion, oppression, discrimination and vulnerabilty. It may be associated with societal attitudes towards a disability, impairment, sexuality or ethnicity. Different people react and respond differently to marginalisation and this is frequently dependent on the personal and social resources available (Burton and Kagan, 2004).

The literature concerning marginalisation is limited despite the fact that nurses often work with marginalised members of society, for example the elderly, the mentally ill and those with a learning disability. Social marginality is defined by Leonard (1984) as:

*Being outside the mainstream of productive activity and/or social reproductive activity.*

Other dictionary definitions define marginalisation as the social process of becoming or being made marginal (especially as a group within the larger society). Marginalisation refers in general to overt or covert acts and trends within societies whereby those perceived as lacking function or desirable traits are excluded from existing social systems of interaction.

Those who have been marginalised often have little control over their lives and the resources that are available to them, for example health-care resources. This, according to Burton and Kagan (2004), is often associated with negative public attitudes towards the marginalised group, leading to stigmatisation and isolation. Isolation can result in withdrawal and this in turn means that the marginalised person will be limited with respect to the contribution they can make to society, leading to a reduction in self-esteem and self-confidence – a vicious circle begins.

## SOCIAL EXCLUSION

The Social Exclusion Unit was established by the UK government in 1997 and works across government departments. The aim of this policy-led unit is to create prosperous, inclusive and sustainable communities. The work of the Social Exclusion Unit includes specific projects to tackle particular issues and wide-ranging programmes to assess past policy and identify future trends.

Social exclusion occurs when people or places suffer from a series of problems such as unemployment, discrimination, poor skills, low incomes, poor housing, high crime, ill health and family breakdown. When such problems combine they can create a vicious cycle. Social exclusion has complex and multidimensional causes and consequences (Social Exclusion Unit, 2004a). Similar to marginalisation, it can also have devastating effects on individual lives.

The Social Exclusion Unit has agreed a number of targets related to the following areas (Social Exclusion Unit, 2004b):

- children and young people
- crime
- employment and opportunity
- health and care
- homes and neighbourhoods
- transport

The list of priorities reflects the government's attempts to bring about 'joined-up' thinking in relation to its policies and practices. Different government policies are meant to pull together with a 'bottom-up' approach (Matthews, 2001).

## THE HOMELESS

Home should not be considered merely a roof over the head, it is a place that provides security, privacy and links to a community and has the potential to act as a support network. However, for some home may also be a place they associate with fear and anxiety. It may be a threatening environment for them where they feel unsafe and at risk and this may be detrimental to their health and wellbeing.

It is difficult to estimate how many people in the UK are homeless; this is primarily due to the hidden nature of the problem. Arrivals into large cities and towns make estimating numbers difficult, some people drift in and out of hostels or other accommodation while others drift in and out of 'sleeping rough'. Estimating data outside of large cities and towns such as London is less robust. The state of 'homelessness' can be temporary and episodic.

In the main, a person is homeless as defined in law (Homelessness Act 2002) if he/she has:

- No accommodation that they are entitled to occupy.
- Accommodation that is available, but it is unreasonable for them to continue to occupy, e.g. because of the risk of violence.
- Accommodation that they are entitled to occupy and it is reasonable to continue to occupy, but is not available to occupy.

It is a mistake to think that homelessness only occurs or has occurred to people who live on the streets or to those who are 'sleeping rough'. The scale of the problem extends beyond this common misconception. The majority of people who are homeless are families or single people. They may be staying with others, for example with friends or relatives, or in temporary accommodation. This can also be detrimental to an individual's health and wellbeing (Diaz, 2005).

Despite the difficulties associated with the ability to quantify the numbers of homeless people, there is some data available. For example, the Office of the Deputy Prime Minister (ODPM) provides data on a quarterly basis regarding the numbers of households that approach local authorities, and those that are given assistance if they meet the requirements stated in legislation that is associated with homelessness, for example the Housing (Homeless Persons) Act 1996 and the amended Homelessness Act 2002. Data is collected by the ODPM to estimate the numbers of people who are sleeping on the streets on any given night.

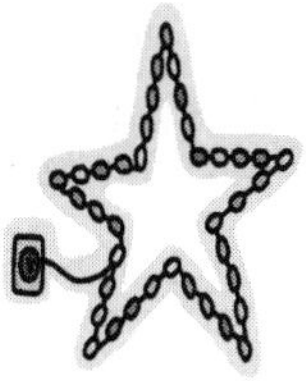

Despite the data the government produces, why do you think this data may not reflect a true account of the situation regarding the homeless?

The following are some of the reasons why the data collected may not be a comprehensive measure of all instances of homelessness:

- There may be a number of people who are legally defined as homeless but may not approach their local authority for assistance.
- People may move from one form of temporary accommodation to another.
- Some may stay with friends.
- The collation of data comes from various sources and the reliability of those sources may be questionable.

## PROBLEMS ASSOCIATED WITH HOMELESSNESS

The most comprehensive survey of the problems of the homeless in the UK was published in 2004 (St Mungo's, 2004). This large-scale survey considered the experiences and challenges faced by 1534 homeless people. Table 9.1 provides key data taken from the St Mungo's survey.

Table 9.2 outlines some specific problems associated with the older homeless population and the general homeless population.

## THE CAUSES OF HOMELESSNESS

Homelessness is often the result of complex interactions between structural and personal factors. They are not exclusively related to housing, and there is no single event that results in homelessness. Events associated with a number of unresolved issues accumulate and this can often result in or lead to homelessness (Centre for the Analysis of Social Exclusion, 2002). Structural factors

**Table 9.1** Key data taken from the older and general homeless population

**Data from the older homeless population – those who are aged 50 years and over**
- 1 in 4 (24%) homeless people are aged over 50 years
- 36% of the people surveyed are parents and over half of them have no contact with their children
- 74% have no next of kin
- As well as their homelessness problem 43% have four or more other problems
- Over 50% have problems associated with alcohol
- 50% have physical problems
- Nearly half of them have mental health problems

**Data gathered from the general homeless population**
- 1 in four have children and 44% of these have no contact with their children
- 50% have no next of kin
- 42% have four or more problems as well as being homeless

*Source*: Adapted from St Mungo's, 2004.

**Table 9.2** Results from data taken from the older and general homeless population in relation to specific issues

| Older homeless population | General homeless population |
|---|---|
| 56% have problems with alcohol and 10% with drugs | 37% have problems with alcohol and 36% with drugs |
| 48% have mental health problems | 40% have mental health problems |
| 47% have problems related to their physical health | 23% have problems related to their physical health |
| 4% have learning disability | 3% have learning disability |
| **Both groups have problems associated with:**<br>• Educational needs<br>• Behaviour (e.g. challenging behaviour, social exclusion)<br>• Relationships (e.g. domestic violence, relationship breakdown)<br>• Employment/unemployment | |

*Source*: Adapted from St Mungo's, 2004.

can be related to the state of the economy, legislation, social trends and the state of the national housing system (Diaz, 2005).

Inclination towards homelessness has been shown to be related to having had or experienced an institutional background, for example having been in care, the armed forces or prison (approximately one third of prisoners lose their housing on imprisonment according to ODPM, 2005a), having experienced family breakdown, sexual and/or physical abuse in childhood or adolescence, or a previous experience of family homelessness. Family conflict is the most common starting point for homelessness (Centre for the Analysis of Social Exclusion, 2002). Factors associated with drug and alcohol misuse, difficulties at school, poor educational attainment, poor physical and mental health and involvement in criminal acts from an early age also play a key role in a person's vulnerability to becoming homeless (Diaz, 2005).

Anderson (2001) points out that low income, unemployment and poverty are universal factors. The unemployed person is unable to pay the mortgage or rent. A result of having a low income can also be an inability to rehouse. Having no fixed address makes finding employment difficult, if not impossible, resulting in further financial hardship – this cycle becomes difficult to break.

## THE IMPACT OF HOMELESSNESS

Disempowerment, isolation and poverty are consequences of homelessness. Those who find themselves homeless may find that they are cut off from social support – formal and informal – as well as access to education and health.

Poor housing and homelessness were recognised as significant causes of ill health in the government report *Saving Lives* (Department of Health, 1999a). Data has already demonstrated that those who are homeless also suffer with

**Table 9.3** Health-related factors associated with being homeless

- Nearly one in 50 homeless people suffers from TB.
- Homeless people are over 40 times more likely not to be registered with a GP than the general public.
- 55% of the homeless have had no contact with a GP in the previous year.
- People in hostels and bed and breakfasts are twice as likely, compared to the general population, to have chronic chest and breathing problems; for those who sleep rough this increases to three times more likely.
- Mental health problems are up to eight times more common in the homeless population.
- Wounds and skin complaints, musculo-skeletal problems and digestive problems are also experienced by the homeless.
- The average age of death of people recorded as homeless on coroners' reports varies between 42 and 53 years of age.
- Because of the effects of rough sleeping on physical and mental health the ageing process is often accelerated. This means that even people in their 50s may exhibit health problems normally associated with an older population.

*Source*: Grenier, 1996; Keyes and Kennedy, 1992.

poor physical and mental health (St Mungo's, 2004). Those who sleep on the street experience the most significant effects of poor health, however the health of children and other adults is also affected by homelessness. The health-related factors in Table 9.3 are associated with being homeless.

Homeless people can often face major barriers in accessing health services, while their life circumstances can mean that they are among those most in need of treatment and care. Homeless people may often leave issues associated with their health untreated until they reach a crisis point and then they need to rely on treatment and care at accident and emergency departments; or they may seek assistance at other primary health services, for example walk-in centres presenting with multiple and entrenched problems. This combination of events can make health problems more expensive to treat; hospital and accident and emergency waiting lists become longer and can lead to people being less able to support themselves and their families in their accommodation. Local authorities and health services must work together to provide accessible and appropriate services if health inequalities and homelessness are to be tackled (ODPM, 2005a). The Office of the Deputy Prime Minister and the Department of Health have issued guidance for all those involved in delivering health services to homeless and vulnerable people on developing shared positive outcomes (ODPM, 2005a).

## ADDRESSING THE HEALTH NEEDS OF HOMELESS PEOPLE

Traditionally health visitors have been seen as working with families with young children. However, they have a much wider public health role, for example working to empower specific groups of people, such as those who are homeless. Health visitors can lead innovative work with homeless people, aiming to assess health needs, improve access to all services, particularly health services, and promote healthy lifestyles. Health visitors work in partnership with a wide range of health and community professionals to evaluate the health needs of individuals, families and communities and then plan and implement strategies to meet them.

Most health visitors working with the homeless are involved in influencing policy in their local areas. The health visitors' public health approach can enable them to be at the interface between relevant services, such as housing, environmental health and the voluntary sector, being pro-active in raising awareness of the difficulties experienced by homeless people in accessing both mainstream and specialist services (ODPM, 2004).

When discharging homeless patients, hospitals should have in place formal discharge policies, thereby ensuring that homeless people are identified on admission and relevant health and homelessness agencies notified when discharge is imminent (ODPM, 2005a). Good practice can be achieved when there is a clear understanding between hospitals and service providers (e.g. social workers and primary care teams) on how appropriate and timely referral and joint working between agencies can be established.

The vast majority of homeless people in the UK are men (Bunce, 2000). Men in general face a number of problems when attempting to access healthcare services (Peate, 2003). For homeless men this is exacerbated even further. Health provision in its current format needs to be addressed in order to provide appropriate and responsive care for this already marginalised and vulnerable group in society (both male and female).

Stereotyping and prejudice must cease if the marginalisation associated with homelessness is to be reduced. All health-care professionals in all health-care settings must address their own attitudes towards the homeless in society. Service provision, using a creative and innovative approach, needs to reflect the needs of this group of the population.

## PRISONERS

In 1999 the government produced a joint policy (the policy was devised by the Joint Prison Services and NHS Executive Working Group) concerning the development and modernisation of primary care in prisons. The policy set out to place primary care provision for prisoners within the context of the wider NHS primary care agenda (Department of Health, 1999a). It was anticipated that the transfer of responsibility for the health care of prisoners in England and Wales to the NHS would happen by April 2006. There are some prisons working in clusters with local primary care trusts making decisions about how best to deliver services locally. Over time the provision of health care has gradually moved from prison officers to registered nurses.

In 2000 HM Prison Service and the NHS Executive produced (HM Prison Service and the NHS Executive, 2000) its deliberation built on the previous work of the Joint Prison Services and NHS Executive Working Group, which led to the establishment of a formal relationship between the NHS and the Prison Service with the prime aim (in England and Wales) of improving the health of prisoners (Department of Health, 2000a). All three prison services in the UK have made strategic decisions to provide health care that reflects what is provided in the wider community. The main resource for health-care provision within the prison services now relies on the registered nurse (RCN, 2001).

## THE PRISON POPULATION

Data regarding the prison population is provided by the Home Office. In 2003 the average prison population in England and Wales was just over 73 000 – the highest annual figure ever recorded (prison population includes prisoners kept in police cells). This number is over 28 000 more than it was in 1993, so there has been an increase of 64 per cent.

There were 69 600 male prisoners and 4400 female prisoners in November 2003. The number of female prisoners has risen at a faster rate than the number of male prisoners. The result of this is that the proportion of males in the prison population fell from 96 per cent in 1997 to 94 per cent in 2003.

White males made up 83 per cent of the male prison population of British nationals in England and Wales in 2003. Black British nationals accounted for 12 per cent. Figures 9.2 and 9.3 provide information related to the prison population.

In Scotland the average daily prison population was 6524 in 2003, a 16 per cent increase since 1993. The average prison population of Northern Ireland was 1160 in 2003, a 40 per cent fall over the same period.

## THE HEALTH-CARE NEEDS OF PRISONERS

The health of the prison population is not only the concern of those who work in prisons, but of all those who are involved in health care. Each day 10 per cent of the prison population report sick. This is nearly eight times more than the numbers of the general population who visit their GP every day. There may be several reasons for this. It may be the result of more general problems, for example the inability of some vulnerable prisoners to cope with prison life. Two-thirds of inmate consultations involve a nurse or a health-care officer.

The main reasons prisoners seek consultations are associated with self-harm, diabetes, asthma, communicable diseases and drug addiction. Sexually transmitted infections, HIV and AIDS are far more prevalent in the prison population than in the general population. Patients within prisons have higher than average rates of mental illness and the most common, according to the RCN (2001), are:

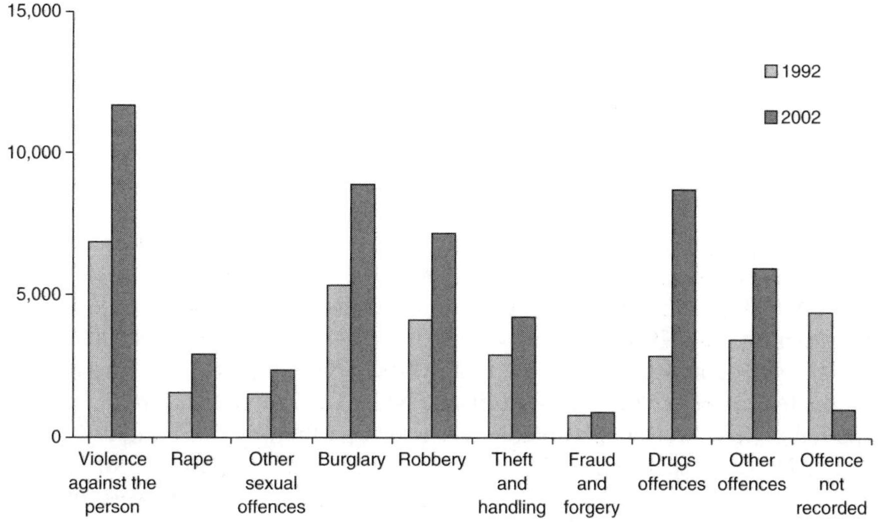


**Figure 9.2** The male prison population under an immediate custodial sentence, 1992–2002
*Source*: Home Office, 2003.

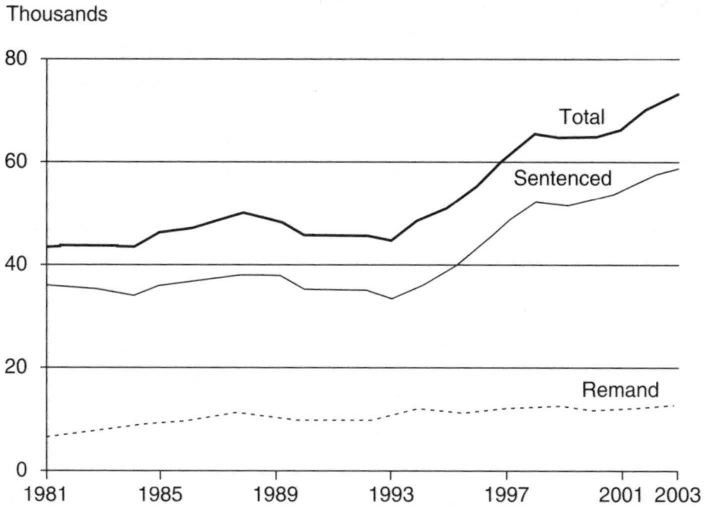


**Figure 9.3** The average prison population in England and Wales
*Source*: Home Office, 2003.

- psychosis
- substance misuse
- depressive illness
- borderline personality disorders

## MENTAL HEALTH ISSUES

Bell (2004) points out that approximately three-quarters of the prison population suffer significant levels of mental illness. The care of patients in prisons with mental health problems does not always meet the same standards experienced by patients in the NHS (Armitage et al., 2002). This is echoed by Reed and Lyne (2000), who demonstrated that the quality of services for prisoners with a mental illness fell far below the standards in the NHS. They report that the prisoners' (patients') lives were unacceptably restricted and therapy was limited.

The National Service Framework for mental health (Department of Health, 1999b) provides a framework for mental health services. This framework, in association with the strategy for modernising mental health services in prisons (Prison Health Task Force and Policy Unit, 2001), provides an outline of the level of primary care services for those patients in prisons who have a mental illness.

## PROVIDING NURSING CARE IN PRISONS

The primary aim of providing patients in prisons with nursing care is to offer quality care. The aims of *The NHS Plan* (Department of Health, 2000b) are:

- To move health care closer to the patient wherever possible.
- To shift the emphasis away from hospital-based treatments.
- More preventive care.
- Better health education, self-awareness and chronic disease management in the community.

These aims apply equally to care provision within prisons as among the general population. The profile and development of primary care in prisons will be further reinforced by the changes in organisational arrangements. A partnership between prison and primary care trusts will provide the resources to deliver improvements to all health services within prisons (Department of Health and HMP, 2002).

Primary care provision in prisons should comprise the following principles of good practice. These principles provide markers for the development of primary care within prisons (Department of Health and HMP, 2002):

- *Fairness* – services should not vary widely in range across the country.
- *Accessibility* – services should be reasonably accessible to people who need them regardless of their age, sex, ethnicity or health status.

- *Responsiveness* – services should reflect users' needs and preferences, and the health and social needs of the local population.
- *Efficiency* – services should be based on research evidence of clinical effectiveness and resources should be used efficiently.

Primary care in the prison service should strive to integrate with the development and planning of services that are occurring within the local primary care trust. Good primary care provision within prisons should eventually become as good as primary care within the community. Just as good primary care in the community integrates with all other health-care activity, so too must primary care in prisons. The interface with other areas of health care is demonstrated in Figure 9.4.

The role of the nurse is complex and multifaceted and this is the same for the nurse working within the prison service. The nurse may need to develop new skills in dealing with the complex needs of the patient in prison. However, he/she must always be cognisant of the fact that the tenets of the professional code (NMC, 2004) apply equally to patients in prisons who, regardless of their conviction, require nursing skills.

Patients in prisons should be entitled to the same level of health care as that provided to society at large. Those who are physically ill, addicted, mentally ill or disabled have the right to be treated, counselled and nursed to the same standards provided to patients within the National Health Service.

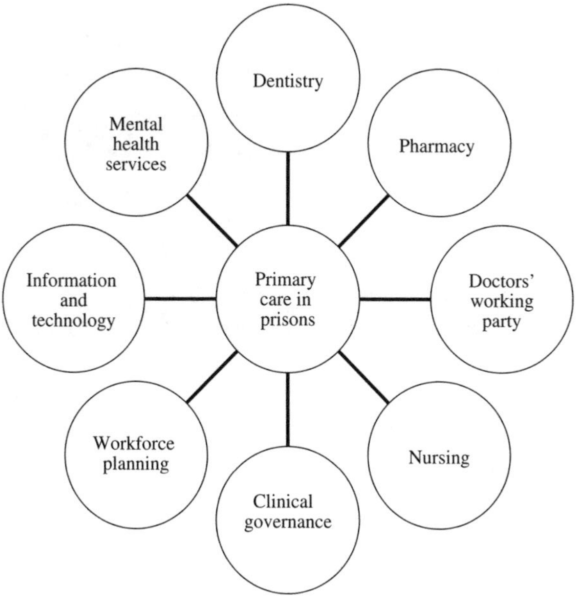


**Figure 9.4** Primary care and the wider health-care agenda
*Source*: Department of Health and HMP, 2002.

## HOMOSEXUALS

The term homosexual means a person who is sexually attracted to persons of the same sex. Homosexuals include males (gays) and females (lesbians). Kinsey et al. (1948) used a homosexual rating scale in an attempt to measure sexual orientation (see Figure 9.5).

It is evident from the early works of Kinsey et al. (1948) that homosexuality for some can be a complex, dynamic and fluid concept. This aspect of the chapter will discuss issues that predominantly concern gay men; however the issues discussed may also apply to lesbians and members of the transsexual and transgendered communities.

Health-care needs of gay men do not differ significantly from those of their heterosexual counterparts. However, there are some issues that are specifically related to gay men that the nurse must understand if he/she is to provide effective, high-quality health care; that is, health care that considers the gay man from a social, physical and emotional perspective (Peate, 2006). The health of men generally is seen as problematic (White and Cash, 2003) and this would also apply to gay men.

The first point of contact with the NHS for many people is with the primary care services; primary care providers are key gatekeepers to health advice and

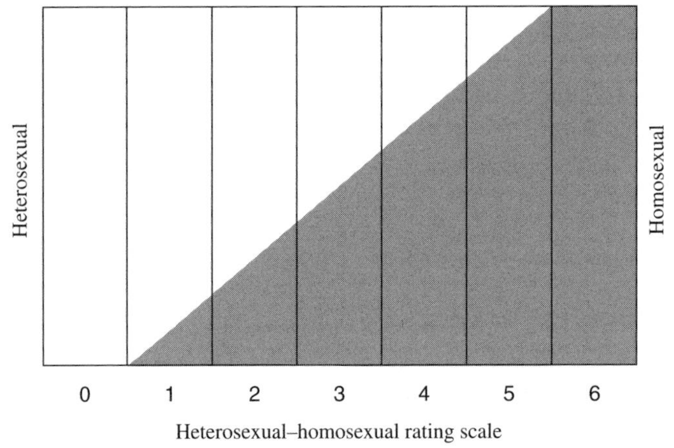


**Figure 9.5** The Kinsey scale
*Source*: Kinsey et al., 1948.
0 – Exclusively heterosexual with no homosexual
1 – Predominantly heterosexual, only incidentally homosexual
2 – Predominantly heterosexual, but more than incidentally homosexual
3 – Equally heterosexual and homosexual
4 – Predominantly homosexual, but more than incidentally heterosexual
5 – Predominantly homosexual, only incidentally heterosexual
6 – Exclusively homosexual

services. Keogh et al. (2004) have considered the treatment gay men receive in primary care – general practice. They have concluded that approximately a third of gay and bisexual men in that study who were registered with a GP said that the staff did not know they had sex with men and that they would be unhappy if the practice did know. These findings appear to capture the challenges some gay men may face in accessing and using health-care provision.

The Royal College of Nursing (RCN, 2003) noted that discrimination, stigma and prejudice exist towards lesbian, gay, bisexual and transgender people. The Nursing and Midwifery Council (NMC, 2004) points out that each registered nurse, midwife or specialist community public health nurse must respect the patient or client as an individual; to do otherwise would be tantamount to professional misconduct.

Within the gay community there are groups within groups, for example gay youths. These youths are a marginalised group, and often there is little opportunity for them to voice their unique needs – they are voiceless (Dootson, 2000). This voicelessness is confounded by the fact that there may be a lack of recognition or acceptance of gay men by some health-care providers. Some health-care providers harbour homophobic attitudes and are unaware of the health-care needs of the vulnerable gay male adolescent (Wells, 1997).

It has been suggested (RCN and UNISON, 2004) that most gay men do not have the necessary confidence to be open and honest about their sexuality, even if this is relevant to their health care. Some gay men fear that the nurse may react in a hostile and judgemental manner and some gay men have experienced hostile and judgemental care. Harbouring such judgemental and hostile attitudes may marginalise and isolate the patient from experiencing good-quality care and support. The result of the inequalities experienced by gay men include:

- Mental health problems, for example higher levels of depression, suicide and self-harm (King and McKeowen, 2003).
- Problems associated with sexual health, for example there is a high prevalence and a high incidence of sexually transmitted infections, such as syphilis.
- There seems to be a higher incidence of eating disorders among gay men (Bloomfield, 2005).
- Substance misuse, for example use and abuse of alcohol (Alcohol Concern, 2004; Dyter and Lockley, 2003).
- The effects of bullying, for example harassment relating to sexual orientation such as homophobic remarks or jokes, offensive comments relating to a person's sexual orientation, threats to disclose a person's sexual orientation to others (King and McKeown, 2003).

## DEFINING TERMS

From the outset the nurse must respect the term that the male chooses to use in order to identify his individual sexuality. Jones (2004) states that gay men are men who have sex with men, however it must be noted that not all men who have sex with men are gay men. This should be borne in mind by the nurse when working with men and when choosing the language that he/she uses.

### ATTITUDES OF HEALTH-CARE PROFESSIONALS

Homophobia in the health service can make health-care provision inaccessible to gay people. Douglas-Scott et al. (2004) state that there is widespread homophobia among health-care professionals, which has a negative impact on a gay man's health outcomes.

Cant (2002) suggests that unwillingness to disclose sexuality to a health-care professional because of a fear of reprisal or disapproval can create difficulties for those gay men who wish to discuss their specific health-care needs in relation to their sexuality. Two barriers to effective communication and possible treatment were noted. First, despite the fact that all the participants in the study had come out – or revealed their sexuality – in many areas of their lives, there was much anxiety and a fear of stigmatisation in relation to doing so and this was specifically related to primary care. The second barrier was associated with the assumption of practitioners (in the primary care practice environments) that all their patients were heterosexual; there was little evidence of any awareness or understanding of gay and bisexual men.

Wells (1997) concludes that attitudes of nurses caring for patients in mental health settings reflect those of the wider society, where 77 per cent were either moderately or severely homophobic. The provision of nursing services, therefore, could be severely compromised by such homophobic attitudes held by nursing staff.

Nurses must address some of the root causes associated with marginalisation, including accessibility to health-care services. Failure to do this may perpetuate the exclusion of gay men. The everyday occurrence of homophobia, be it implicit or explicit, will affect the gay man's self-confidence, self-worth and emotional wellbeing. Homophobia in nursing can be an extreme violation of the individual's human right to receive care that is adequate, professional and compassionate (Christensen, 2005).

## ANTIDISCRIMINATORY PRACTICE

Practice that aims to acknowledge the sources of a person's oppression and works with them to reduce these oppressions is antidiscriminatory practice (Carter and Green, 2002). The nurse must bear in mind the issues that the patient sees as oppressive when planning care.

Thurgood (2004) recommends that patients have access to trained interpreters in the patient's preferred language, that they be given the choice of the gender and ethnicity of the person working with them, and where relevant, as far as is possible, the involvement of religious and cultural organisations, in an attempt to reduce the effects of discriminatory practice.

When providing care using an antidiscriminatory approach, the nurse engages with the patient and considers the social, cultural, legal, political and economic influences associated with care provision. The nurse mobilises and utilises resources to achieve planned outcomes of nursing care that respect the patient and prevent oppression and discrimination.

Oppression and discrimination of patients and communities can have a negative impact on patient outcomes. Discrimination causes suffering to many individuals, weakens the cohesiveness of society, it can and does increase social exclusion, denying our society the talents of individuals who are discriminated against. Identifying the factors underlying discrimination and oppression, addressing the issues such as sexism, racism and ageism, can enhance care (Thompson, 2001).

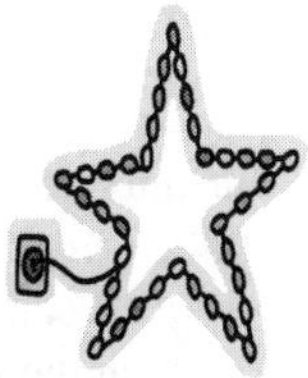

Can you think of any legislation that may focus on the prevention of discrimination or legislation that may enhance antidiscriminatory practice?

Table 9.4 provides a list of some key aspects of legislation that aim to prevent the incidence of discrimination.

In Britain the introduction of antidiscrimination legislation occurred in the 1960s and the two initial Acts were the Race Relations Acts 1965 and 1968. Ten years later other antidiscriminatory legislation was introduced:

- Race Relations Act 1976.
- Equal Pay Act 1970.
- Sex Discrimination Act 1975.

People in Britain suffer from various forms of discrimination (Better Regulation Task Force, 1996) in relation to:

- age
- sexual orientation
- transsexualism
- religion
- nationality
- geographical location

Much progress has been made over the last 20 years to address discrimination and oppression. However, it must be recognised that much discrimination

**Table 9.4** Some key antidiscrimination legislation and international obligations

| Legislation | Year | Areas Covered |
|---|---|---|
| Equal Pay Act | 1970 | The EqPA gives an individual a right to the same contractual pay and benefits as a person of the opposite sex in the same employment, where the man and the woman are doing: • like work; or • work rated as equivalent under an analytical job evaluation study; or • work that is proved to be of equal value. |
| Sex Discrimination Act (as amended) | 1975 | The SDA (which applies to women and men of any age, and children) prohibits sex discrimination against individuals in the areas of employment, education and the provision of goods, facilities and services and in the disposal or management of premises. |
| Race Relations Act (*) | 1976 | The RRA makes it unlawful to treat a person less favourably than another on racial grounds. These cover grounds of race, colour, nationality (including citizenship), and national or ethnic origin. |
| Disability Discrimination Act | 1995 | The DDA prohibits discrimination against disabled people in the areas of employment, the provision of goods, facilities, services, access to premises, education; and provides for regulations to improve public transport to be made. |
| Sex Discrimination (Gender Reassignment) Regulations | 1999 | These regulations are a measure to prevent discrimination against transsexual people on the grounds of sex in pay and treatment in employment and vocational training. They effectively constitute a provision to extend the Sex Discrimination Act, insofar as it refers to employment and vocational training, to include discrimination on gender reassignment grounds. |
| Employment Equality (Sexual Orientation) Regulations | 2003 | These regulations outlaw discrimination (direct discrimination, indirect discrimination, harassment and victimisation) in employment and vocational training on the grounds of sexual orientation. These regulations apply to discrimination on grounds of orientation of persons of the same sex (lesbians and gays), the opposite sex (heterosexuals) and the same and opposite sex (bisexuals). |
| Employment Equality (Religion or Belief) Regulations) | 2003 | These regulations outlaw discrimination (direct discrimination, indirect discrimination, harassment and victimisation) in employment and vocational training on the grounds of religion or belief. The regulations apply to discrimination on grounds of religions, religious belief or similar philosophical belief. |

**Table 9.4** *Continued*

| Legislation | Year | Areas Covered |
|---|---|---|
| Equal Treatment Directive (76/207) amended by Directive (2002/73) | 1976 and 2002 | This provides that there shall be no discrimination on grounds of sex in access to employment including promotion, vocational training and working conditions. |
| Pregnant Workers Directive (92/85) | 1992 | This requires minimum measures to improve the health and safety at work of pregnant women and women who have recently given birth and are breastfeeding, including a right to maternity leave. |
| Employment Rights Act | 1996 | The ERA covers, among other matters, the rights:<br>• not to be unfairly dismissed;<br>• to maternity leave and paid time off for antenatal care;<br>• to parental leave; and<br>• to unpaid time off for dependants. |
| Humans Rights Act | 1998 | The Human Rights Act came fully into force on 2 October 2000 and gives further effect in the UK to rights contained in the European Convention of Human Rights. The Act:<br>• makes it unlawful for a public authority (e.g. government department, local authority or the police) to breach human rights, unless an Act of Parliament meant it could not have acted differently.<br>• means that cases can be dealt with in a UK court.<br>• says that all UK legislation must be given a meaning in relation to Convention rights, if that is possible. |
| Working Time Regulations | 1998 | These contain provisions regulating working time including:<br>• a limit of an average 48 hours work per week (though individual workers can agree to waive this).<br>• daily and weekly rest entitlements and rest breaks.<br>• special provisions relating to night work. |
| Maternity and Parental Leave Regulations (as amended) | 1999 | These contain the detail of the rights to maternity and parental leave contained in the Employment Rights Act 1996 (ERA). They also prescribe the circumstances in which a dismissal will be automatically unfair for the purposes of the ERA, if the dismissal is for a reason related to pregnancy, childbirth, maternity leave, or parental leave. |

**Table 9.4** *Continued*

| Legislation | Year | Areas Covered |
|---|---|---|
| Employment Act | 2002 | A wide-ranging package, covering dispute resolution in the workplace, improvements to employment tribunal procedures, including the introduction of an equal pay questionnaire, provisions to implement the Fixed Term Work Directive, a new right to time off for union learning representatives, work-focused interviews for people receiving working-age benefits and some data protection provisions. The Act also gives parents of children under six, or disabled children under 18, the right to request flexible working, with a requirement on employers to seriously consider their requests. It also gives rights for fathers and adoptive parents to paid time off for the first time, and improved existing maternity rights. |

*Source*: Adapted from Women and Equality Unit, 2003.
*Note*: (*) There are various Race Relations Acts and regulations that have been published and amended.

still exists. Discrimination exists directly and indirectly; it may be intended and unintended. A commitment to diversity and equal opportunities is fundamental to a successful, modern, pluralistic and civilised society. There is a need for nurses to address the continuing discrimination that many patients experience.

It is not easy to provide care on the basis of equality and with respect to social justice. There are issues that compound nondiscriminatory practice (Thompson, 2001) and working in large, complex organisations that are steeped in political activity (implicit or explicit) can often act as an impediment to change.

Nursing functions (occurs) within the context of various sets of power relations:

- legislative powers
- professional powers
- powers the state holds
- powers associated with class, race and gender

The nurse must consider care provision from a personal, cultural and structural perspective. A longer-term strategic approach is needed; however, this approach must include shorter-term aims that can go towards providing important improvements and advances. No one formula has been produced to provide solutions to the issues raised – there are no quick-fix tactics available.

Thompson (2001) suggests that most of the discrimination inherent in social work can be seen as unintentional; this may also be true of discriminatory practice that occurs in nursing. There may be a lack of awareness as opposed to a deliberate attempt to oppress or discriminate. It is important, therefore, that nurses have the opportunity to undertake awareness guidance sessions so that examples and issues associated with discrimination can be raised. This type of approach may enhance individual and collective consciousness and encourage individuals and groups to challenge and confront discriminatory activity.

Failure to address social injustice and inequality is tantamount to professional misconduct. It must be central to the work of the nurse. Good practice must have embedded within it antidiscriminatory policies. This kind of practice challenges values and assumptions and allows the nurse to think about taken-for-granted presumptions. Being open and critical to your own practice is a major step towards providing antidiscriminatory nursing care.

## CONCLUSIONS

There are certain sociocultural determinants or factors that can influence a person's health and wellbeing, either in a positive or negative direction. They have the ability to influence the patient's ability to carry out the activities of living. Sociocultural factors are wide and varied; they can be considered from a social, economic, environmental and political perspective. What they are and the effects they have on individuals are also wide and varied. Being aware of these determinants may help the nurse provide care that is individual and holistic.

Marginalised or oppressed societies are societies that nurses come into contact with on a day-to-day basis. Three particular groups have been discussed in this chapter in order to illustrate the effects of marginalisation on those who are oppressed. Marginalisation and the modes in which it operates are complex. It can result in social isolation and withdrawal, leading to low self-esteem and lack of self-confidence.

In an attempt to reduce the effects of marginalisation on the individual and the wider society, the nurse is encouraged to provide antidiscriminatory care. It has been noted that the provision of care that is antidiscriminatory is complex and always hard to achieve, however the nurse should strive to achieve this. One of the root causes of marginalisation and discrimination is an unwillingness or an inability to adapt services to meet the needs of those groups who are marginalised and oppressed.

The marginalised and oppressed deserve good-quality nursing care. This should not be dependent on whim and fancy, it must be based on a concerted effort by all agencies and health-care professionals involved in the patient's care in an attempt to address the inequalities in health.

The motivation required to provide care to the oppressed should be based on a desire to see people treated fairly and also the knowledge that care provided is successful, both socially and financially, from an individual and community perspective.

## REFERENCES


Alcohol Concern (2004) *Gay and Lesbian People's Fact Sheet*. Alcohol Concern. London.

Anderson, I. (2001) *Pathways through Homelessness: Towards a Dynamic Analysis*. University of Stirling. Scotland.

Armitage, C., Fitzgerald, G. and Cheong, P. (2002) 'Prison in-reach mental health nursing'. *Nursing Standard*. Vol 17, No 26, pp 40–42.

Bell, A. (2004) 'The sad state of mental health in prison'. *British Journal of Health Care Management*. Vol 10, No 6, p 185.

Better Regulation Task Force (1996) *Anti Discriminatory Legislation*. Better Regulation Task Force. London.

Bloomfield, S. (2005) *Eating Disorders and Men: The Facts*. Eating Disorders Association. Norwich.

Bunce, D. (2000) 'Problems faced by homeless men in obtaining health care'. *Nursing Standard*. Vol 14, No 34, pp 43–45.

Burton, M. and Kagan, C. (2004) 'Marginalization' in Nelson, G. and Prilleltensky, I. (eds) *Community Psychology: In Pursuit of Liberation and Well-being*. Palgrave. Basingstoke. Ch 14 pp 291–308.

Cant, B. (2002) 'An exploration of the views of gay and bisexual men in one London borough of both their primary care needs and the practice of primary care practitioners.' *Primary Health Care Research and Development*. Vol 3, No 2, pp 124–130.

Carter, S. and Green, A. (2002) 'Body image and sexuality' in Hogston, R. and Simpson, P.M. (eds) (2nd edn) *Foundations of Nursing Practice: Making the Difference*. Palgrave. Basingstoke. Ch 7 pp 238–261.

Centre for the Analysis of Social Exclusion (2002) *Routes into Homelessness*. Centre for the Analysis of Social Exclusion. London.

Christensen, M. (2005) 'Homophobia in nursing: A concept analysis'. *Nursing Forum*. Vol 40, No 2, pp 60–71.

Department of Health (1999a) *Saving Lives: Our Healthier Nation*. The Stationery Office. London.

Department of Health (1999b) *A National Service Framework for Mental Health*. Department of Health. London.

Department of Health (2000a) *Report of the Working Group on Nursing in Prisons: Summary and Key Recommendations*. Department of Health. London.

Department of Health (2000b) *The NHS Plan: A Plan for Investment, A Plan for Reform*. The Stationery Office. London.

Department of Health and Her Majesty's Prison Service (2002) *Developing and Modernising Primary Care in Prisons*. Department of Health. London.

Diaz, R. (2005) *Housing and Homelessness*. Shelter. London.

Dootson, L.G. (2000) 'Adolescent homosexuality and culturally component nursing.' *Nursing Forum*, Vol 35, No 3, pp 13–21.

Douglas-Scott, S., Pringle, A. and Lumsdaine, C. (2004) *Sexual Exclusion – Homophobia and Inequalities: A Review*. UK Gay Men's Health Network. London.

Dyter, R. and Lockley, P. (2003) *Drug Misuse Amongst People from the Lesbian, Gay and Bisexual Community: A Scoping Study*, Home Office. London.

Grenier, P. (1996) *Still Dying for a Home*. Crisis. London.

Heath, H. and McCormack, B. (2002) 'Nurses, the body and body work' in Heath, H. and White, I. (eds) *The Challenge of Sexuality in Health Care*. Blackwell. Oxford. Ch 5 pp 66–86.

Her Majesty's Prison Service and the NHS Executive (2000) *Nursing in Prisons: Report by the Working Group Considering the Development of Prison Nursing, With Particular Reference to Health Care Officers*. Department of Health. London.

Holland, K. (2003) 'An introduction to the Roper, Logan and Tierney model for nursing, based on activities of living' in Holland, K., Jenkins, J., Solomon, J. and Whittam, S. (eds) *Applying the Roper, Logan and Tierney Model in Practice*. Churchill Livingstone. Edinburgh. Ch 1 pp 3–22.

Home Office (2003) *Prison Statistics: England and Wales*. HMSO. Norwich.

Joint Prison Services and NHS Executive Working Group (1999) *The Future Organisation of Prison Health Care*. Department of Health. London.

Jones, M. (2004) 'Working with gay men' in Society of Sexual Health Advisors. *The Manual for Sexual Advisors*. SSHA. London. Ch 34 pp 326–338.

Keogh, P., Weatherburn, P., Henderson, L., Reid, D., Dodds, C. and Hickson, F. (2004) *Doctoring Gay Men: Exploring the Contribution of General Practice*. Sigma Research. London.

Keyes, S. and Kennedy, M. (1992) *Sick to Death of Homelessness: An Investigation into the Links Between Homelessness, Health and Mortality*. Crisis. London.

King, M. and McKeowen, E. (2003) *Mental Health and Social Wellbeing of Gay Men, Lesbians and Bisexuals in England and Wales*. MIND. London.

Kinsey, A.C., Pomeroy, W.B. and Martin, C.E. (1948) *Sexual Behaviour in the Human Male*. Saunders. Philadelphia.

Lehtinen, V., Riikonen, E. and Lahtinen, E. (1997) *Promotion of Mental Health on the European Agenda*. National Research and Development Centre for Welfare and Health. Helsinki.

Leonard, P. (1984) *Personality and Ideology: Towards a Materialist Understanding of the Individual*. Macmillan. London.

Matthews, H. (2001) *Children and Community Regeneration: Creating Better Neighbourhoods*. Save the Children. London.

Nursing and Midwifery Council (2004) *The NMC Code of Professional Conduct: Standards for Conduct, Performance and Ethics*. NMC. London.

Office of the Deputy Prime Minister (2004) *Homelessness and Health. Information Sheet Number 2: Health Visiting Services*. ODPM. London.

Office of the Deputy Prime Minister (2005a) *Homelessness and Health. Information Sheet Number 4: Hospital Discharge*. ODPM. London.

Office of the Deputy Prime Minister (2005b) *Sustainable Communities: Settled Homes; Changing Lives*. ODPM. London.

Peate, I. (2003) *Men's Sexual Health*. Whurr. London.

Peate, I. (2006) 'Caring for gay men 1: Specific health needs'. *Practice Nurse*. Vol 17, No 2, pp 64–68.

Prison Health Task Force and Policy Unit (2001) *Changing the Outlook: A Strategy for Developing and Modernising Mental Health Services in Prison*. HMP and Department of Health. London.

Reed, J.L. and Lyne, M. (2000) 'Inpatient care of mentally ill people in prison: Results of a year's programme of semi-structured inspections'. *British Medical Journal.* Vol 320, No 7241, pp 1031–1034.

Roper, N., Logan, W.W. and Tierney, A.J. (1996) (4th edn) *The Elements of Nursing: A Model for Nursing Based on the Activities of Living.* Churchill Livingstone. Edinburgh.

Royal College of Nursing (2001) *Caring for Prisoners: Guidance for Nurses.* RCN. London.

Royal College of Nursing (2003) *The Nursing Care of Lesbian and Gay Male Patients or Clients: Guidance for Nursing Staff.* RCN. London.

Royal College of Nursing and UNISON (2004) *Not 'Just' a Friend.* RCN/UNISON. London.

St Mungo's (2004) *St Mungo's Big Survey into the Problems and Lives of Homeless People.* St Mungo's. London.

Sarafino, E.P. (2006) (5th edn) *Health Psychology: Biopsychosocial Interactions.* John Wiley & Sons Ltd. New Jersey.

Smith R. (1999) 'Medicine and the marginalised'. *British Medical Journal.* Vol 319, pp 1589–1590.

Social Exclusion Unit (2004a) *Tackling Social Exclusion: Taking Stock and Looking to the Future.* Social Exclusion Unit. London.

Social Exclusion Unit (2004b) *The Drivers of Social Exclusion: A Review of the Literature for the Social Exclusion Unit in the Breaking the Cycle Series.* Social Exclusion Unit. London.

Taylor, C., Lillis, C. and LeMone, P. (2005) (5th edn) *Fundamentals of Nursing: The Art and Science of Nursing Care.* Lippincott. Philadelphia.

Taylor, J. and Muller, D. (1995) *Nursing Adolescents: Research and Psychological Perspectives.* Blackwell. Oxford.

Thompson, N. (2001) (3rd edn) *Anti-Discriminatory Practice.* Palgrave. Basingstoke.

Thurgood, M. (2004) 'Engaging clients in their care and treatment' in Norman, I. and Ryrie, I. (eds) *The Art and Science of Mental Health Nursing: A Textbook of Principles and Practice.* Open University. Milton Keynes. Ch 22 pp 649–664.

Wells, A. (1997) 'Homophobia and nursing care'. *Nursing Standard.* Vol 12, No 6, pp 41–42.

White, A. and Cash, K. (2003) *The State of Men's Health Across 17 European Countries.* The European Men's Health Forum. Belgium.

Wight, D. and Henderson, M. (2004) 'The diversity of young people's sexual behaviour' in Duffy, M. and Burtney, E. (eds) *Young People and Sexual Health: Social, Political and Individual Contexts.* Palgrave. London.

Women and Equality Unit (2003) *Key Anti-Discrimination Legislation and International Obligations.* Department of Trade and Industry. London.

# 10 Evaluating Nursing Care and Patient Satisfaction

The final aspect of a systematic approach to nursing care is evaluation, which has been discussed briefly in Chapter 6. This chapter focuses on the nurse's ability to evaluate and document the outcomes of nursing interventions.

Emphasis is placed on the need to evaluate and document nursing care regularly in response to nursing interventions. There is a call to encourage the patient to collaborate actively with the evaluation and monitoring of care interventions.

It is vital that the nurse uses a repertoire of skills to respond to a change in the patient's condition after any nursing intervention. This is important as the prioritisation of care may change or need to be reconsidered in the light of the response made. The use of critical thinking is encouraged, as this will enable the nurse to solve unique and complex problems that may arise during the evaluation stage. The chapter will also encourage the nurse to become a skilled reflective practitioner. Knowledge and insight are provided in order for the nurse to use this repertoire of skills.

## EVALUATION

Evaluating the effectiveness of nursing care is necessary for developing a sound knowledge base to guide practice. There has been an increase in the emphasis on evaluation and evidence-based practice in health care (Swage, 2004; Donaldson, 2004). The critical and regular use of evidence as the basis for the provision of nursing care and health-care practice has emerged as a key principle reflecting current health-care provision (see Offredy, Chapter 8 in this text).

Nurses, as members of the health-care team, are concerned with evaluation in a variety of guises. Nurses measure patient outcome achievements and evaluate how they have helped groups of patients achieve specific outcomes. For example, a nurse may carry out the dressing of a wound with expert skill, however if that intervention does not help the patient reach his/her desired outcome, then the activity may not be meaningful. Taylor et al. (2005) suggest that the aim of nursing evaluation is to assess the overall quality of care.

In Chapter 6 it was stated that there are five stages associated with the nursing process:

- assessing
- diagnosing
- planning
- implementing
- evaluating

All five stages need to be seen as ongoing activities as opposed to one-off events. Evaluation is a fluid and dynamic activity. This is also true of the evaluatory stage of the nursing process.

Evaluation affects and is affected by all other aspects of the nursing process (Fitzpatrick, 2002). Freiheit (2004) suggests that without evaluation, the nursing process has not been completed. Hogston (2002) makes the point that in reality, although the evaluation stage is seen as the last stage of the nursing process, it is also the beginning of the process. Evaluation completes the process and examines the outcome(s).

Smith et al. (2004) suggest that evaluation is examination of the outcome of nursing interventions, or the extent to which the anticipated outcomes or goals were achieved. They propose that three questions are asked:

- Was the goal achieved?
- What parts of the goal were not achieved?
- Was client behaviour modified?

They also add that there are five classic elements of evaluation (see Table 10.1).

Evaluation, according to Gega (2004), is often associated with outcomes in relation to certain criteria. She continues and states that this is concerned with whether a problem has improved and goals have been met against certain criteria. The objective of evaluation should be clearly stated in the nursing care plan.

**Table 10.1** The five classic elements of evaluation

| Element | Example |
|---|---|
| Identifying evaluative criteria and standards | What you are looking for when you are evaluating care, for example what was the proposed goal/aim/outcome |
| Collecting data to determine if these criteria and standards have been met | Measuring, observing and communicating |
| Interpreting and summarising the findings | Making clinical judgements |
| Documenting your judgement | Being accountable for your actions |
| Terminating, continuing or modifying the plan | Reassessment |

*Source*: Adapted from Smith et al., 2004.

Depending on the response of the patient (and the nurse should be guided by the patient's responses) to the interventions, the patient and nurse may:

- Discontinue the care plan as each goal has been achieved.
- Alter and amend the plan of care in the light of the evaluation, consider factors that may have prevented the patient from achieving the desired outcomes. Check to see if the care plan is specific and clear, and whether the goals are realistic and achievable.
- Reconsider time frames if more time is needed for the goals to be achieved.

The skills associated with the evaluation stage of the nursing process will be similar to those used in the assessment stage (Freiheit, 2004):

- communicate
- measure
- observe

Alabaster (2003) states that this lends meaning to the previous stages. Examples of achieving the goals set can be decided, for example if a patient has moved along the dependence–independence continuum, demonstrating an ability to become more independent as a result of the nursing interventions (see Figure 10.1).

Situational variables will play an important part in determining if goals have been met as a result of nursing interventions or other variables at play, for example the patient's emotional state, medical interventions or the interventions of other health-care professionals such as therapists. There are a number of factors that can influence the achievement or nonachievement of a goal that has been set.

While evaluating the care the patient has received, Alabaster (2003) makes the important point that the evaluation stage also allows the nurse to evaluate him/herself. She states that all nurses cannot be all things to all people. They may need to develop their own strategies for coping with issues that may arise and give the nurse cause for concern, such as the considerable physical and emotional stressors placed on the nurse in a therapeutic nursing relationship. Evaluation does not only involve a nurse, it does and should involve the patient and, if appropriate, the patient's family and other members of the health-care team (Slevin, 2003). Overlooking the patient's response to care interventions should be avoided. No area of care provision should be exempt from this, where of course this is achievable. Involving the patient and the family will empower them and allow them to voice their opinions about actual or potential problems concerning their health.

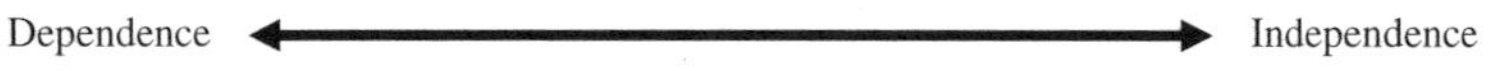


**Figure 10.1** The dependence–independence continuum

Alfaro-LeFevre (2004) suggests that when evaluation is carried out beforehand the nurse is able to 'check out' the interventions and make any alterations or amendments early. This early intervention could be called a formative approach to evaluation. An evaluation that occurs at the end of the interaction, the final aspect (e.g. discharge of the patient), might be deemed summative evaluation.

While it has been stated that evaluation is an ongoing process, there may be a policy where you work that requires you to evaluate, for example, at the beginning and end of each shift or every 24 hours. In some long-term facilities, for example residential care homes, the interval between evaluations may be extended. You must remember, however, that you should evaluate the care of the patient whenever his/her condition dictates, and in some instances that may be more often than the policy in your place of work suggests.

Recall from Chapter 6 that the components of a measurable goal should comprise the following, using the mnemonic **STAMP**:

**S**pecific – the goal must be specific with details and avoid being vague.
**T**ime element – time limits should be applied. The time limits will depend on the goal set, e.g. whether it is a long-term goal or a short-term goal. The target date or time for achievement should be specified when possible.
**A**chievable – the goal must be realistic for the patient and the situation he/she finds him/herself in.
**M**easurable – the proposed intervention should be measurable.
**P**atient centred – 'The patient will. . . .'

Critical questioning is needed during the evaluation phase. This would include the following approach: 'How well did the patient accomplish the goal(s) set?' as well as: 'What could he/she/we have done differently?' and: 'Is this aspect of the care plan now complete and is the problem no longer a concern for the patient?'

An objective approach is required if care is to be modified in any way, as opposed to an emotional or subjective approach.

## TECHNIQUES

In order to evaluate care to the best of your ability you must be an effective communicator, as already discussed. You have to be able to communicate verbally and nonverbally as well as possessing practised skills of observation. Being in possession of these skills will allow you to work with the patient in order to gain as much important information as you can concerning the nursing interventions that have been carried out to resolve the patient's problems. Therefore the nurse must use therapeutic communication to encourage the patient to disclose data that is necessary to evaluate care.

Freiheit (2004) alerts the nurse to be sensitive to changes in relation to the patient's physiological condition, emotional status and behaviour. Changes in respect to these issues can often be subtle, therefore the nurse must be alert and use his/her communication skills to the best of his/her ability to elicit any changes. The judicial use of all five senses – hearing, smelling, feeling, seeing and touching – will be needed when ascertaining clues about the patient's state of health. The nurse should be aware of his/her nonverbal and verbal communication skills. Being conscious of these issues sets a scene that will encourage the patient and his/her family to share comments, be these positive and/or negative (Freiheit, 2004).

Both subjective and objective approaches are used when assessing the patient's health status. A description of the patient's feelings and objective data related to measurable facts are required. The nurse must avoid becoming defensive regarding the feedback the patient gives him/her about care. Employing such a manner may prevent the patient voicing his/her true feelings and being open. This kind of approach can place patients in a position where they feel they have to say what they think the nurse wants to hear, or refuse to participate in evaluatory activities.

## SUBJECTIVE AND OBJECTIVE METHODS

Being able to separate information that the patient or his/her family offers you into subjective and objective categories is difficult. It is important, however, to do this as this helps with critical thinking, as each category complements and clarifies the other.

For example, a patient says to you: 'I feel like my heart is pounding, it feels like it is racing.' The data the patient is providing you with is subjective data.

When you take the patient's pulse you find it is tachycardic at 160 beats per minute. This data is objective, measurable data.

In the scenario above the two categories, subjective and objective, do indeed complement each other. The data you have observed and measured – a pulse rate of 160 beats per minute – confirms what the patient is feeling, 'pounding, racing'.

There are situations, however, where what the patient tells you and what you observe or measure differ.

For example, the patient tells you in response to your question about how they are feeling: 'I feel fine' (subjective data).

You observe that the patient has a respiratory rate of 30 breaths per minute, is cold and clammy and is cyanotic (objective data).

In this scenario the subjective data given to you and the objective data observed are at odds with each other; what you are being told is not the same as what you are observing. In this situation you will have to do more investigating to determine why there may be inconsistencies in order to obtain a full picture of all of the issues that might be occurring.

**Table 10.2** Some examples of subjective data

| |
|---|
| I feel sick and anxious |
| I have a headache |
| I have a gripping vice-like pain across my chest |
| I feel everyone is talking about me |
| My tracheotomy tube is burning like fire |
| I wish my mum were here |
| I can't manage any more |

**Table 10.3** Some examples of objective data

| |
|---|
| Glasgow coma scale score 6 |
| Heart rate 82 beats per minute |
| Vomited 120 ml of vomitus |
| Has a blood pressure of 130/65 mm/hg |
| Mucous membranes cyanotic |
| The patient has an Hb of 8.3 g/dl |
| Passed 200 ml of diarrhoea |

### SUBJECTIVE DATA

Subjective data can be anything the patient or the patient's family says or communicates to you, for example their main complaint. See Table 10.2 for some examples of subjective data.

### OBJECTIVE DATA

Objective data is factual. This data is data that you can clearly observe or measure, for example vital signs, laboratory test results. Table 10.3 outlines some examples of objective data.

There are some patient groups who may have difficulty expressing their responses to nursing interventions and their treatment, for example the paediatric patient. When this is the case, Potts and Mandelo (2002) point out that you may only be able to gather objective data to help you determine if the outcomes or goals have been achieved.

## CRITICAL THINKING AND EVALUATION

Critical thinking can be defined in many ways (Lipe and Beasley, 2004). Fundamentally, it involves asking questions; it is thinking with a purpose.

A more detailed definition is provided by the Foundation for Critical Thinking (2005):

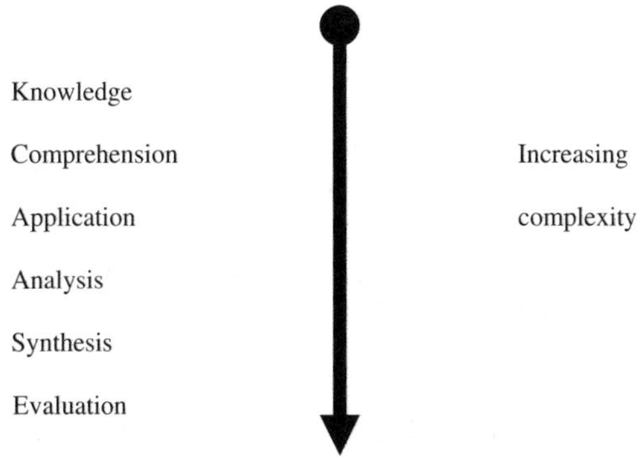


**Figure 10.2** Bloom's taxonomy
*Source*: Bloom, 1956.

> *Critical thinking is that mode of thinking – about any subject, content, or problem – in which the thinker improves the quality of his or her thinking by skillfully taking charge of the structures inherent in thinking and imposing intellectual standards upon them.*

Sometimes the terms critical thinking, problem solving and decision making are used synonymously. While there are similarities, they are different and should be treated differently. There is further discussion of this later in the chapter.

Critical thinking requires the use of higher thinking abilities. One particular model (and one of the earliest models of critical thinking) is that of Bloom (1956); see Figure 10.2.

There have been, and will continue to be, changes occurring within health care and the organisation of health care:

- Technology continues to advance and with it comes an attempt to prolong an individual's life span.
- There is greater demand by the patient and patient organisations for quality care.
- Lengths of stay in hospitals have been reduced.
- Cost containment is a reality and health expenditure continues to rise.
- Disease processes and management are becoming more complex.
- We have an ageing population.

These ongoing and complex changes need to be acknowledged by nurses if they are to address the health-care needs of the nation in an effective manner. To maintain personal accountability in this ever-changing environment, the nurse must become engaged in higher-level thinking, accompanied with an increasing ability to apply sound reasoning to problems that emerge.

When evaluating care it has to be remembered that this does not occur in a vacuum, it occurs among and within the changes cited above. Oermann et al. (2000) expect that the nurse does or will have to provide skilled multidimensional nursing care, often in an unfamiliar setting. Examples could be within the domain of nurse prescribing and the growing field of telenursing. The result of this will be that the nurse needs to develop his/her skills in order to practise as a safe and effective practitioner in these unfamiliar environments. A nurse must be prepared to take on and assimilate new information in a constantly changing clinical environment.

Very often the nurse is confronted with enormous amounts of information on a daily basis that has to be absorbed and managed in an attempt to identify problems and provide solutions to the problems. Decisions need to be made and choices taken as to what approach is to be adopted, bearing in mind that there may not be a single, correct response to dilemmas that arise. These 'new', ever-changing health-care situations will require nurses who apply critical thinking approaches to care planning and, in particular, the evaluation of care that has been delivered (Fowler, 1998).

Colucciello (1997) suggests that in order to deal with day-to-day, simple and complex situations faced by nurses, they must make use of critical thinking to examine these issues and challenges. Using critical thinking can help to determine if the information obtained during the assessment phase was appropriate and also articulated in a meaningful manner.

Developing and honing critical thinking requires effort and commitment. Ulsenheimer et al. (1997) are of the opinion that anyone can master the ability to become a critical thinker. As a novice nurse you will need help to develop your skills in relation to critical thinking. Benner (1984) speaks about becoming an expert nurse. She details the nurse's journey from novice to expert nurse and has identified five stages of development (see also Dreyfus and Dreyfus, 1980 and Table 10.4).

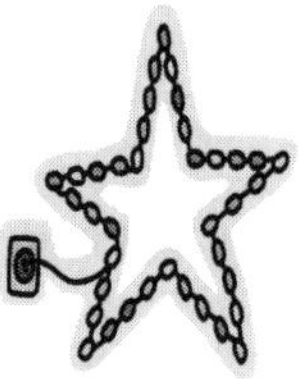

Think about you and your practice. Where would you place yourself on the scale in Table 10.5?

Evaluating nursing care using a critical thinking approach allows the nurse to have a broader outlook, consider creative solutions and ultimately bring about improvements. In contrast, having discovered discrepancies in care as a result of evaluation and failing to act on these inconsistencies and irregularities can result in inequitable, poor-quality and even dangerous nursing care (Tanner, 2000).

**Table 10.4** From novice to expert nurse

| Level | Characteristic |
|---|---|
| Expert | This nurse need no longer rely on an analytical principle, rule, guideline or maxim to connect her/his understanding of the situation to an appropriate action. The expert nurse has an enormous background of experience, and has the ability to zero in on the accurate region of the problem without wasteful consideration of a large range of unfruitful, alternative diagnoses and solutions. This nurse operates from a deep understanding of the total situation. The expert is no longer aware of features and rules; his/her performance becomes fluid, flexible and highly proficient. However, the expert will still use analytical tools when appropriate. Analytical tools are required for those times when the expert gets a wrong grasp of the situation and then finds that events and behaviours are not occurring as expected. |
| Proficient | At this level the nurse perceives situations in total as opposed to fragmented parts or aspects – can now see the 'bigger picture'. Performance is guided by principles and tenets. This nurse understands situations as a whole because he/she perceives their meaning in terms of long-term goals. The proficient nurse learns from experience, e.g. what typical events to expect in any given situation and how plans might need to be modified in response to these events. The proficient nurse can now recognise when the expected normal picture does not materialise. This holistic approach improves the nurse's decision making; it becomes less laboured as the nurse now has a perspective on which of the many existing attributes and aspects in the present situation are the important ones – he/she has experienced it many times before. The proficient nurse uses maxims as guides that the competent or novice performer would perceive as unintelligible nuances of the situation; they can mean one thing at one time and then another thing later. |
| Competent | The nurse who has been deemed competent has been experiencing nursing practice in various forms for approximately two or three years. Competence comes about when the nurse begins to see his/her actions in terms of long-range goals or plans of which he/she is consciously aware. The competent nurse when working with complex problems applies considerable conscious, abstract and analytical thinking. They have become efficient and organised, beginning to trust their own judgement. The competent nurse does not as yet possess the speed and flexibility of the proficient nurse but he/she is able to cope with and manage the many eventualities associated with clinical nursing. The competent nurse lacks the experience to recognise a situation in terms of an overall picture or the most salient and most important points. |
| Advanced beginner | The performance of the advanced beginner is marginally acceptable; he/she has experienced real situations enough to note, or to have pointed out to them by a teacher/mentor, the recurring meaningful situational components of the experiences. The advanced beginner tends to formulate and use principles to guide their actions. This nurse relies very much on the use of protocols to guide him/her. The principles are based on experience. |

**Table 10.4** *Continued*

| Level | Characteristic |
|---|---|
| Novice | Novice nurses (beginners) have had no experience of the situations in which they are expected to perform. They are taught rules that will help them perform. The rules are applied universally as they are not context dependent. The novice's behaviour (in situations where they have no experience) is limited and inflexible. The novice nurse may ask: 'Tell me what I need to do and I'll do it.' He/she is rule dependent. He/she matches actual cases with textbook descriptions. |

*Source*: Adapted from Benner, 1984; Dracup and Bryan-Brown, 2004.

**Table 10.5** From novice to expert nurse – your own level

| Level | Your assessment (tick) |
|---|---|
| Novice | |
| Advanced beginner | |
| Competent | |
| Proficient | |
| Expert | |

## PROBLEM SOLVING, DECISION MAKING AND CRITICAL THINKING

Problem solving, just like the nursing process, is a systematic approach that aims to result in the formation of solutions (Hogston, 2002). Taylor et al. (2005) suggest that there are seven approaches to problem solving (see Figure 10.3).

While the nurse works throughout the day with the patient, in the hospital or in the patient's own home, he/she is confronted with several problems that arise concerning the health of the patient. When the problems have been identified by the nurse he/she then consciously applies a problem-solving approach to the issues.

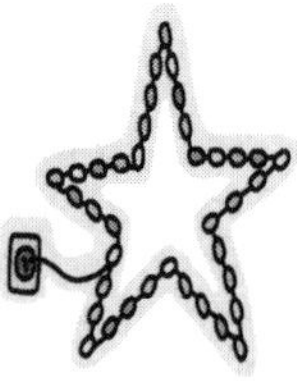

Think about a problem you may have experienced in your own life. How did you:

- Know the problem existed.
- Define the problem.

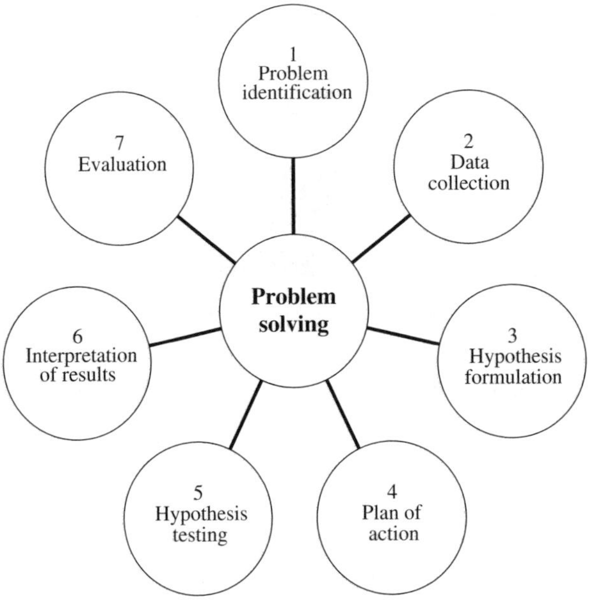


**Figure 10.3** The seven-step problem-solving approach
*Source*: Taylor et al., 2005.

- Decide on possible solution(s) to solve the problem.
- Eventually choose a solution from the various options available.
- Know you had resolved the problem – how did you evaluate it?

Think about the above points and then compare them to the seven-step problem-solving approach in Figure 10.3. While the steps in Figure 10.3 are often used in strict scientific settings, they are also used by nurses when working with patients in the form of the nursing process. The problem-solving approach is a process, a series of stages that have to be experienced in order to achieve an outcome or goal.

While problem solving involves processes, decision making asks that choices be made from the options that are available. Not all decisions are the result of a problem: priority setting is a feature of decision making (Lipe and Beasley, 2004). Critical thinking is an integral aspect of the decision making process. Having been presented with alternative option(s) the nurse then evaluates these options, arrives at a conclusion and makes a selection (Ellis and Hartley, 2000). Clinical decision making is discussed in more detail in Chapter 11.

Those involved in critical thinking have to deal with data and be able to separate the data into two categories – the irrelevant and the pertinent. Clusters of data are then formed and analysed, patterns appear and solutions to problems may emerge (Lipe and Beasley, 2004; Alfaro-LeFevre, 2004).

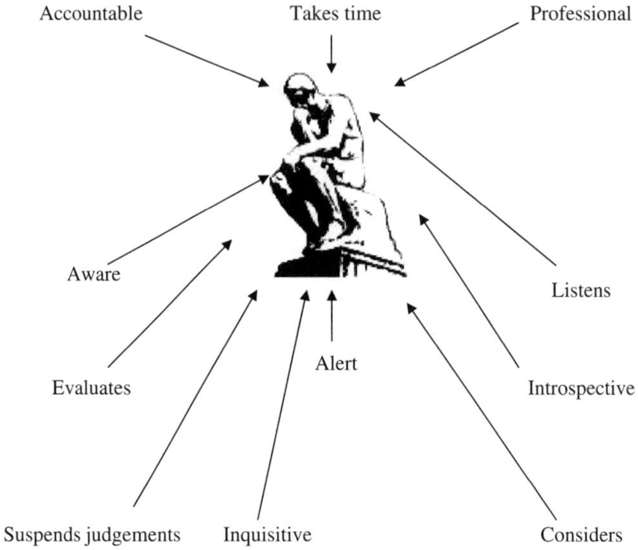


**Figure 10.4** The skills associated with critical thinking

Evaluation of care will mean that the nurse has to critically analyse each of the goals set, or the outcome decided on, as well as all other aspects of the nursing care plan, including the data collection stage and also the care that has been implemented (Seaback, 2001). The nurse needs to use the mechanisms associated with critical thinking to analyse and make judgements. Evaluation of care will only be as good as the plan of care and the goals set. According to Smith et al. (2004) the plan of care provides the basis for evaluation. Each of the classic elements described in Table 10.1 requires the nurse to apply critical thinking when determining if the patient has/will achieve the goals set.

## CHARACTERISTICS OF THE CRITICAL THINKER

The critical thinker has many characteristics. They are neither gullible nor dogmatic. The most distinctive features of the critical thinker's attitude are open mindedness and scepticism (Carroll, 2005). Table 10.6 outlines some characteristics associated with a critical thinker.

Those who are unable to think critically often approach problems in the following ways:

- muddled
- disorganised
- producing complicated or vague solutions
- ready to give up when they face the first difficulty
- approaching the problem in an over-simplified manner

**Table 10.6** Critical thinking skills with examples

| Skill | Example |
|---|---|
| Interpretation | Understands and expresses meaning or significance of a variety of experiences, situations, data, events, judgements, conventions, beliefs, rules, procedures or criteria |
| Analysis | Identifies the potential and actual inferential relationships among statements, questions, concepts, descriptions or other forms of representation intended to express belief, judgement, experiences, reasons, information or opinion |
| Evaluation | Assesses the credibility of statements, outcomes of care or other representations that are accounts or descriptions of a person's perception, experience, situation, judgement, belief or opinion |
| Explanation | States the results of one's reasoning; is able to justify that reasoning and can provide a reasoning in the form of cogent arguments for action taken or omissions |
| Self-regulation | Self-consciously monitors his/her cognitive activities, the elements used in those activities, and the results determined particularly by applying skills in analysis and evaluation to his/her own inferential judgements with a view towards questions, confirming, validation or correcting reasoning or results |
| Inference | Ability to draw reasonable conclusions; to form conjectures and hypotheses; to consider relevant information and to extract the consequences flowing from data, statements, principles, evidence, judgements, beliefs, opinions, concepts, descriptions, questions or other forms of representation |

*Source*: Adapted from Ulsenheimer et al., 1997; Alfaro-LeFevre, 2004; Carroll, 2005.

To become an effective critical thinker, Doenges et al. (2002) suggest the nurse requires the following:

- cognition
- psychomotor skills
- affective skills
- a comprehensive knowledge base
- insight and knowledge related to the nursing process
- the ability to anlayse data

Figure 10.4 encapsulates the skills associated with critical thinking.

Nurses use critical thinking on a daily basis when assessing, diagnosing, planning, implementing and evaluating care. The skills associated with critical thinking can be developed by the novice nurse and used in order to identify best practice and also practice that needs further consideration.

## REFLECTIVE PRACTICE

Reflection is a process within which the nurse can think about and achieve a better knowledge of his/her practice. There are various ways and models to use to help the nurse reflect on practice and the method chosen will depend on each individual's preference. Models such as Kolb (1984); Gibbs (1988); Atkins and Murphy (1994); and Johns (2000) are available to help guide the nurse and structure the reflective process. These models prompt the user to ask questions and relive events, in order to confront, resolve and understand experiences gained through clinical practice (Savage, 2003).

This aspect of the chapter provides guidelines only, in an attempt to provide an overview of how to reflect. Some examples of reflective models and tools that are available to guide this process are provided, in such a way that reflective activity can support the development of the personal and professional portfolio (see Chapter 6). Reflective practice has the ability to underpin good professional nursing practice, as reflection is an opportunity to review progress to date and help the nurse identify areas of practice that he/she may need to develop further, as well as those areas of practice that may have already been successfully developed (Driscoll and Teh, 2001). In certain circumstances reflection can force the nurse to face strange and uncomfortable facts about his/her practice, him/herself and the place where he/she works (Bulman and Burns, 2000).

During your programme of study to become a registered nurse you may be required to produce a portfolio of practice. Often this portfolio requires you to include a piece of reflection, after or during each clinical placement you have experienced. One of the requirements may be that the reflective account has to be related to situations you have experienced during your clinical work, for example where you feel you have learnt something that is of value to you for your nursing practice and ultimately your future nursing career. Experiences you choose to reflect on may be positive experiences, for example where something has gone well; or even a negative experience that you feel requires you to think back about what has happened. You may be required, in relation to your reflective accounts, to identify what you have learnt from the experience and how this relates to the theoretical component of your programme. Lyons (1999) suggests that structured reflection is often used to assess and evaluate student performance.

## CONCLUSIONS

The final stage of the nursing process – evaluation – can in some respects also be considered as the first stage of the process. Evaluation is interwoven with all other aspects of the nursing process. Without evaluation of care having taken place the process of nursing has not been completed. There are several aims associated with evaluation, for example whether the patient has progressed or not in relation to the goal or outcome originally set.

Evaluation also enables the nurse to make judgements concerning nursing actions implemented. In order to enable the patient to achieve his/her outcomes or goals, the nurse is able to consider the results of nursing actions critically. This chapter has encouraged the nurse to use the skills associated with critical evaluation, since applying these skills can encourage creative and innovative nursing care. The outcome of effective evaluation will provide direction for the care plan and enable the nurse to alter or draw to a close the care that has been planned and provided.

As the patient progresses to a higher level of wellbeing, revision and modifications to the plan of care are necessary. Documenting these changes is needed to ensure that the nursing team are aware of any modified care interventions that may be required. Documentation also provides the evidence supporting your interventions. Chase (1997) states that failure to document the evaluatory aspects of the process is providing less than adequate documentation of professional nursing outcomes.

The skills required to evaluate care are essentially similar to the skills required to assess the patient. The nurse needs the skills of observation, to possess effective communication skills and be able to measure outcomes objectively. The whole process is a mutually ongoing one, working with the patient, the patient's family, other nurses and other health-care professionals.

There is a link and a relationship between patient satisfaction and quality assurance and evaluation. The outcomes of evaluation can inform nurses and nurse managers about how care can be improved and built on. A structure, process and outcome approach can allow important decisions to be made in how care is managed and delivered, which may have an impact on the quality of care delivered.

Reflective practice is central to evaluation. The nurse should endeavour to reflect on all aspects of care provision, the organisation he/she works in, and above all to be able to reflect on him/herself. There are many models of reflection available and the choice of model will depend on the individual's preferences.

Finally, evaluation has the potential to enhance professional accountability. It could be said that evaluation is a way of professionally self-checking your actions. Professional accountability is related to your being able to account for your actions and omissions and being able to explain your nursing actions.

## REFERENCES

Alabaster, E.S. (2003) 'The chronically ill person' in Alexander, M.F., Fawcett, J.N. and Runciman, P.J. (eds) (2nd edn) *Nursing Practice Hospital and Home: The Adult.* Churchill Livingstone. Edinburgh.Ch 32 pp 945–962.

Alfaro-LeFevre, R. (2002) (5th edn) *Applying Nursing Process: Promoting Collaborative Care*. Lippincott. Philadelphia.

Alfaro-LeFevre, R. (2004) (3rd edn) *Critical Thinking in Nursing: A Practical Approach*. Saunders. Philadelphia.

Atkins, S. and Murphy, K. (1994) 'Reflective practice'. *Nursing Standard*. Vol 8, No 39, pp 49–56.

Benner, P. (1094) *From Novice to Expert*. Addison-Wesley. Menlo Park.

Bloom, B. (1956) *Taxonomy of Educational Objectives: The Classification of Educational Goals Handbook One: Cognitive Domains*. McKay. New York.

Bulman, S. and Burns, C. (2000) *Reflective Practice in Nursing: The Growth of the Nurse Practitioner*. Blackwell Science. Oxford.

Carroll, R.T. (2005) (2nd edn) *Becoming a Critical Thinker*. Pearson. New York.

Chase, S.K. (1997) 'Charting critical thinking: Nursing judgments and patient outcomes'. *Dimensions of Critical Care Nursing*. Vol 16, No 2, pp 100–111.

Colucciello, M. (1997) 'Critical thinking skills and dispositions of baccalaureate nursing students – A conceptual model for evaluation'. *Journal of Professional Nursing*. Vol 13, No 4, pp 236–245.

Doenges, M.E., Moorhouse, M.F. and Geissler-Murr, A.C. (2002) (6th edn) *Nursing Care Plans: Guidelines for Patient Care*. Davis. Philadelphia.

Donaldson, L. (2004) 'Clinical governance: A quality concept' in van Zwanenberg, T. and Harrison, J. (eds) (2nd edn) *Clinical Governance in Primary Care*. Radcliffe Medical Press. Oxford. Ch 1 pp 3–16.

Dracup, K. and Bryan-Brown, C.W. (2004) 'From novice to expert to mentor: Shaping the future'. *American Journal of Critical Care*. Vol 13, No 6, pp 448–450.

Dreyfus, S.E. and Dreyfus, H.L. (1980) *A Five-Stage Model of the Mental Activities Involved in Directed Skill Acquisition*. University of California. Berkeley.

Driscoll, J. and Teh, B. (2001) 'The potential of reflective practice to develop individual orthopaedic nurse practitioners and their practice'. *Journal of Orthopaedic Nursing*. Vol 5, pp 95–103.

Ellis, J.R. and Hartley, C.L. (2000) *Managing and Coordinating Nursing Care*. Lippincott. Philadelphia.

Fitzpatrick, J. (2002) 'The nursing shortage revisited: Focus on patient outcomes'. *Applied Nursing Research*. Vol 15, No 3, p 117.

Foundation for Critical Thinking (2005) *Miniature Guide to Critical Thinking Concepts and Tools*. Foundation for Critical Thinking. Dillon Beach.

Fowler, L.P. (1998) 'Improving critical thinking in nursing practice'. *Journal for Nurses in Staff Development*. Vol 14, No 4, pp 183–187.

Freiheit, H. (2004) 'Evaluation' in Daniel, R. (ed.) *Nursing Fundamentals: Caring and Clinical Decision Making*. Thompson. New Jersey. Ch 15 pp 279–290.

Gega, L. (2004) 'Problems. goals and care planning' in Norman, I. and Ryrie, I. (eds) *The Art and Science of Mental Health Nursing: A Textbook of Principles and Practice*. Open University Press. Milton Keynes. Ch 23 pp 665–678.

Gibbs, G. (1988) *Learning by Doing: A Guide to Teaching and Learning Methods*. Further Education Unit, Oxford Polytechnic. Oxford.

Hogston, R. (2002) 'Managing nursing care' in Hogston, R. and Simpson, P.M. (eds) (2nd edn) *Foundations of Nursing Practice: Making the Difference*. Palgrave. Basingstoke. Ch 1 pp 1–25.

Johns, C. (2000) *Becoming a Reflective Practitioner: A Reflective and Holistic Approach to Clinical Nursing Practice Development and Clinical Supervision*. Blackwell Science. Oxford.

Kolb, D.A. (1984) *Experiential Learning: Experience as the Source of Learning and Development*. Prentice Hall. New Jersey.

Lipe, S.K. and Beasley, S. (2004) *Critical Thinking in Nursing: A Cognitive Skills Workbook*. Lippincott. Philadelphia.

Lyons, J. (1999) 'Reflective education for professional practice: Discovering knowledge from experience'. *Nurse Education Today*. Vol 19, pp 29–34.

Oermann, M., Truesdell, S. and Ziolkowski, L. (2000) 'Strategy to assess, develop and evaluate critical thinking'. *Journal of Continuing Education in Nursing*. Vol 31, No 4, pp 155–160.

Potts, N. and Mandelo, B. (2002) *Pediatric Nursing: Caring for Children and Their Families*. Delmar. New York.

Savage, S. (2003) 'Maintaining professional standards' in Hinchliff, S., Norman, S. and Schober, J. (eds) (4th edn) *Nursing Practice and Health Care*. Arnold. London. Ch 3 pp 49–75.

Seaback, W.W. (2001) *Nursing Process Concepts and Application*. Delmar Thompson. Albany.

Slevin, O. (2003) 'Problem solving frameworks: The nursing process approach' in Basford, L. and Slevin, O. (eds) (2nd edn) *Theory and Practice of Nursing: An Integrated Approach to Caring Practice*. Nelson Thornes. Cheltenham. Ch 24 pp 447–469.

Smith, S.F., Duell, D.J. and Martin, B.C. (2004) *Clinical Nursing Skills: Basic to Advanced Skills*. Pearson. New Jersey.

Swage, T. (2004) (2nd edn) *Clinical Governance in Health Care Practice*. Butterworth Heinemann. Edinburgh.

Tanner, C.A. (2000) 'Critical thinking: Beyond nursing process'. *Journal of Nursing Education*. Vol 39, No 8, pp 338–339.

Taylor, C., Lillis, C. and Le Monde, P. (2005) (5th edn) *Fundamentals of Nursing: The Art and Science of Nursing Care*. Lippincott. Philadelphia.

Ulsenheimer, J.H., Bailey, D.W., McCullough, E., Thornton, S. and Warden, E.W. (1997) 'Thinking about thinking'. *Journal of Continuing Education in Nursing*. Vol 28, No 4, pp 150–156.

# 11 Clinical Decision Making

In this chapter the theoretical components associated with decision making are discussed. Decision-making tools and models are described and considered and their relevance to clinical practice is outlined. Much debate is presented about the decision-making process and how important it is for the nurse to understand how decisions are made. Sound clinical judgement is vital if care is to be effective and, above all, safe. Emphasis is placed on the consequences of the outcome of the clinical decision made.

The types of decisions nurses make will be considered in the light of the expanding and developing roles that nurses are undertaking. Various approaches to decision making are discussed. The pros and cons of using the bottom-up or top-down approach are examined. The factors influencing clinical decision making are outlined and described.

The hypothetico-deductive and intuitive approaches to clinical decision making are outlined; both approaches have a place in clinical decision making. There are decision-making tools available that may help (and in some instances hinder) the nurse when faced with complex clinical decisions, and this chapter considers the decision-making tree.

While it is acknowledged that there are several factors that can help the nurse to arrive at a sound decision, there are also some barriers to effective clinical decision making and these are described. Finally, the reader is offered some dos and don'ts in respect of clinical decision making.

## DECISION MAKING

As individuals we make decisions on a daily basis, we are always faced with making decisions, and we approach decision making in various ways – consciously or subconsciously. Pesut and Harman (1999) provide a definition of decision making: it is the consideration and selection of interventions from a repertoire of actions that will result in the achievement of a desired outcome. Another, simpler definition is one provided by Etherington (2003), who suggests that decision making means fitting together the pieces to obtain a full picture in order for the nurse to determine care priorities. Decisions may be made consciously or unconsciously, with or without a framework. We may consider options and then list factors that are important and will enable us to make a choice or a decision, and ultimately opt for what we think is going to be the right decision. There are some decisions that are hurried and others

**Table 11.1** Some factors that may be taken into consideration when making a decision

- What is the decision that needs to be made? Make a definition.
- What do you need to know in order to make the decision? This is the aim.
- What needs to be borne in mind? These are the criteria.
- Work out what the options may be.
- Are there any decision-making tools that need to be used?
- Review the decision.

that need time; we may need to deliberate on the decision being made. Roberto (2005) suggests that the key to good decision making is maintaining a balance between disagreement and agreement. The right decision is more likely to occur if all options have been thoroughly explored and thought through.

The decision that is being made may be either an individual or group decision. The outcome of the decision can be almost instantaneous or it may take a little longer or a lot longer. Table 11.1 demonstrates some of the factors that may be involved when making a decision.

Think about the following decisions you may make on daily basis:

- What clothes to wear.
- What television programme to watch.
- Deciding what to eat.
- Where to go on holiday.

Table 11.2 demonstrates how the factors cited in Table 11.1 may be applied to what television programme you wish to watch.

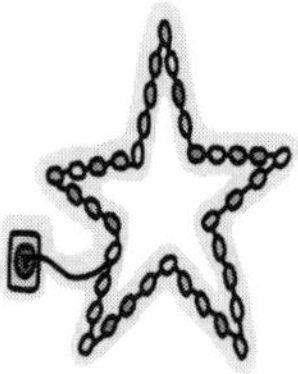

Now think about applying the factors in Table 11.1 to how you would decide to choose a restaurant for a meal with group of fellow students; the occasion is that you have all just successfully finished your second year.

You might have included some of the following:

- Cost.
- Location.
- Type of food, e.g. is there a vegetarian option, do they serve Halal food.

**Table 11.2** Application of the factors to be taken into account when deciding what television programme to watch

| Factor | Consideration |
|---|---|
| What is the decision that needs to be made? | What programme is to be watched |
| What do you need to know in order to make the decision? | Who is involved, just one person or several people? |
| Work out what the options may be. | Programmes may clash, do you have the option to record programmes that clash?<br>How much time do you have available?<br>How many television channels are available?<br>What are the choices of programme available?<br>Your personal preferences and those of others, e.g. comedy or soap operas.<br>Are there some programmes that may be unsuitable, e.g. there may be young children who are also watching.<br>Who pays the television licence, as they may have the final say? |
| Are there any decision-making tools that need to be used? | None. |
| Review the decision | Was the programme enjoyable?<br>Would you view something different next time?<br>Is there anything in the decision-making process you would do differently? |

- Previous experience of the alternatives available.
- Recommendations from others.
- Whether you will all be able to make it on the same night and at the same time.
- Whether the restaurant has a table available for you.
- Whether the restaurant has the capacity to seat you all.

The factors that you need to consider in this example will be very different to the factors associated with sitting alone and choosing a television programme. In the example of the television programme, there is only one party that needs to be satisfied – you. The added issues for consideration associated with the choice of restaurant are that you are not alone, and the decisions you make will affect others. This is exactly the same with any clinical decision you make: in clinical practice the consequences of the decision will have an impact on and for others, be they patients or other fellow health-care workers.

## CLINICAL DECISION MAKING

It has already been stated in this text that the provision of high-quality, effective nursing care is complex. Clinical decision making is also a complex process; often nurses are required to make decisions quickly and with information or data that is incomplete.

Clinical decisions and judgements are made concerning the needs of the patient and also regarding the most appropriate interventions that are required to address these needs and meet goals and outcomes that have been agreed on. Clinical decisions help nurses to describe how they assign meaning to problems being faced by patients, with the ultimate aim of eliminating or alleviating the problem. Muir (2004) states that nurses make important clinical decisions on a daily basis and that these decisions have the potential to have an effect on the patient's health and the actions of the health-care professional.

The role and function of the nurse have expanded over the years and as nursing practice continues to expand nurses will be required to take on and make complex clinical decisions. Nurses are taking over work in clinical areas that had hitherto been deemed the domain of the doctor, and as a result of this they will need help and support when making decisions (Department of Health, 2001b). Clinical decision making should also include patients: they should be encouraged to become equal partners (Department of Health, 2001a). Despite this, little research or empirical study has been undertaken into the decision-making role of the patient (Doherty and Doherty, 2005). The nurse of today, and more importantly the nurse of tomorrow, requires autonomous decision-making skills if he/she is to encourage the patient to participate in the decision-making process.

*Fitness for Practice* (UKCC, 1999) was a report that was commissioned by the now defunct United Kingdom Central Council for Nurses, Midwives and Health Visitors; this report is also known as the Peach Report. The commission was established to evaluate the results of the new education system for nurses, which was known as Project 2000, and also to make recommendations for change. Key recommendations made in the Peach Report are outlined in Table 11.3.

The Peach Report identified that some qualifying students were ill prepared for practice (Garrett, 2004). Boney and Baker (1997) suggested that some registered nurses appear to lack the skills required to make effective decisions. These findings tended to reflect the widely held concerns of some service staff that newly qualified nurses did not possess the practice skills or levels of competence expected of them by future employers.

The recommendations do not only concern helping the student to acquire nursing practice skills, but are also concerned with assisting students to apply their theoretical knowledge within the practice setting, thereby helping them to acquire the decision-making skills needed to function as a registered nurse. Clinical decision making is explicitly mentioned in the report.

**Table 11.3** Some of the recommendations of the Peach Report

| Concerns about | Recommendations |
|---|---|
| Practical skills | The introduction of practical skills and clinical placements early in the Common Foundation Programme, the first part of any degree or diploma, which should be reduced from 18 months to one year.<br>A period of at least three months supervised clinical practice towards the end of the course.<br>Longer student placements with agreed outcomes.<br>A review of the four branches of nursing (adult, mental health, learning disabilities and children's nursing). |
| Relationship between universities and the health service | The involvement of health service providers in the recruitment and selection of students.<br>Purchasers of education, university departments and service providers to resolve together the ownership of, and responsibility for, practice-based education.<br>The development of exchanges and secondments between universities and the hospitals, joint appointments, a more clearly defined role for lecturer-practitioners and more of them. |
| To address concerns about a lack of flexibility | Greater flexibility in entry to nursing programmes to attract more recruits with a wider range of skills and abilities, widening the entry gate at all levels.<br>The Accreditation of Prior (Experiential) Learning to be used so that students with relevant experience, such as health-care assistants, can have programmes tailored to suit their needs.<br>An expansion of graduate preparation for nursing and midwifery.<br>Students who decide to leave at the end of the new Common Foundation Programme should gain academic and practice credits for that year and can re-enter the programme at a later point. |

*Source*: UKCC, 1999.

Clinical decision making and problem solving have long been recognised as key components of effective and safe nursing practice. Elements associated with critical thinking are also required. Critical thinking skills were addressed in Chapter 10. Alfaro-LeFevre (2004) is a major exponent of critical thinking in nursing and Redding (2001) has examined critical thinking in nurse education.

Roberts et al. (1993) assert that while problem-solving ability is acknowledged as critical if the nurse is to maintain effective clinical practice, to that date it retains a marginal place in nurse education curricula; this, it is suggested, is also true today. Nurse educationalists have a role to play in ensuring that students are provided with opportunities to develop and enhance their problem-solving and clinical decision-making skills.

Garrett (2005) suggests that the pre-registration nursing curriculum focuses throughout on the development of problem-solving abilities. However, he adds that clinical decision-making skills are often developed in the workplace under the supervision and guidance of registered nurses and clinical mentors. The development of clinical decision-making skills has become an important focus for nurse education (Garrett, 2005). Thompson (2001) concurs and states that decision making by nurses is now firmly established, not only in practice and policy-making arenas but also within educational disciplines.

Kriariksh and Anthony (2001) have suggested that there is evidence to support an association between the quality of patient care and the nurse's decision-making ability. Harbison (2001) adds that clinical governance and quality decision making go hand in hand. One way to enhance patient care is to increase the nurse's participation in decision making regarding nursing interventions.

Making a clinical decision is different to making a decision generally, as the consequences of the decision being made must be given much thought. It is imperative, therefore, that the nurse makes the correct clinical decision (Robinson, 2002). As with decision making in general, the nurse uses several approaches to arriving at the decision.

Nearly every aspect of health care is associated with uncertainty and this is also true when making health-related decisions. Nurses have to be aware of this and deal with this uncertainty in their decision making. The construction and implementation of evidence-based policies and practice will impinge on how they do this, and also on the quality of decision making.

## WHAT ARE THE CLINICAL DECISIONS THAT NURSES ARE MAKING?

Thompson et al. (2000) have identified the decisions that nurses make. The decisions range from consulting with another health-care professional regarding a patient's dietary needs to deciding to refer another patient with 'niggling' chest pain to a doctor.

Contemporary nursing practice is expanding. There is a wide range of new and extended nursing roles being developed (RCN, 2005a). This means that nurses are taking on more responsibility and with this comes more opportunity to make more clinical decisions.

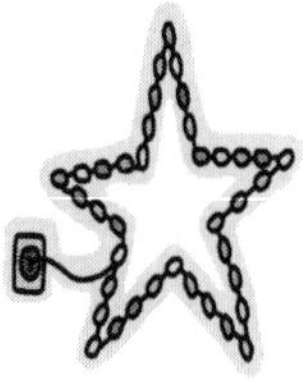

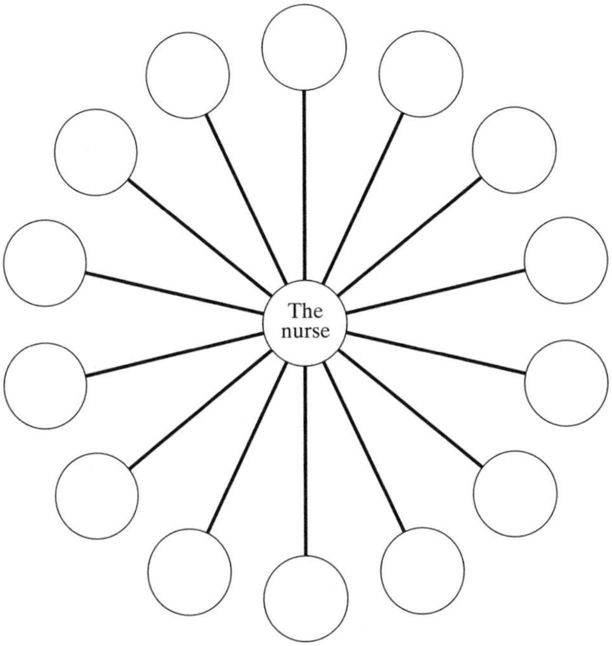


**Figure 11.1** New nursing roles

Take some time to think about the expanding and developing roles that nurses are taking on in order to provide the patient with more effective health care. In Figure 11.1 fill in what you think those roles might be.

In 2004 the RCN (Ball, 2005) conducted a study asking nurses who were employed in advanced specialist roles about their jobs and what their role entails. Analysis of the data determined that the role of the advanced specialist fell into three main categories (see Table 11.4).

To perform as a competent registered nurse high-level clinical decision making is required. This is amplified when taking on extended and developing nursing roles. The RCN (2005b) suggests that one aspect associated with the role of nurse practitioner is the ability to make professionally autonomous decisions for which the nurse is accountable.

It is very difficult, if not impossible, to list the clinical decisions a nurse makes in clinical practice. Attempting to formulate such a list would have to take into account the myriad of activities and the various contexts of care in which the nurse practises. Thompson et al. (2000) observed the decisions being made by a staff nurse working on a medical ward in a three-hour period (see Table 11.5). Compare the list in Table 11.5 with your list of roles you have identified above.

**Table 11.4** Different activities associated with the role of the advanced specialist nurse, falling into three categories

| Category | Example |
|---|---|
| **Case management** | Developing plans with others<br>Coordinating programmes of care<br>Admitting/discharging patients |
| **Diagnosis** | Undertaking physical examination<br>Making diagnoses<br>Screening patients<br>Ordering investigations |
| **Organisational activity** | Leadership<br>Educating staff<br>Initiating research |

*Source*: Ball, 2005.

**Table 11.5** Some of the decisions made by a staff nurse in a three-hour period

- Decision regarding a dressing.
- Decision to discharge a patient after blood results are deemed normal.
- Shared decision making with a bed manager regarding bed management.
- Decision to check that a patient has signed a consent form.
- Decides to move a patient who had chemotherapy into a side room.
- Decision to seek advice from a dietician regarding the dietary needs of a diabetic patient.
- Decision regarding what information she needs to impart to a relative about a patient's condition.
- Decides on the appropriateness of meals for various diabetic patients at lunchtime.
- Decides on the optimal balance of skills during lunch breaks for staff.
- Decides to call a doctor regarding a patient and aspirin.
- Makes a decision to refer a patient to the palliative care clinical nurse specialist.
- Decides to place a patient on a pressure-relieving mattress.
- Decides to give analgesics to a patient who has requested pain relief.
- Decides to refer a patient who has niggling chest pain to a doctor.
- Decides what advice should be given to a colleague regarding the taking of a wound swab.
- Decides to refer a patient who has a sore mouth to the clinical nurse specialist.
- Decides not to discharge a patient who should have been discharged.
- Decides to contact the colonoscopy clinic for advice regarding the dietary requirements for a patient who is to have an endoscopy.

*Source*: Adapted from Thompson et al., 2000.

The decisions this staff nurse made equated to one decision every 10 minutes over the three-hour period (Thompson et al., 2000). It is evident that nurses are continually making decisions; often it might be suggested the nurse may not be aware that he/she is making these decisions.

## TOP-DOWN AND BOTTOM-UP APPROACHES TO DECISION MAKING

The top-down approach to decision making occurs when there is a centralised management structure in place, and in general decisions are made by senior managers. Those who are further down the chain of command are expected to carry out these decisions, despite having little, if any, input into the process. In the decentralised or bottom-up approach the decisions are formulated by those who are most knowledgeable about the concerns being deliberated, those who are closest to where the impact of the decision is felt most.

The decentralised approach encourages and enhances an individual's accountability, placing the responsibility for the decision-making process at the door of those who have made it – the nurses working with the patient. Nurses are accountable both personally and professionally for any decision they make and subsequently act on (Muir, 2004). The NMC (2004) makes this very clear in the code of professional conduct.

Most organisations blend both centralised and decentralised approaches. For example, centralised decisions may be linked with strategic economic issues and manpower planning, and the decentralised approach is often related to clinical issues, such as the introduction of new or innovative procedures (Taylor et al., 2005).

## THE DECISION-MAKING PROCESS

The nurse needs an understanding of the decision-making process in order to make the most appropriate health-care decisions (Thompson and Dowding, 2002). There are many models available that outline the decision-making process or the steps that are involved in the decision-making process. Bryans and McIntosh (1996) suggest that most of the theory associated with decision making comes from the field of psychology. Models and theories will reflect the context in which they are being used.

One mnemonic that may be used to help remember the various stages is **BRAND**:

**B**enefits of the action.
**R**isks in the action.
**A**lternatives to the prospective action.
**N**othing – doing nothing.
**Decision.**

More formal descriptions of the steps involved in the decision-making process have also been devised, for example a four-stage process developed by Elstein et al. (1978); see Table 11.6. A more complex model that has seven stages associated with it has been developed by Carnevali et al. (1984); see Table 11.7.

**Table 11.6** Elstein et al.'s four-stage approach to clinical decision making

| | |
|---|---|
| 1 | Cue acquisition. |
| 2 | Hypothesis generation. |
| 3 | Cue interpretation. |
| 4 | Hypothesis evaluation. |

*Source*: Elstein et al., 1978.

**Table 11.7** A more complex seven-stage approach to clinical decision making

| | |
|---|---|
| 1 | Exposure to pre-encounter data. |
| 2 | Entry to the data search field and shaping the direction of data gathering. |
| 3 | Coalescing of cues into clusters and chunks. |
| 4 | Activating possible diagnostic explanations (hypothesis). |
| 5 | Hypothesis and data-directed search of the data field. |
| 6 | Testing diagnostic hypothesis for goodness of fit. |
| 7 | Diagnosis. |

*Source*: Carnevali et al., 1984.

**Table 11.8** Carroll and Johnson's alternative seven-stage model

| | |
|---|---|
| 1 | Recognition. |
| 2 | Formulation. |
| 3 | Alternative generation. |
| 4 | Information search. |
| 5 | Judgement or choice. |
| 6 | Action. |
| 7 | Feedback. |

*Source*: Carroll and Johnson, 1990.

Carroll and Johnson (1990), in relation to their model, state that not all stages of the model must be followed through in their sequential order. The stages of the model may repeat and backtrack in a complex manner. The seven stages of this model can be seen in Table 11.8.

Tschikota (1993) considers the elements of decision making, and in her study she identifies six elements:

- cue
- hypothesis
- knowledge base
- nursing intervention
- search
- assumption

Tschikota (1993) describes and defines each element and provides an example (see Table 11.9).

**Table 11.9** Elements of the decision-making process

| Element | Definition | Example |
|---|---|---|
| Cue | A piece of information or data | Patients provide nurses with pieces of information all of the time. It may be something they say or do, signs and symptoms, or it could be information gained from the patient when undertaking a nursing history. Other pieces of information might be the information or data provided by the patient's vital signs, e.g. his/her respiratory rate or temperature. Other data may include laboratory values, for example blood results or the results of an investigatory procedure such as renal function tests.<br>This element of the decision-making process involves the gathering of preliminary information. It can occur prior to meeting the patient, e.g. the gathering of the patient's name, age and address from records or when meeting the patient. This stage is also known as the cue acquisition stage. |
| Hypothesis | A proposed possibility or a projected likelihood. Often the word 'might' is used at this stage, for example what might it be that concerns the patient? Other words used are 'probably', 'if', 'could be', 'maybe' or 'perhaps'. The hypothesis made is tentative: 'What might be the patient's problems?' | The number of hypotheses generated is generally between four and six.<br>'Probably croup.'<br>'Could be a chest infection.'<br>'May be paranoid schizophrenia.'<br>'If we increase the rate of oxygen it might change the oxygen saturation.' |
| Knowledge base | The information gained is used to support any statements made by the subject. The information – correct or incorrect – is used as a rationale for proposed action. | 'Because the patient has tachycardia and pyrexia he/she probably has an infection.'<br>'Because the patient is hypotensive and tachycardic he/she is probably hypovolaemic.'<br>'Because the patient is hypertensive and bradycardic he/she may have raised intracranial pressure.' |
| Nursing intervention | Any proposed nursing activity. | 'Place the patient flat.'<br>'Elevate the limbs.' |

**Table 11.9** Elements of the decision-making process

| Element | Definition | Example |
|---|---|---|
| Search | A desire to search for additional or supplementary information concerning the situation. | 'I think we need to know what the patient's cardiac enzymes are.' 'Do we know what might have exacerbated this condition – what was the patient doing prior to becoming so breathless?' |
| Assumption | A conclusion, where there is insufficient information or data to make a definitive judgement. This may lead the nurse to search for more supplementary information concerning the situation. | 'I believe the patient has a urinary tract infection as she has dysuria, haematuria, proteinuria, is tachycardic and has a pyrexia.' 'I think the patient is experiencing hallucinations as his behaviour suggests he is talking to an imagined thing, he has told me he feels he is being followed.' |

*Source*: Adapted from Thompson and Dowding, 2002; Thompson, 1998; Tschikota, 1993.

**Table 11.10** The nursing process aligned to the decision-making process

| Stage of the nursing process | Elements in decision making |
|---|---|
| Assessment | Information is collected and **cues** acted on |
| Diagnosing | The nurse makes a tentative diagnosis – **formulates a hypothesis** |
| Planning | **Nursing knowledge** is used to plan care in order to ameliorate or reduce the impact the problem may have for the patient |
| Implementation | The nurse carries out the care planned using **nursing interventions.** While carrying out care the nurse is constantly **searching** for other cues to either confirm or refute the tentative diagnosis that has been made in the earlier stage |
| Evaluation | The nurse makes **assumptions** during this stage where there is insufficient information or data evaluating his/her judgement. This may lead the nurse to search for more evidence or information concerning the situation. |

## THE NURSING PROCESS AND CLINICAL DECISION MAKING

The nursing process, as already outlined, is a framework that represents ways in which nurses work. Nurses use the nursing process to help them solve problems and to make decisions. Recall that the nursing process is only a representation of what nurses actually do in practice; the same is true of the clinical decision-making process. The five phases of the nursing process can align closely to the elements of decision making; see Table 11.10.

## RATIONAL AND INTUITIVE DECISION MAKING

There are many models/frameworks that have been devised to attempt to describe decision-making processes (Muir, 2004). Two key competing or opposing conceptual frameworks are:

- the analytical framework (hypothetico-deductive)
- the intuitive framework

Decision making using an analytical, rational approach is sometimes also referred to as the hypothetico-deductive approach. This approach assumes that actions are a result of rational and logical thought, for example information processing (Thompson et al., 2000). Tanner (1987) (see Table 11.11) suggests that the hypothetico-deductive approach is based on certain presuppositions.

When using the hypothetico-deductive approach the individual relies on guiding principles, rules and guidelines (Fonteyn and Ritter, 2000). Taylor (2000) suggests that nurses use this approach when they gather data from the patient. Carnevali et al.'s (1984) complex seven-stage approach to clinical decision making (see Table 11.7) is an example of a model that employs the hypothetico-deductive approach. Carroll and Johnson's (1990) alternative seven-stage model is a more flexible model that allows the nurse to approach decision making in a nonlinear fashion (Muir, 2004). This approach relies on the capacity of memory, both long and short term. The person making the decision relies on their memory to recall information that has been stored there in an attempt to problem solve.

The competing framework is the intuitive framework. Carper (1978) suggests that intuition is often seen as an alternative explanation for the ways in which the nurse makes a decision. Various definitions of intuition are available, just as there are various definitions and terms for the hypothetico-deductive approach (Thompson and Dowding, 2002). Benner (1984) defines intuition as understanding that is based on experience; this is acknowledged by other health-care professionals as clinical judgement. Benner and Tanner

**Table 11.11** Assumptions associated with clinical decision making when using a hypothetico-deductive approach

- Action is the outcome of rational and logical thought.
- The strategies employed in clinical decision making are generalisable to all situations.
- A clinical situation can be broken down into its essential elements.
- It is possible to explain and formalise the knowledge used in clinical decision making.
- Explaining the thinking processes of and knowledge used in clinical decision making will enhance the quality of the decision.

*Source*: Adapted from Tanner, 1987.

(1987) suggest that it is intuition that distinguishes the expert nurse from the novice nurse and they define intuition as understanding without rationale. There are other ways of describing intuition:

- gut reaction/feeling
- sixth sense
- a hunch
- an inner prompting

The expert nurse does not need to rely on analytical principles to connect their understanding of the situation to appropriate actions. Intuition, therefore, can be said to be linked to the nurse's experience and Taylor et al. (2005) suggest it allows the nurse to be creative.

Buckingham and Adams (2000) consider heuristics as an alternative to intuition. Heuristics, according to Thompson and Dowding (2002), is defined as 'rules of thumb'. Individuals develop particular strategies to process large amounts of information efficiently. Often they need to use shortcuts to manage and process these large amounts of information, determining the relevant and irrelevant. According to Cioffi (2001), the shortcuts used are based on previous experiences and recall of past usual patterns or presentations.

Buckingham and Adams (2000) suggest that intuition is predominantly associated with pattern recognition and experience and often occurs at the unconscious level, whereas the use of an analytical approach may occur at a more conscious level. It is difficult to account for decisions that have been made using an intuitive approach, and when used alone there is a danger of increased risk. Intuition can become trial and error. The safest approach, according to Taylor et al. (2005), is the logical approach, but this stifles 'thinking outside of the box' ideas. Alfaro-LeFevre (2004) promotes the bringing together of the hypothetico-deductive and intuitive approaches.

The differences between the two competitive frameworks is summarised in Hamm's cognitive continuum (see Figure 11.2). This diagrammatic representation depicts and acknowledges the differences between the two frameworks.

## DECISION-MAKING TOOLS

Sometimes when a nurse makes a decision the outcome is certain. At other times, however, when the nurse makes the decision he/she may not have all of the information available to ensure a good outcome (Kelly-Heidenthal, 2004). This certainty versus uncertainty can be improved if the nurse uses a decision-making tool to enhance the potential outcome of a given situation.

Decision-making tools can only help and guide the nurse when faced with complex options and potential outcomes. Decision trees (sometimes referred to as decision analytic models) provide different options, including chance events and potential outcomes. They also include probabilities and likelihoods

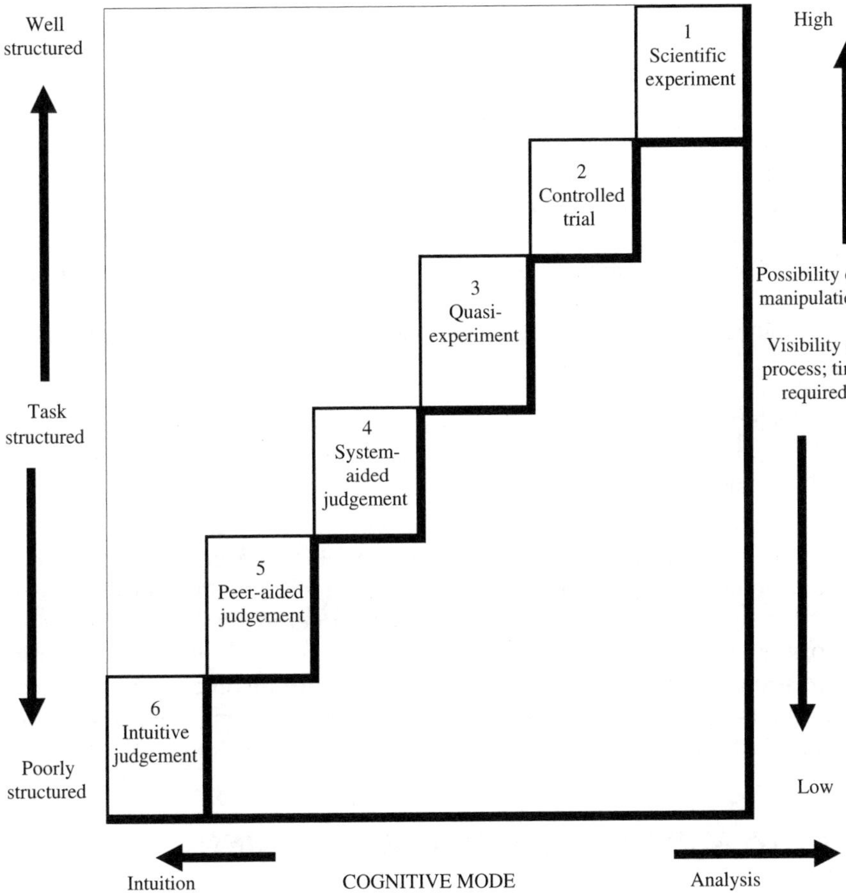


**Figure 11.2** Hamm's cognitive continuum
*Source*: Hamm, 1988. Reproduced with permission of Cambridge University Press.

of a chance event occurring; this is often expressed as a numerical value (Dowding and Thompson, 2002; RCN, 2004).

There are several advantages to using a decision-making tool such as a decision tree. In complex situations this approach makes explicit the important issues that need to be given consideration; sometimes these considerations are often implicit and may otherwise go unnoticed or ignored. However, the content of the decision tree will only be as good as the assumptions that the creator has chosen to include in it. The probability values may not always be based on objective measurement, instead subjective values may be included. The probability of an event occurring (or not), therefore, may be under- or even over-estimated. Acknowledging the strengths and weaknesses of decision-making trees can help the nurse to decide if he/she needs to use one.

## BARRIERS TO EFFECTIVE CLINICAL DECISION MAKING

Despite the fact that nurses are involved in making decisions at various levels in various contexts, there are barriers to decision making in practice. If nurses are to continue to enhance patient care, and it has been demonstrated that one way in which this can occur is through making effective decisions, then it is necessary for the nurse to understand what the barriers to effective clinical decision making may be. There are many factors that have the potential to influence the decision-making process. It is also true that there are many other factors that are barriers to effective clinical decision making.

The following could be considered barriers to effective clinical decision making:

- inadequate skills
- emotional difficulties
- lack of opportunity
- dependence on others

As your nursing skills develop and grow, and as you become more competent and confident, the factors listed above may diminish and you will become proficient at making effective decisions. Hoffman et al. (2004) point out that one of the key barriers to clinical decision making is lack of participation in the decision-making process. You will become more involved in this process as your nursing career progresses. As a student you must make clear any anxieties or fears you might have about making clinical decisions.

## THE DOS AND DON'TS OF DECISION MAKING

Becoming a proficient clinical decision maker comes with experience and learning. Learning takes place once you have been exposed to various scenarios related to patient care. Table 11.12 provides some dos and don'ts associated with decision making.

## CONCLUSIONS

This chapter has provided a brief introduction to the complex theories associated with clinical decision making. Nurses in various situations make a range of decisions. These decisions can be made consciously or subconsciously, using various forms and types of knowledge, often under difficult circumstances.

Clinical decision making is an essential component of the role of the professional nurse. Nurses who make clinical decisions must also be prepared to accept responsibility and be prepared to be held accountable for the consequences of those decisions, or the failure to make a decision. In order to do

**Table 11.12** Some dos and don'ts of decision making

| Dos | Don'ts |
|---|---|
| Try to gather good pertinent information prior to making a decision. | Make snap decisions. |
| Use all relevant information to the best of your ability, 'think outside the box'. | Make decisions for the sake of making them; avoid wasting your time making decisions that do not have to be made. |
| Take time to consider the pros and cons of the issue being dealt with. | Feel that there is a right or wrong decision, decisions are choices among alternatives. |
| Try not to allow decisions to be made to build up and accumulate – make decisions as you go along. | Procrastinate about making a decision. |
| Delay or revise a decision as you feel necessary – trust yourself and do not be afraid to do this. | Regret making a decision. |
| Remember that any decision you make will have consequences and ramifications. | Rush, pre-empt and jump to a conclusion. |
| Avoid basing decisions on 'the way things are always done here'. | Make decisions in order to justify any decision you have made earlier. |
| | Be forced or coerced into making a decision. |

this the factors that affect the decision making and decision makers must be understood.

The outcome of effective decision making results in finding solutions, providing safe and effective nursing care and the provision of an individual, holistic approach to care. There has been an established association between patient outcomes and nurses' decision making and as such one way to enhance patient care is to increase and enhance the nurse's ability to make effective decisions.

## REFERENCES

Alfaro-LeFevre, R. (2004) (3rd edn) *Critical Thinking in Nursing: A Practical Approach.* Saunders. Philadelphia.

Ball, J. (2005) *Maxi Nurses: Advanced and Specialist Nursing Roles.* Royal College of Nursing. London.

Benner, P. (1984) *From Novice to Expert: Excellence and Power in Clinical Nursing Practice.* Addison-Wesley. Menlo Park.

Benner, P. and Tanner, C.A. (1987) 'Clinical judgment: How expert nurses use intuition'. *American Journal of Nursing.* Vol 87, No 1, pp 23–31.

Boney, J. and Baker, J.D. (1997) 'Strategies of teaching clinical decision-making'. *Nurse Education Today.* Vol 17, pp 16–21.

Bryans, A. and McIntosh, J. (1996) 'Decision making in community nursing: An analysis of the stages of decision making as they relate to community nursing assessment practice'. *Journal of Advanced Nursing.* Vol 24, pp 24–30.

Buckingham, C. and Adams, A. (2000) 'Classifying clinical decision making: Interpreting nursing intuition, heuristics and medical diagnosis'. *Journal of Advanced Nursing.* Vol 32, No 4, pp 981–989.

Carnevali, D.L., Mitchell, P.H., Woods, N.F. and Tanner, C.A. (1984) *Diagnostic Reasoning in Nursing.* Lippincott. Philadelphia.

Carper, B. (1978) 'Fundamental patterns of knowing in nursing'. *Advances in Nursing Science.* Vol 1, No 1, pp 13–23.

Carroll, J.S. and Johnson, E.J. (1990) *Decision Research: A Field Guide.* Sage. Newbury Park.

Cioffi, J. (2001) 'Heuristics, servants to intuition, in clinical decision making in emergency situations'. *International Journal of Nursing Studies.* Vol 38, No 5, pp 591–599.

Department of Health (2001a) *The Expert Patient.* Department of Health. London.

Department of Health (2001b) *Learning from Bristol: The Report of the Public Inquiry into Children's Heart Surgery at the Bristol Royal Infirmary 1984–1995.* Department of Health. London.

Doherty, C. and Doherty, W. (2005) 'Patients' preferences for involvement in clinical decision making within secondary care and the factors that influence their preferences'. *Journal of Nursing Management.* Vol 13, pp 119–127.

Dowding, D. and Thompson, C. (2002) 'Decision analysis' in Thompson, C. and Dowding, D. (eds) *Clinical Decision Making and Judgement in Nursing.* Churchill Livingstone. Edinburgh. Ch 8 pp 131–145.

Elstein, A.S., Shulman, L.S. and Sprafka, S.A. (1978) *Medical Problem Solving: An Analysis of Clinical Reasoning.* MIT Press. Cambridge.

Etherington, L. (2003) 'Nursing the patient in the accident and emergency department' in Brooker, C. and Nichol, M. (eds) *Nursing Adults: The Practice of Caring.* Mosby. Edinburgh. Ch 30 pp 923–945.

Fonteyn, M. and Ritter, B. (2000) 'Clinical reasoning in nursing' in Higgs, J. and Jones, M. (eds) *Clinical Reasoning in the Health Professions.* Cambridge University Press. Cambridge.

Garrett, B. (2005) 'Student nurses' perceptions of clinical decision-making in the final year of adult nursing studies'. *Nurse Education Practice.* Vol 5, pp 30–39.

Hamm, R.M. (1988) 'Clinical intuition and clinical analysis: Expertise and the cognitive continuum' in Dowie, J. and Elstein, A. (eds) *Professional Judgement: A reader in Clinical Decision Making.* Cambridge University Press. Cambridge. Ch 3 pp 78–105.

Harbison, J. (2001) 'Clinical decision making in nursing: Theoretical perspectives and their relevance to practice'. *Journal of Advanced Nursing.* Vol 35, No 1, pp 126–133.

Hoffman, K., Duffield, C. and Donoghue, J. (2004) 'Barriers to clinical decision-making in nurses in Australia'. *Australian Journal of Advanced Nursing.* Vol 21, No 3, pp 8–13.

Kelly-Heidenthal, P. (2004) *Essentials of Nursing Leadership and Management.* Delmar. New York.

Kriariksh, M. and Anthony, M.K. (2001) 'Benefits and outcomes of staff nurses' participation in decision making'. *Journal of Nursing Administration.* Vol 31, No 1, pp 16–23.

Muir, N. (2004) 'Clinical decision making: Theory and practice'. *Nursing Standard.* Vol 18, No 36, pp 47–52.

Nursing and Midwifery Council (2004) *The NMC Code of Professional Conduct: Standards for Conduct, Performance and Ethics.* NMC. London.

Pesut, D.J. and Harman, J. (1999) *Clinical Reasoning: The Art and Science of Critical and Creative Thinking.* Delmar. New Jersey.

Redding, D.A. (2001) 'The development of critical thinking among students in baccalaureate nursing education'. *Holistic Nursing Practice.* Vol 15, No 4, pp 57–64.

Roberto, M. (2005) *Why Great Leaders Don't Take Yes for an Answer: Managing Conflict and Consensus.* Wharton School Publishers. Pennsylvania.

Roberts, J.D., While, A.E. and Fitzpatrick, J.M. (1993) 'Problem solving in nursing practice: Application, process, skill acquisition and measurement'. *Journal of Advanced Nursing.* Vol 18, pp 886–891.

Robinson, D.L. (2002) (2nd edn) *Clinical Decision Making: A Case Study Approach.* Lippincott. Philadelphia.

Royal College of Nursing (2004) *Clinical Practice Guidelines for the Assessment and Prevention of Falls in Older People.* RCN. London.

Royal College of Nursing (2005a) *Maxi Nurses: Nurses Working in Advanced and Extended Roles Promoting and Developing Patient-Centred Health Care.* RCN. London.

Royal College of Nursing (2005b) *Nurse Practitioners: An RCN Guide to the Nurse Practitioner Role, Competencies and Programme Approval.* RCN. London.

Tanner, C. (1987) 'Theoretical perspectives for research in clinical judgment' in Hannah, K.J., Reimer, M., Mills, W.C. and Letourneau, S. (eds) *Clinical Judgment and Decision Making: The Future with Nursing Diagnosis.* John Wiley & Sons Ltd. New York. Ch 3 pp 21–28.

Taylor, C. (2000) 'Clinical problem-solving in nursing: Insights from the literature'. *Journal of Advanced Nursing.* Vol 33, No 4, pp 842–849.

Taylor, C., Lillis, C. and Le Monde, P. (2005) (5th edn) *Fundamentals of Nursing: The Art and Science of Nursing Care.* Lippincott. Philadelphia.

Thompson, C. (1998) 'A conceptual treadmill: The need for "middle ground" in clinical decision making theory in nursing'. *Journal of Advanced Nursing.* Vol 30, No 5, pp 1222–1229.

Thompson, C. (2001) 'Clinical decision making in nursing: Theoretical perspectives and theory relevance to practice – A response to Jean Harbison'. *Journal of Advanced Nursing.* Vol 35, No 1, pp 134–137.

Thompson, C. and Dowding, D. (2002) 'Decision making and judgment in nursing – An introduction' in Thompson, C. and Dowding, D. (eds) *Clinical Decision Making and Judgement in Nursing.* Churchill Livingstone. Edinburgh. Ch 1 pp 1–20.

Thompson, C., McCaughan, D., Cullen, N., Thompson, D.R. and Mulhall, A. (2000) *Nurses' Use of Research Information in Clinical Decision Making: A Descriptive Analytical Study – Final Report.* NHS Research and Development. London.

Tschikota, S. (1993) 'The clinical decision making process of student nurses'. *Journal of Nursing Education.* Vol 32, No 9, pp 389–398.

United Kingdom Central Council (1999) *Fitness to Practise, Nursing and Midwifery Education. Report of the UKCC's Commission for Nursing and Midwifery Education.* UKCC. London.

# III Care Management

# 12 Quality Care and Risk Management

Quality assurance and risk management strategies are required to provide the public with protection in order to maintain a safe environment. Clinical governance and risk management strategies are key features of this chapter. The chapter provides an understanding of the principles and policies used to maintain a safe environment. The need to recognise and the appropriate way to report situations that are potentially unsafe for patients and others are also discussed.

Clinical governance cannot be achieved in isolation. There are national structures in place that will support local developments and initiatives, for example the National Service Frameworks and the National Institute for Health and Clinical Excellence. The role and function of these supporting structures are described. Clinical audit, a quality improvement process that has become a central aspect of clinical governance and the clinical audit cycle, is outlined.

Risk is an unavoidable aspect of all of our lives and this is also true when considering the provision of health care: mistakes and errors do occur. The purpose and function of risk management and risk management strategies are briefly described. The safe and effective management of drug treatment is chosen as one aspect of clinical governance. Some practical tips are provided in order to minimise the likelihood of mistakes occurring when administering medicines.

This chapter will draw on some of the content of Chapter 8 and describes the nurse's responsibility to apply relevant principles to ensure the safe and effective administration of therapeutic substances.

## KEY MATTERS

There is a need to define some of the terms used when discussing quality and risk management in relation to the provision of health-care services. This aspect of the chapter will concentrate primarily on terms associated with and used within the field of quality assurance; it will also consider the various definitions associated with risk management. Often quality and risk cannot be separated as each has implications for the other – they complement each other. An artificial split will be made in this chapter in order to provide the reader with information.

## CLINICAL GOVERNANCE

Clinical governance is a relatively new term within the NHS. There are other terms used alongside it, for example:

- quality assurance
- clinical audit
- quality enhancement
- clinical effectiveness
- evidence-based practice

Since its inception in 1948 the NHS has been reinvented in many ways. At its inception the NHS was a state-run entity, bureaucratic with highly centralised systems (Better Regulation Taskforce, 2001). The intention was to provide identical structures and functions for all of the organisations that comprised the NHS. The contemporary NHS aims to move to a more decentralised, innovative service with a clear remit to enhance and improve patient care. The new NHS is concerned with ensuring that structures and processes meet local needs, recognising and respecting diversity, while at the same time working with common definitions of good quality and good clinical care (Scrivens, 2005).

The ethos of the NHS that was central to its setting up will prevail nevertheless. In 1948 hospital provision (at that stage the NHS was only concerned with hospital care) was to be made available for every citizen. The service was to be made available at the earliest moment, when the necessary provision was to be made regardless of any financial consideration (Beveridge, 1942). The new NHS then was to be free to all at the point of provision.

The twenty-first-century NHS is to become a service that is responsive to individual and local needs and must therefore decentralise its provision and be devolved. One way of making this move towards devolution is to change the way health services are managed and run. Centralised services fail to provide care that is patient centred, and do not recognise that patients are individuals with local and individual needs. Care needs to be delivered in a meaningful manner to the people who pay for it – the patients and the public.

The introduction of clinical governance was seen as one way of achieving this meaningful approach to health-care provision. In 1997 *The New NHS: Modern and Dependable* (Department of Health, 1997) was produced with a plan to modernise health-care provision within ten years. Clinical governance is an integral part of the ten-year plan to improve the quality of care (Department of Health, 1999a). One key component of this document (a White Paper) was to bring about major improvements in the quality of care delivered to patients from a clinical perspective. For the first time statutory duties were enforced on NHS providers regarding the quality of care they offer (Department of Health, 2000b). A formal responsibility for quality has now been placed on every health organisation in the UK through arrangements for clinical governance at local level.

Clinical governance is central to quality. There are many different interpretations of what clinical governance means. Clinical governance can be defined as (Department of Health, 1998):

> *A framework through which NHS organisations are accountable for continuously improving the quality of their services and safeguarding high standards of care by creating an environment in which excellence in clinical care will flourish.*

The overall aim of clinical governance is to strengthen and build on existing systems of quality assurance across a range of services. Clinical governance has the ability to liberate and enable clinicians to lead the health-care agenda in order for patients to benefit. These opportunities bring with them added responsibility and increased accountability (Heard, 2000).

Kehoe (2005) notes that clinical governance and the drive for clinical governance arose through untoward incidents, mainly medical in origin, such as the problems at Bristol. The Bristol inquiry was undertaken to investigate children's heart surgery at the Bristol Royal Infirmary between 1984 and 1995 and highlighted the importance of clinical governance (Department of Health, 2002). The outcome of these improper incidents such as Bristol led to an increased focus on the competence and performance of health-care professionals.

Clinical governance is a complex activity. The RCN (2003) provides a number of key principles that underpin the implementation of clinical governance:

- Clinical governance must be focused on improving the quality of patient care.
- Clinical governance should apply to all health care wherever it is being delivered.
- Clinical governance demands true partnership between all health professionals, between clinical staff and managers, and between patients and clinical staff.
- Public and patient involvement is an essential requirement for effective clinical governance.
- Nurses have a key role to play in the implementation of clinical governance.
- An improvement-based approach to quality health care creates an enabling culture that celebrates success and learns from mistakes.
- Clinical governance applies to all health-care staff. It needs to be defined and communicated clearly so that all staff understand its relevance to their work.

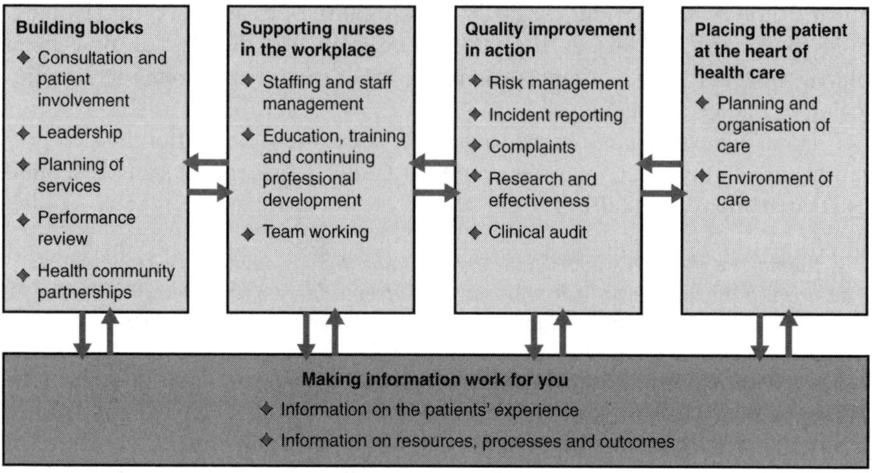


**Figure 12.1** Key themes associated with clinical governance
*Source*: RCN, 2003. Reproduced with the kind permission of the Royal College of Nursing Clinical Governance: An RCN Resource (2005).

- Clinical governance does not replace individual clinical judgement or professional self-regulation; it complements these and provides a framework in which they can operate.

Figure 12.1 provides a diagrammatic representation of the key themes associated with clinical governance.

Clinical governance places the responsibility for the quality of care on both organisations and individuals working within those organisations. Although the emphasis is on joint responsibility, the nurse must not forget that exercising individual accountability is paramount within a multiprofessional clinical environment. Clinical governance extends to all NHS services (Department of Health, 2001) and is everybody's business not just those who excel at it or those who are poor at it.

It is not possible to achieve clinical governance in isolation. Structures need to be in place to support it, as well as ensuring that there are common standards and the common public ethos is ensured. National structures are in place to underpin local clinical governance initiatives.

## NATIONAL SERVICE FRAMEWORKS

The National Service Frameworks (NSFs) set national standards. They are long-term strategies with the aim of improving specific areas of care and have time frames with measurable goals attached to them. They provide strategies that support their implementation and delivery at local level. The NSFs were launched in 1998 and have so far addressed the following specific areas of care:

- mental health (established 1999)
- paediatric intensive care (established 1999)
- coronary heart disease (established 2000)
- cancer (established 2000)
- older people (established 2001)
- diabetes (established 2001)
- renal (established 2004)
- children (established 2004)
- long-term conditions (established 2005)

## NATIONAL INSTITUTE FOR HEALTH AND CLINICAL EXCELLENCE

The National Institute for Clinical Excellence (NICE), as it was originally called, is an independent organisation charged with the responsibility to provide national guidance on the promotion of good health and the prevention and treatment of ill health. In 2005 this organisation merged with the Health Development Agency and is now known as the National Institute for Health and Clinical Excellence (it retains its acronym NICE). Guidance is published on many topics, for example depression in younger people (NICE, 2005a) and pressure ulcer management (NICE, 2005b).

## NHS PERFORMANCE ASSESSMENT FRAMEWORK

This service was created in response to the government's policy to make information about the quality of health-care services available to the public. The framework monitors service delivery against plans for improvement, thus the performance of the NHS (in essence) is assessed (NHS Executive, 1999).

## COMMISSION FOR HEALTH IMPROVEMENT

CHI (Commission for Health Improvement) was key in ensuring that local clinical governance arrangements were reviewed. It was superseded by the Healthcare Commission in 2004, the legal name for which is the Commission for Health Care Audit and Inspection. One of the significant roles of this body is the ability to intervene if shortcomings and problems have been identified (Roberts, 2005). Its role (in England) is to:

- inspect
- inform
- improve

## CLINICAL AUDIT

Clinical audit is a quality improvement process that seeks to improve patient care and outcomes through a systematic review of care against the explicit criteria and the implementation of change. Clinical audit is at the heart of clinical governance; it is a multidisciplinary, multi-agency and multiprofessional working approach (Sasaru et al., 2005).

To provide the best care in a competent manner it is important that the processes and procedures used by the NHS to deliver care are the most appropriate in relation to the service(s) being delivered. Research and development activity and the evidence gathered in order to provide evidence-based practice (see Chapter 8) aim to increase the sum of academic knowledge. They do this by establishing facts that can then be generalised to a given population and will provide the nurse with the information he/she needs to do the job well – in the best, most effective way possible. Clinical audit has the potential to monitor how well the job is being done and to ensure that standards are being maintained (Maughan and Conduit, 1999). According to Sasaru et al. (2005) clinical audit asks: 'How does the care that we provide compare with established standards for practice?' It cannot increase the sum of knowledge, nor can it provide evidence that can be generalised to a population as research does.

Kehoe (2005) suggests that clinical audit is:

- A tool to assist when implementing clinical governance.
- A means of checking that things are being done correctly.
- An activity that involves clinicians (nurses) and users of the service (patients).
- A means of ensuring that the treatments used have been shown by research to be effective.

He also adds that audit is not:

- A means of demonstrating that a type of treatment works.
- An excuse to collect endless data.
- An activity exclusively for the audit department.
- An activity that always works.

### THE AUDIT CYCLE

Audit as a concept is not new and has been used by the NHS for many years, for example nursing audit and medical audit (Burke and Lugon, 1999). Quality assurance has also been used in the past (Morrell and Harvey, 1999), and this was said to be an attempt at deciding what should be, and comparing that with reality, identifying gaps and taking action (Pearson, 1987).

Clinical audit is designed as a cycle of change. Actions are taken following a review of existing practices. Several cycles (models) have been suggested

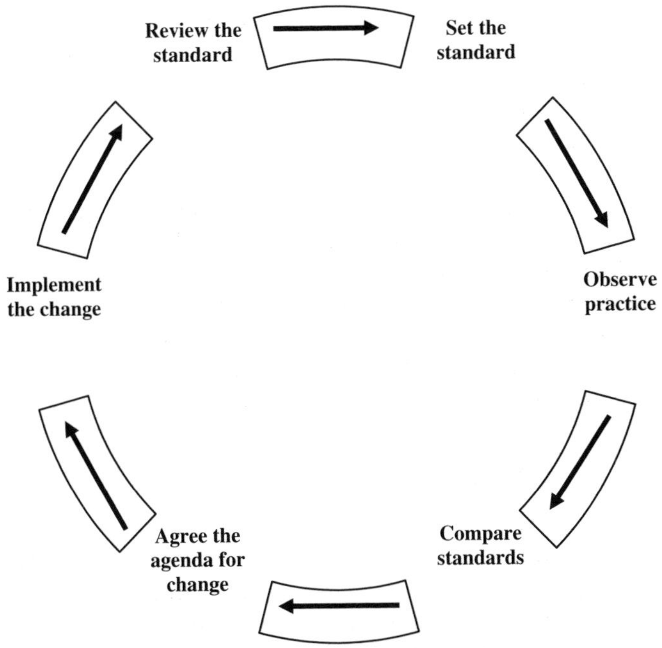


**Figure 12.2** Audit cycle
*Source*: Sasaru et al., 2005.

over the last decade, which can be very simple or very detailed and complex. However, Saunders (2003) points out that the concept of audit is remarkably uncomplicated, but it is also a powerful tool for change. The type of model used will depend on local conditions and requirements. The key to ensuring that audit is successful is to ensure that a systematic approach is used and that planning and preparation are carried out in advance. Kehoe (2005) and Sasaru et al. (2005) provide more details concerning planning and preparation for an audit. Audit is a continuous, cyclical process (see Figure 12.2).

## SET THE STANDARD

Some standards already exist and have been predetermined, for example the standards outlined in the NSFs. The NICE also provides guidance that the nurse can use to formulate standards. Benchmark statements have also been provided (Modernisation Agency, 2003); these statements concern aspects of fundamental care such as oral hygiene, which allow nurses to compare benchmark statements with current practice. Where no standards have been preset or no guidance exists, then standards may need to be formulated locally using a multidisciplinary approach. One approach (and there are several approaches available) to standard setting that has been used before by the nurse is structure (what you need), process (what you do) and outcome (what you expect) (Royal College of Nursing, 1990; Sasaru et al., 2005).

## OBSERVE PRACTICE

Current practice is observed by gathering data associated with, for example, everyday or usual practice, nursing and case-notes data, and patient satisfaction surveys. Data-collection tools are often forms or documents and each clinical area/trust will have its own documentation for doing this. This stage of the process must be given careful consideration as the documentation used must yield the data required. Some trusts employ specific individuals to gather this data and then analyse it.

## COMPARE STANDARDS

When the data has been collected it needs to be analysed. Data collected, according to Sasaru et al. (2005), should say with enough accuracy to what extent the care measured matched the standard set. Both standards – the standard set (e.g. the NSF) and the standards being delivered (care being provided) – are compared and contrasted.

## AGREE THE AGENDA FOR CHANGE

If there is a discrepancy between the standards set (the set criteria) and the care delivered, then an action plan must be formulated to address the shortcomings and improve the service. If care provided is seen as an example of good practice, then similarly a plan must also be agreed to ensure that good practice is maintained and, where appropriate, replicated. The implementation of change is needed at this stage of the process. Management of change must be done with an understanding of the situation.

Action plans or audit reports are needed; they are best formulated using a multidisciplinary approach. The plan must be written, presented and fed back into clinical practice and to others in a way that is clear and realistic. Dissemination in this manner will help to ensure that whatever new practices or changes are required are understood by all of those involved. Time frames are needed as well as measurable criteria to determine success. This is similar to the setting of goals described in Chapter 6.

## IMPLEMENT CHANGE

This stage requires that the changes needed are implemented. Change is central to clinical audit. Staff may need support or supervision to ensure this is carried out effectively and there are many interventions that can be used to facilitate the change process. It may be appropriate to provide a programme of staff development to ensure that the action plans are addressed and implemented.

REVIEW STANDARDS

The cycle is completed when change, as indicated by audit, has been implemented (Saunders, 2003). Sasaru et al. (2005) see this aspect of the cycle as the closing of the loop. Review should be undertaken to ensure that standards are maintained and are still appropriate – this means the cycle may need to be repeated and revisited once the action plan has been implemented.

## QUALITY AND THE INDEPENDENT SECTOR

While there has been an explicit and concerted effort over the years to enhance the quality of care provided by the NHS, the same applies to the independent sector. The Independent Healthcare Association (IHA) requires that all member organisations demonstrate the quality of their services by achieving a recognised quality award. The Health Quality Service (HQS) is an independent charity that sets organisational standards and makes assessments to determine if the standards have been met.

Assessment of services is conducted by a team of experienced health-care professionals. During the assessment documentation is reviewed, staff are interviewed and practices observed. Successful achievement of the standards set allows the independent facility accreditation for three years.

The Commission of Social Care Inspectorate carries out local inspections of all social-care organisations – public, private and voluntary – against national standards and publishes reports. The general aims of inspections are to check compliance with standards and regulations (Healthcare Commission, 2005).

The principles applying to clinical governance in the NHS are applied equally across the independent sector. The creation of the Care Standards Act 2000 demonstrated this (RCN, 2003).

## RISK ASSESSMENT

Most of the care delivered within the NHS is of a high quality. Serious incidents and failures are uncommon when related to the high numbers of patients requiring care provided daily in hospitals and in the community (Department of Health, 2000a). Clinical governance provides NHS organisations with powerful authority to focus on adverse health-care occurrences.

Mistakes and errors do occur and when they occur they can have devastating consequences for patients and their families. Every day over one million people are treated successfully in the NHS (National Patient Safety Agency, 2004). However, it is estimated that in the NHS over 850 000 adverse incidents occur per year (Department of Health, 2000a). The umbrella term 'clinical governance' includes all things that help to maintain high standards of patient care and this includes, therefore, the identification and prevention of risks to the welfare of the patient. Patients expect care that is safe and of such quality as is consonant with good practice based on sound evidence (Department of Health, 2002).

Improving quality includes a range of activities, and some of these have already been discussed, for example providing care that is based on the best available evidence and clinical audit. It also includes the management of risk, the reporting of incidents (actual and near misses) and the management of complaints.

## RISK MANAGEMENT

Risk management is a central feature of clinical governance. It aims to reduce the risk of adverse incidents by recognising risks, assessing risks and putting in place strategies to reduce or contain risks that have been identified (Amos and Snowden, 2005).

As with several important concepts related to health care, there are many ways to define key terms and the definition of risk is not excluded from this. Risk is often associated with probability or chance (Douglas, 1992), but increasingly it is being linked with danger and hazards (Alaszewski, 2003). The Performance and Innovation Unit (2002) maintains the approach that risk is associated with hazard and adds that it is something to be avoided. Another definition offered by the University of Manchester (1996) is that risk is the possibility of beneficial and harmful outcomes and the likelihood of their occurrence in a stated time scale.

The final definition moves from a negative connotation to a more balanced approach, citing both harm and benefit as potential outcomes. Risk according to the Centre for Business Performance (1999) is not only about bad things happening, it is also about good things *not* happening. Risk must be minimised if harmful and unwanted outcomes are to be avoided; however, risk is an essential aspect of health-care provision, encountered on a daily basis. Health care is a risky activity (NHS Executive, 1993).

Risk taking occurs on a daily basis for all of us, in our own everyday lives. We gamble with risk daily, and this is the same for nurses.

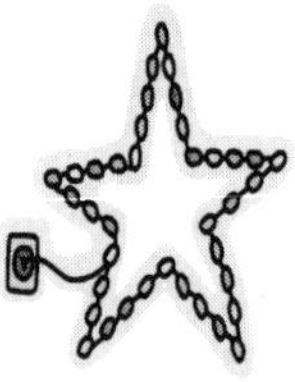

Take some time to think of the risks you take on a daily basis. Think about what they are and how you gambled with the potentially harmful or beneficial results that could be the result of taking those risks.

There may have been several very different things in your list. Did it include any of the following?

- Crossing the road.
- The first time you decided to taste sushi.
- The risks you took when taking up nurse education.
- The risks you took when having unsafe sex.
- The risks you took when having a general anaesthetic.

The fact is that risks are a part of life. We should aim to contain them in our personal lives and also when working with patients. It may be impossible, and even undesirable, to reduce risk taking to zero (Amos and Snowden, 2005). Risks must be managed and tolerated.

Risk management is about reducing the likelihood of patients coming to harm and creating a safe environment for both patients and staff. NHS organisations must ensure that they adhere to and comply with all applicable legislation. Staff must all feel they are able to (and encouraged to) report risks, incidents and near misses. Arrangements must be in place for this to occur and policy and procedures applicable to the reporting of risks, incidents and near misses should be clarified, as detailed in Department of Health (1999b).

Davies (1999) suggests that acceptable risks are those that are not significant enough to be considered unreasonable. Good risk management helps to reduce hazards and builds confidence for innovation and creativity to occur (Scrivens, 2005).

Risk management, according to the National Audit Office (2000), is said to address all of the processes that are involved in the identification, assessment and judgement of risks as well as the monitoring and reviewing of progress. All activities related to risk can be subjected to risk management. The following are risks that may be subjected to risk management:

- Corporate issues.
- Financial matters.
- Clinical activity.
- Nonclinical activity.

Risk management utilises a systematic approach when identifying and assessing reduction of risk to both patients and staff (NHS Executive, 1999; Scrivens, 2005).

Amos and Snowden (2005) suggest that there are three stages associated with a dynamic approach to risk management:

- Risk identification or recognition.
- Risk assessment and analysis.
- Risk management and reduction.

There are several risk-assessment tools available. However, risk-assessment tools are only as good as the nurse who is conducting the assessment (see for example Chapter 6 in this text). In Chapter 6 the Waterlow scale (Waterlow, 1985) was given as an example of a risk-assessment tool. Other tools are also available, for example tools that assess the risk of future violence occurring. This kind of tool was produced in response to an increase in violence associated with patients with a mental illness. Suicide-prediction scales have also been published. Murphy et al. (2005) describe the use of the dynamic risk-assessment and management system for people with a learning disability and offending behaviours. When risk-assessment tools are used they often predict the probable degree of risk to the patient. When this has been established, the nurse then needs to put into place actions to alleviate the risk, or prevent the risk from becoming any greater.

## THE ADMINISTRATION OF MEDICINES

It has been said many times in this chapter that improving the quality of care is at the heart of clinical governance. Safe and effective drug treatment is also a part of clinical governance. A prescribed medicine is the most common treatment provided for patients in the NHS. In primary care in England, GPs issue more than over 600 million prescriptions per year; in hospitals this figure is estimated to be as many as 200 million (Department of Health, 2004).

Most medications are prescribed and administered safely in the UK. However, errors do occur and the effects can be upsetting and the consequences serious for all concerned: the patient, his/her family, the prescriber, the dispenser and the administrator. The errors that do occur can be prevented (Department of Health, 2004). The government aims to reduce the number of serious medication errors by 40 per cent (Department of Health, 2000a). Guidance has been prescribed nationally and locally to help ensure that errors are avoided, for example the law (statute), local Trust drug policies and the NMC's *Guidelines for the Administration of Medicines* (NMC, 2002a; see Appendix 12.1). Medication errors can render the nurse prone to civil liability and in certain instances criminal prosecution.

As a student nurse the standards enshrined in the NMC's code of conduct (2004a) also apply to you. At all times you must work only within the level of your understanding and competence and always under the direct supervision of a registered nurse or midwife (NMC, 2002b). This must also apply during the administration of medicines or while assisting with the drug round. As a student you are responsible for your actions or omissions, but as you are not yet registered with the NMC you cannot be answerable for them: the registered nurse or midwife who is supervising your practice is ultimately accountable for your actions or omissions. You must not forget, however, that you are and may be required to be answerable to your educational institution's policies, procedures and rules. Furthermore, you also remain accountable in law for your actions or omissions.

The NMC (2002b) state that as a student you should not participate in any procedure for which you have not been fully prepared or in which you are not being adequately supervised. Should you ever find yourself in this position, you must make this known to your supervisor as quickly as possible. You must always work within the policies and procedures that apply in the area of care where you are working (NHS or independent sector, health or social care) as well as follow the advice provided by your educational institution. Additional sources of information and references should be accessed and used as required.

Registered nurses are accountable for their actions and omissions when administrating medications and, as such, they take full responsibility for any errors that they may make. There are many reasons for drug errors occurring, for example increasing demands being made on the nurse, overwork and stress (Copping, 2005). Parish (2003) suggests that in some instances drug errors can occur as a result of complacency. Other causes of medication errors are related to distractions and a prescriber's illegible handwriting (Mayo and Duncan, 2004).

Registered nurses are reminded by the NMC (2002a) that they must exercise professional judgement and apply their skills and knowledge to the various situations that may emerge during medicine administration. This advice is irrespective of the environment in which the registered nurse is practising.

## PRESCRIBING, DISPENSING AND ADMINISTRATION OF MEDICINES: AN OVERVIEW

There are many government and other agencies involved in the prescribing, dispensing and administration of medicines. These agencies may be concerned with the licensing and manufacturing of medicines for human use. The pharmacist is an invaluable source of advice if the nurse needs to confirm or validate the content of a prescription, but there are other relevant bodies that may be just as resourceful.

### Prescribing

Who can prescribe medications? There are a several mechanisms available for the prescribing of medicines (Modernisation Agency, 2005). In certain instances after consultation with doctors, pharmacists and other health-care professionals the following registered health-care professionals may, so long as they remain within the confines of the law, prescribe medications using a patient group directive:

- nurses, midwives and health visitors
- paramedics
- optometrists
- chiropodists
- radiographers
- physiotherapists
- pharmacists
- dieticians
- occupational therapists
- prosthetists and orthoptists
- speech and language therapists

Each of the health-care professionals cited above must be deemed competent, appropriately qualified and educated to use a patient group directive.

### Dispensing

Fewer errors occur with the dispensing of medications than with the prescribing of them (Department of Health, 2004). Nurses may dispense drugs in exceptional circumstances, but this must be done in line with hospital policy and with the written instructions of a registered medical practitioner – a doctor. In some areas, dispensing of drugs is seen as the nurse's extended role. If this is the case the nurse must practise this activity under the directions of a doctor (Department of Health, 2004). The public has a right to know that the nurse will carry out this duty with the same reasonable skill expected of a pharmacist.

### Administration

Nurses administer medicines in a variety of settings to a variety of patients: those who are mentally ill or those at the extremes of age, for example neonates and the elderly. Administration can take place in the patient's home, in residential homes and on hospital wards. The administration of medicines is therefore a fundamental and important nursing activity.

Prior to administering medications the nurse must ensure that he/she is familiar with policy and regulations, locally and nationally, that govern medicine administration. Principles surrounding medicine administration can be found in the NMC's *Guidelines for the Administration of Medicines* (NMC, 2002a). Regardless of whether a prescription has been hand written or electronically generated, the nurse must ensure that it contains the details stated in Table 12.1.

Telephone orders are not acceptable for a previously unprescribed drug. However, in exceptional circumstances when the medicine has been previously prescribed and the authorised prescriber is unable to issue a new prescription,

**Table 12.1** Principles advocated by the NMC associated with prescribed medicines

- The prescription is based on informed consent, with the patient's informed consent and awareness of the purpose of the treatment.
- Be clearly written, typed or computer generated and be indelible.
- Clearly identify for who the medication is intended.
- When the dosage of medication is related to the patient's weight this must be recorded on the prescription sheet.
- The substance to be prescribed must be clearly specified and include the generic or brand name of the medication, the form of medication, strength, dose, frequency, start and finish dates and the route of administration.
- Be signed by the authorised prescriber.
- The prescription must not be for a substance to which the patient is known to be allergic.
- Prescribed controlled drugs must state the dosage and the number of dosage units and the total course. If this is a prescription in an outpatient or community setting the prescription must be in the authorised prescriber's own handwriting, signed and dated. There are some exceptions to this handwritten rule.

*Source*: Adapted from NMC, 2002a.

but there is a need to alter the dose, telephone alterations may be acceptable. The preferred method is to use other methods of communicating the change, for example email or fax. The change that has been agreed must be reflected in the writing of a new prescription within 24 hours (NMC, 2002a).

## REDUCING RISKS ASSOCIATED WITH DRUG ADMINISTRATION

In high-risk areas there is a responsibility to minimise the potential for a drug error occurring, for example in paediatric settings such as special care baby units, and in those clinical areas where large quantities of controlled drugs are administrated, for example operating theatres, cardiac care units and intensive therapy units (Department of Health, 2004).

Medication errors (the terms medication and drug error are often used interchangeably) are said to account consistently for between 10 and 20 per cent of all adverse events. Aside from the danger to patients, these errors cost the NHS a considerable amount of money. It is therefore of value to make concerted efforts to reduce the numbers and types of errors caused by maladministration. Research is currently being undertaken to understand more about how medication errors occur and the best way to prevent them (Department of Health, 2004).

O'Shea (1999) has undertaken a literature review associated with factors that contribute to medication errors. One of the aims of the review was to determine what a drug error was – to define it. The findings demonstrate that there is no consistent definition of drug error that can be agreed between health-care professionals. A medication error is defined by the Department of

Health (2004) as any preventable event that may cause or lead to inappropriate medication use or patient harm while the medication is in the control of a health-care professional, patient or consumer. Medication errors can be the result of professional practice, products, procedures, environment or systems – they are preventable (Department of Health, 2004). Errors can occur at all stages associated with the production, prescribing, dispensing and administration of medications, which includes labelling, packaging and the communication the nurse has with the patient regarding his/her medication.

Drug errors can be related to miscalculation of doses, overdosing and underdosing. Often, however, drug errors are not the result of isolated incidents: they may be the product of an accumulation of incidents that are complex and multifaceted (Preston, 2004). There are some areas of practice that are deemed high risk and these have been highlighted previously. Likewise there are some particular drug groups that have also been deemed high risk (Department of Health, 2004):

- anaesthetic agents
- anticoagulants
- chemotherapeutic medications
- any drug delivered via the intravenous route
- methotrexate
- opiates
- potassium chloride

The nurse should also be aware of drugs that have been involved most commonly in 'wrong drug', 'wrong strength' dispensing errors. These drugs can be found in Table 12.2.

The nurse must ensure that he/she understands the reasons why a particular drug is being given and the therapeutic dose that should be prescribed. The nurse must ensure that he/she is up to date regarding pharmacological developments. Calculation errors occur commonly in paediatric settings where

**Table 12.2** Most common 'wrong drug', 'wrong dose' errors that occur

| | |
|---|---|
| Amiloride | Amlodipine |
| Fluoxetine | Paroxetine |
| Hydralazine | Hydroxyzine |
| Carbamazepine | Carbimazole |
| Omeprazole 10 mg | Omeprazole 20 mg |
| Atenolol 100 mg | Atenolol 50 mg |
| Morphine sulphate tablets (MST) 10 mg | Morphine sulphate tablets (MST) 30 mg |
| Paroxetine 20 mg | Paroxetine 30 mg |
| Warfarin 3 mg | Warfarin 5 mg |
| Diazepam 2 mg | Diazepam 5 mg |
| Co-codamol 30/500 | Co-codamol 8/500 |

*Source*: Department of Health, 2004.

doses used can vary widely according to the weight of the child (Department of Health, 2004).

It is essential that when calculating drug doses for any patient, the nurse should make certain that he/she employs meticulous methods to do this. Any confusion or concerns should be raised and clarified with a senior member of staff prior to administration. If you are in doubt about any aspect of the prescription or administration of the medication, then you must carefully exercise your professional judgement; you may decide not to administer the medication.

Good record keeping is also a part of good, safe drug administration. You must ensure that your records are up to date and meet the requirements of your employing authority and that you also adhere to the guidelines and standards produced by the NMC (NMC, 2004b).

Prior to the administration of any drug the nurse must ensure that this is the:

- right drug
- right dose
- right route
- right time
- right patient

## DRUG ERRORS

To err is human and mistakes do happen. Hackel et al. (1996) suggest that the number of drug errors that are acknowledged and reported is not a true reflection of reality; many more, they state, go unreported. The reasons some go unreported may be associated with a fear of reprisal from managers and worry about how colleagues may react. There may also be loss of self-esteem if a nurse reports an error (Pape, 2001; Arndt, 1994).

The nurse who has made a drug error, made known the error and dealt with it promptly should be supported in identifying how the error occurred, and how it may be prevented in the future. A 'no blame' culture should be established in the organisation in order to ensure that learning takes place from the error(s) made.

## SOME EXPRESSIONS AND TERMS USED IN RELATION TO MEDICATIONS

- *Patient specific direction* – a traditional written instruction from a nurse prescriber, dentist or doctor for medicines to be supplied or administered to a named person.
- *Patient group direction* – a written instruction for the supply or administration of a medicine where the patient may not be individually identified before presenting for treatment.

- *Nurse Prescriber's Formulary* – The formulary used by district nurse and health visitor prescribers. This formulary contains medicines and certain types of dressings and appliances relevant to community nursing and health visiting practice. The district nurse and health visitor prescribers must have undertaken a period of education to enable them to prescribe from the formulary.
- *Nurse Prescriber's Extended Formulary* – this formulary is used for independent prescribing by nurses and lists the medical conditions that nurses can prescribe for, and the medicines they can prescribe. All first-level registered nurses may legally train to prescribe from the Nurse Prescriber's Extended Formulary, however they must have had a minimum of three years' post-registration experience. This formulary may be extended in the near future. Before a suitably trained nurse can independently prescribe using the Nurse Prescriber's Extended Formulary, he/she must register his/her prescribing qualification with the NMC.
- *P* – pharmacy-only medicines, medicines sold or supplied at registered pharmacy premises by or under the personal supervision of a pharmacist. The pharmacist must be present before a P medicine can be sold.
- *POM* – prescription-only medicines, medicines sold or supplied at registered pharmacy premises by or under the personal supervision of a pharmacist *but* in accordance with the authorised practitioner's prescription. The pharmacist must be present before a POM medicine can be sold. This kind of medicine requires a prescription to be produced.
- *GSL* – general sales list medicines can be sold from a wider range of premises, for example general shops and supermarkets, but the premises must be lockable and can be closed to exclude the public. All medicines sold must be pre-packed and are sold in smaller quantities. These medicines are deemed safer than P medicines.
- *OTC* – over the counter, a generic term that covers GSL and P medicines.

## REPORTING SITUATIONS THAT ARE POTENTIALLY UNSAFE

As a student of nursing it has already been emphasised that you are neither accountable nor answerable to the NMC. You do, however, have a responsibility to make known any situations that you find or consider unsafe in an attempt to protect the patient and others. These situations do not only concern medication errors but concern any unsafe, or potentially unsafe, practice.

There are local policies and procedures (as well as the policies and procedures your university produces) that must be adhered to if you wish to make a complaint or raise a concern about the quality, and ultimately the safety, of patient care. You should raise the matter immediately with the person supervising you or another appropriate person, for example your trade union or tutors at your university.

Being aware of errors that have occurred and taking steps to rectify them will add to current awareness of the cases of medication errors. This in time will provide examples of good practice.

If you are asked to write a report or statement regarding the incident that concerns you, you must seek advice from a more senior member of staff in the clinical area or from staff at your university. Reports and statements must be factual. It is important to be as accurate as possible, use a chronological approach, write the statement as soon after the event has occurred as possible and always ensure you keep a copy.

## CONCLUSIONS

Every day more than one million patients are treated safely and successfully in the NHS. However, the complexity of contemporary health care brings with it risk, and the consequence sometimes, no matter how hard staff work to prevent incidents arising, is harm to the patient.

When the idea of clinical governance was first introduced it challenged traditional ways of thinking, the culture within the health service and the attitudes held by some of those who worked there. It has become an opportunity for nurses and other health-care professionals to improve care provision for all who use health-care services. Clinical governance, described as a framework that provides NHS organisations with the tools to become accountable for continuously improving the quality of their services and safeguarding the public, is central to the 'new NHS'. Today's NHS is moving towards a more decentralised, innovative service with a clear remit that aims to enhance and improve patient care. Central to the new NHS is that structures and processes meet local needs, recognising and respecting diversity, but at the same time working with common definitions of good quality and good clinical care.

Clinical audit is a quality-improvement process that seeks to improve and enhance patient care and outcomes through a systematic review of care against the explicit criteria and the implementation of change. It is at the heart of clinical governance and is a multidisciplinary, multi-agency and multiprofessional working approach to quality enhancement.

Risk management is a crucial component of clinical governance. Risk management aims to reduce the risk of adverse incidents. Risk taking is evident in most clinical situations and its occurrence is unlikely to be reduced to zero. Risk management is not confined to clinical care only, it also occurs in other areas of the health service, for example in health finance and the wider corporate arena.

Clinical governance is about improving the quality of all the services provided to the patient. Quality in this respect is not just restricted to the clinical aspects of care; it encompasses and includes the quality of life and the overall patient experience (Department of Health, 2000a).

## REFERENCES

Alaszewski, A. (2003) 'Risk, clinical governance and best value: Restoring confidence in health and social care' in Pickering, S. and Thompson, J. (eds) *Clinical Governance and Best Value: Meeting the Modernisation Agenda*. Churchill Livingstone. Edinburgh. Ch 10 pp 171–182.

Amos, T. and Snowden, P. (2005) 'Risk management' in James, A., Worrall, A. and Kendall, T. (eds) *Clinical Governance in Mental Health and Learning Disability Services*. Gaskell. London. Ch 12 pp 174–203.

Arndt, M. (1994) 'Medication errors. Research into practice: How drug mistakes affect self-esteem'. *Nursing Times.* Vol 90, No 15, pp 27–30.

Better Regulation Taskforce (2001) *Annual Report 2000–2001*. Better Regulation Taskforce. London.

Beveridge, W. (1942) *Social Insurance and Allied Services*. His Majesty's Stationery Office. London.

Burke, C. and Lugon, M. (1999) 'Clinical audit and clinical governance' in Lugon, M. and Secker-Walker, J. (eds) *Clinical Governance: Making It Happen*. Royal Society of Medicine. London. Ch 6 pp 61–76.

Centre for Business Performance (1999) *Implementing Turnbull*. The Institute of Charted Accountants. London.

Copping, C. (2005) 'Preventing and reporting drug administration errors'. *Nursing Times.* Vol 101, No 33, pp 32–34.

Davies, M. (1999) 'A simple approach to the management of service risk in a local mental health service'. *Psychiatric Bulletin.* Vol 23, pp 649–651.

Department of Health (1997) *The New NHS: Modern and Dependable*. Department of Health. London.

Department of Health (1998) *A First Class Service Quality in the New NHS*. Department of Health. London.

Department of Health (1999a) *Clinical Governance: Quality in the New NHS*. Department of Health. London.

Department of Health (1999b) *The Public Disclosure Act 1998: Whistleblowing in the NHS, HSC1999/198*. Department of Health. London.

Department of Health (2000a) *An Organisation with a Memory: Report of an Expert Group on Learning from Adverse Events in the NHS Chaired by the Chief Medical Officer*. Department of Health. London.

Department of Health (2000b) *The NHS Plan: A Plan for Investment, A Plan for Reform*. Department of Health. London.

Department of Health (2001) *Clinical Governance in Community Pharmacy: Guidelines on Good Practice for the NHS*. Department of Health. London.

Department of Health (2002) *Learning from Bristol: The Department of Health's Response to the Report of the Public Inquiry into the Children's Heart Surgery at the Bristol Royal Infirmary 1984–1995*. The Stationery Office. London.

Department of Health (2004) *Building a Safer NHS for Patients: Improving Medication Safety. A Report by the Chief Pharmaceutical Officer*. Department of Health. London.

Douglas, M. (1992) *Risk and Blame: Essays in Cultural Theory*. Routledge. London.

Hackel, R., Butt, L. and Banister, G. (1996) 'How nurses perceive medication errors'. *Nursing Management.* Vol 27, No 1, pp 31–34.

Healthcare Commission (2005) *Inspection Manual: Independent Health Care.* Healthcare Commission. London.

Heard, S. (2000) 'Clinical governance: An opportunity or Pandora's box?' in Scotland, A.D. (ed.) *Clinical Governance: One Year On*. Quay Books. Salisbury. Ch 1 pp 1–7.

Kehoe, R.F. (2005) 'Clinical audit' in James, A., Worrall, A. and Kendall, T. (eds) *Clinical Governance in Mental Health and Learning Disability Services*. Gaskell. London. Ch 15 pp 224–236.

Maughan, B. and Conduit, A. (1999) 'Clinical risk in primary care' in Wilson, J. and Tingle, J. (eds) *Clinical Risk Modification: A Route to Clinical Governance?* Butterworth. Heinemann. Ch 6 pp 103–116.

Mayo, A.M. and Duncan, D. (2004) 'Nurses' perception of medicine errors.' *Nurse Management.* Vol 27, No 1, pp 31–34.

Modernisation Agency (2003) *Essence of Care: Patient-Focused Benchmarks for Clinical Governance*. Modernisation Agency. London.

Modernisation Agency (2005) *Medicine Matters: A Guide to Current Mechanisms for the Prescribing, Supply and Administration of Medicines*. Modernisation Agency. London.

Morrell, C. and Harvey, G. (1999) *The Clinical Audit Handbook: Improving the Quality of Health Care*. Bailliere Tindall. London.

Murphy, L., Cox, L. and Murphy, D. (2005) 'Users' views of a dynamic risk assessment system'. *Nursing Times.* Vol 1010, No 33, pp 35–37.

National Audit Office (2000) *Supporting Innovation: Managing Risk in Government Departments*. National Audit Office. London.

National Health Service Executive (1993) *Risk Management in the NHS*. Department of Health. London.

National Health Service Executive (1999) *The NHS Performance Assessment Framework*. Department of Health. London.

National Institute for Health and Clinical Excellence (2005a) *Depression in Children and Young People: Identification and Management in Primary, Community and Secondary Care*. NICE. London.

National Institute for Health and Clinical Excellence (2005b) *The Prevention and Treatment of Pressure Ulcers*. NICE. London.

National Patient Safety Agency (2004) *Introduction: Seven Steps to Patient Safety*. National Patient Safety Agency. London.

Nursing and Midwifery Council (2002a) *Guidelines for the Administration of Medicines*. NMC. London.

Nursing and Midwifery Council (2002b) *An NMC Guide for Students of Nursing and Midwifery*. NMC. London.

Nursing and Midwifery Council (2004a) *The NMC Code of Professional Conduct: Standards for Conduct, Performance and Ethics*. NMC. London.

Nursing and Midwifery Council (2004b) *Guidelines for Records and Record Keeping*. NMC. London.

O'Shea, E. (1999) 'Factors contributing to medication errors: A literature review'. *Journal of Clinical Nursing.* Vol 8, No 5, pp 496–504.

Pape, T.M. (2001) 'Searching for the final answer: Factors contributing to medical administration errors'. *Journal of Continuing Education in Nursing.* Vol 32, No 4, pp 152–160.

Parish, C. (2003) 'Complacency to blame for transfusion mistakes'. *Nursing Standard.* Vol 17, No 45, p 8.

Pearson, V. (1987) *Nursing Quality Measurement: Quality Assurance Measures for Peer Review*. John Wiley & Sons Ltd. Chichester.

Performance and Innovation Unit (2002) *Performance and Innovation Unit Project: Risk and Uncertainty*. Performance and Innovation Unit. London.

Preston, R.M. (2004) 'Drug errors and patient safety: The need for a change in practice'. *British Journal of Nursing.* Vol 13, No 2, pp 72–78.

Roberts, G.W. (2005) 'The quality agenda in health and social care' in Clouston, T.J. and Westcott, L. (eds) *Working in Health and Social Care*. Elsevier. Edinburgh. Ch 8 pp 119–130.

Royal College of Nursing (1990) *The Dynamic Standard Setting System*. RCN. London.

Royal College of Nursing (2003) *Clinical Governance: An RCN Resource Guide*. RCN. London.

Sasaru, R., Sheward, Y. and Sasaru, S. (2005) 'Audit in allied health professional practice' in Clouston, T.J. and Westcott, L. (eds) *Working in Health and Social Care.* Elsevier. Edinburgh. Ch 10 pp 145–160.

Saunders, M. (2003) 'Audit: The beginning and the end of the change cycle' in Pickering, S. and Thompson, J. (eds) *Clinical Governance and Best Value: Meeting the Modernisation Agenda*. Churchill Livingstone. Edinburgh. Ch 8 pp 131–147.

Scrivens, E. (2005) *Quality, Risk and Control in Health Care*. Open University Press. Buckingham.

University of Manchester (1996) *Learning Materials on Mental Health Risk Assessment.* School of Psychiatry and Behavioural Sciences. Manchester.

Waterlow, J. (1985) 'A risk assessment card'. *Nursing Times.* Vol 81, No 49, pp 51–55.

## APPENDIX 12.1 GUIDELINES FOR THE ADMINISTRATION OF MEDICINES

Because of the many changes that have taken place in relation to medicines management and the way health care is developed in the United Kingdom, the advice previously given by the regulatory body on the administration of medicines has been reviewed. *Guidelines for the administration of medicines* replaces the 1992 document *Standards for the administration of medicines*. It was revised by the NMC in April 2002 and again in August 2004. Many of its principles remain of equal relevance today, for example:

> The administration of medicines is an important aspect of the professional practice of persons whose names are on the Council's register. It is not solely a mechanistic task to be performed in strict compliance with the written prescription

of a medical practitioner. It requires thought and the exercise of professional judgement . . .

Many government and other agencies are involved in medicines management from manufacture, licensing, prescribing and dispensing, to administration. An extensive range of guidance on these issues is provided by the relevant bodies. . . . One of the best sources of advice locally is usually your pharmacist.

As with all NMC guidance, this booklet is neither intended to be a rule book nor a manual. Nor is it intended to cover every single situation that you may encounter during your career. Instead, it sets out a series of guidelines or principles that we hope will enable you to think through the issues and to apply your professional expertise and judgement in the best interests of your patients. It will also be necessary to develop and refer to additional local policies or protocols to suit local needs. Within the document, the word 'patient' is used for convenience to refer to a person receiving medication, irrespective of the environment in which they are residing.

## PRINCIPLES IN RELATION TO THE PRESCRIPTION

As a registered nurse, midwife or specialist community public health nurse, you are accountable for your actions and omissions. In administering any medication, or assisting or overseeing any self-administration of medication, you must exercise your professional judgement and apply your knowledge and skill in the given situation. When administering medication against a prescription written manually or electronically by a registered medical practitioner or another authorised prescriber, the prescription should:

- Be based, whenever possible, on the patient's informed consent and awareness of the purpose of the treatment.
- Be clearly written, typed or computer-generated and be indelible (please refer to the NMC's *Guidelines for records and record keeping*).
- Clearly identify the patient for whom the medication is intended.
- Record the weight of the patient on the prescription sheet where the dosage of medication is related to weight.
- Clearly specify the substance to be administered, using its generic or brand name where appropriate and its stated form, together with the strength, dosage, timing, frequency of administration, start and finish dates and route of administration.
- Be signed and dated by the authorised prescriber.
- Not be for a substance to which the patient is known to be allergic or otherwise unable to tolerate.
- In the case of controlled drugs, specify the dosage and the number of dosage units or total course; if in an outpatient or community setting, the prescription should be in the prescriber's own handwriting; some prescribers are

subject to handwriting exemption but the prescription must still be signed and dated by the prescriber.

Instruction by telephone to a practitioner to administer a previously unprescribed substance is not acceptable. In exceptional circumstances, where the medication has been previously prescribed and the prescriber is unable to issue a new prescription, but where changes to the dose are considered necessary, the use of information technology (such as fax or e-mail) is the preferred method. This should be followed up by a new prescription confirming the changes within a given time period. The NMC suggests a maximum of 24 hours. In any event, the changes must have been authorised before the new dosage is administered.

## PRESCRIBING BY NURSES, MIDWIVES AND SPECIALIST COMMUNITY PUBLIC HEALTH NURSES

The *Medicinal Products: Prescription by Nurses Act 1992* and subsequent amendments to the pharmaceutical services regulations allow health visitors and district nurses, who have recorded their qualification on the NMC register, to become nurse prescribers. The preparation for this new area of practice is also included in the appropriate programmes to enable newly-qualified health visitors and district nurses to prescribe. Practitioners whose prescribing status is denoted on the register and who are approved within their employment setting may prescribe from the *Nurse Prescribers' Formulary*. Nurse, midwife and specialist community public health nurse prescribers must comply with the current legislation for prescribing and be accountable for their practice.

## PATIENT GROUP DIRECTIONS (GROUP PROTOCOLS)

Changes to medicines legislation, which came into effect in August 2000, clarify the law in relation to the supply or administration of medicines under patient group directions. You must follow the guidance supplied by your government health department regarding implementation. A patient group direction is a specific written instruction for the supply and administration of a named medicine or vaccine in an identified clinical situation. It applies to groups of patients who may not be individually identified before presenting for treatment. Patient group directions are drawn up locally by doctors or, if appropriate, by dentists, pharmacists and other health professionals. They must be signed by a doctor or dentist and a pharmacist, both of whom should have been involved in developing the direction, and must be approved by the appropriate health care body.

## DISPENSING

If, under exceptional circumstances, you are required to dispense, there is no legal barrier to this practice. However, this must be in the course of the business of a hospital and in accordance with a doctor's written instructions. In a dispensing doctor's practice, nurses may supply to patients under a particular doctor's care, when acting under the directions of a doctor from that practice.

Dispensing includes such activities as checking the validity of the prescription, the appropriateness of the medicine for an individual patient, assembly of the product, labelling in accordance with legal requirements and providing information leaflets for the patient.

If you, as a registered nurse, midwife or specialist community public health nurse, are engaged in dispensing, this represents an extension to your professional practice. The patient has the legal right to expect that the dispensing will be carried out with the same reasonable skill and care that would be expected from a pharmacist.

## PRINCIPLES FOR THE ADMINISTRATION OF MEDICINES

In exercising your professional accountability in the best interests of your patients, you must:

- Know the therapeutic uses of the medicine to be administered, its normal dosage, side effects, precautions and contra-indications.
- Be certain of the identity of the patient to whom the medicine is to be administered.
- Be aware of the patient's care plan.
- Check that the prescription, or the label on medicine dispensed by a pharmacist, is clearly written and unambiguous.
- Have considered the dosage, method of administration, route and timing of the administration in the context of the condition of the patient and co-existing therapies.
- Check the expiry date of the medicine to be administered.
- Check that the patient is not allergic to the medicine before administering it.
- Contact the prescriber or another authorised prescriber without delay where contra-indications to the prescribed medicine are discovered, where the patient develops a reaction to the medicine, or where assessment of the patient indicates that the medicine is no longer suitable.
- Make a clear, accurate and immediate record of all medicine administered, intentionally withheld or refused by the patient, ensuring that any written entries and the signature are clear and legible; it is also your responsibility to ensure that a record is made when delegating the task of administering medicine.
- Where supervising a student in the administration of medicines, clearly countersign the signature of the student.

Some drug administrations can require complex calculations to ensure that the correct volume or quantity of medication is administered. In these situations, it may be necessary for a second practitioner to check the calculation in order to minimise the risk of error. The use of calculators to determine the volume or quantity of medication should not act as a substitute for arithmetical knowledge and skill.

It is unacceptable to prepare substances for injection in advance of their immediate use or to administer medication drawn into a syringe or container by another practitioner when not in their presence. An exception to this is an already established infusion which has been instigated by another practitioner following the principles set out above, or medication prepared under the direction of a pharmacist from a central intravenous additive service and clearly labelled for that patient.

In an emergency, where you may be required to prepare substances for injection by a doctor, you should ensure that the person administering the drug has undertaken the appropriate checks as indicated above.

Midwives should refer to the NMC's *Midwives rules and standards* for specific additional information.

## AIDS TO SUPPORT COMPLIANCE

Self-administration from dispensed containers may not always be possible for some patients. If an aid to compliance is considered necessary, careful attention should be given to the assessment of the patient's suitability and understanding of how to use an appropriate aid safely. However, all patients will need to be regularly assessed for continued appropriateness of the aid.

Ideally, any compliance aid, such as a monitored dose container or a daily/weekly dosing aid, should be dispensed, labelled and sealed by a pharmacist.

Where it is not possible to get a compliance aid filled by a pharmacist, you should ensure that you are able to account for its use. The patient has a right to expect that the same standard of skill and care will be applied by you in dispensing into a compliance aid as would be applied if the patient were receiving the medication from a pharmacist. This includes the same standard of labelling and record keeping. Compliance aids, which are able to be purchased by patients for their own use, are aids that are filled from containers of dispensed medicines. If you choose to repackage dispensed medicines into compliance aids, you should be aware that their use carries a risk of error.

## SELF-ADMINISTRATION OF MEDICINES

The NMC welcomes and supports the self-administration of medicines and the administration of medication by carers wherever it is appropriate. However, the essential safety, security and storage arrangements must be available and, where necessary, agreed procedures must be in place.

For the hospital patient approaching discharge, but who will continue on a prescribed medicines regime on the return home, there are obvious benefits in adjusting to the responsibility of self-administration while still having access to professional support. It is essential, however, that where self-administration is introduced, arrangements are in place for the safe and secure storage of the medication, access to which is limited to the specific patient.

Where self-administration of medicines is taking place, you should ensure that records are maintained appropriate to the environment in which the patient is being cared for.

It is also important that, if you are delegating this responsibility, you ensure that the patient or carer/care assistant is competent to carry out the task. This will require education, training and assessment of the patient or carer/care assistant and further support if necessary. The competence of the person to whom the task has been delegated should be reviewed periodically.

## COMPLEMENTARY AND ALTERNATIVE THERAPIES

Complementary and alternative therapies are increasingly used in the treatment of patients. Registered nurses, midwives and specialist community public health nurses who practise the use of such therapies must have successfully undertaken training and be competent in this area (please refer to *The NMC code of professional conduct: standards for conduct, performance and ethics*). You must have considered the appropriateness of the therapy to both the condition of the patient and any co-existing treatments. It is essential that the patient is aware of the therapy and gives informed consent.

## MANAGEMENT OF ERRORS OR INCIDENTS IN THE ADMINISTRATION OF MEDICINES

It is important that an open culture exists in order to encourage the immediate reporting of errors or incidents in the administration of medicines. If you make an error, you must report it immediately to your line manager or employer.

Registered nurses, midwives and specialist community public health nurses who have made an error, and who have been honest and open about it to their senior staff, appear sometimes to have been made the subject of local disciplinary action in a way that might discourage the reporting of incidents and, therefore, be potentially detrimental to patients and the maintenance of standards.

The NMC believes that all errors and incidents require a thorough and careful investigation at a local level, taking full account of the context and circumstances and the position of the practitioner involved. Such incidents require sensitive management and a comprehensive assessment of all the circumstances before a professional and managerial decision is reached on the appropriate way to proceed. If a practising midwife makes or identifies a drug error or incident, she should also inform her supervisor of midwives as soon as possible after the event.

The NMC supports the use of local multi-disciplinary critical incident panels, where improvements to local practice in the administration of medicines can be discussed, identified and disseminated.

When considering allegations of misconduct arising from errors in the administration of medicines, the NMC takes great care to distinguish between those cases where the error was the result of reckless or incompetent practice or was concealed, and those that resulted from other causes, such as serious pressure of work, and where there was immediate, honest disclosure in the patient's interest. The NMC recognises the prerogative of managers to take local disciplinary action where it is considered to be necessary but urges that they also consider each incident in its particular context and similarly discriminate between the two categories described above.

## LEGISLATION

There are a number of pieces of legislation that relate to the prescribing, supply, storage and administration of medicines. It is essential that you comply with them. The following is a summary of those that are of particular relevance.

## MEDICINES ACT 1968

This was the first comprehensive legislation on medicines in the United Kingdom. The combination of this primary legislation and the various statutory instruments (secondary legislation) on medicines produced since 1968 provides the legal framework for the manufacture, licensing, prescription, supply and administration of medicines. Among recent statutory instruments of particular relevance to registered nurses, midwives and specialist community public health nurses is *The Prescription Only Medicines (Human Use) Order 1997, SI No 1830*. This consolidates all previous secondary legislation on prescription-only medicines and lists all of the medicines in this category. It also sets out who may prescribe them. The sections on exemptions are of particular relevance to midwives, including those in independent practice, and to nurses working in occupational health settings. The *Medicines Act 1968* classifies medicines into the following categories:

### Prescription-only Medicines (POMs)

These are medicines that may only be supplied or administered to a patient on the instruction of an appropriate practitioner (a doctor or dentist) and from an approved list for a nurse prescriber. The pharmacist is the expert on all aspects of medicines legislation and should be consulted.

### Pharmacy-only Medicines

These can be purchased from a registered primary care pharmacy, provided that the sale is supervised by the pharmacist.

### General Sale List Medicines (GSLs)

These need neither a prescription nor the supervision of a pharmacist and can be obtained from retail outlets. Generally, no medication should be administered without a prescription. However, local policies or patient group directions should be developed to allow the limited administration of medicines in this group to meet the needs of patients.

## MISUSE OF DRUGS ACT 1971

This prohibits the possession, supply and manufacture of medicinal and other products, except where such possession, supply and manufacture has been made legal by the *Misuse of Drugs Regulations 1985*. The legislation is concerned with controlled drugs and categorises these into five separate schedules. As a registered nurse, midwife or specialist community public health nurse, you should be particularly familiar with the regulations concerning schedule 2 medicines such as morphine, diamorphine and pethidine, and schedule 3 drugs such as barbiturates. If you are responsible for the storage or administration of controlled drugs, you should be aware of the content of the *Misuse of Drugs Regulations 1985* and the *Misuse of Drugs (Safe Custody) Regulations 1973*. Queries are often raised in relation to prescriptions for schedule 2 medicines (controlled drugs). The legislation states that the prescription should:

- Be in ink or such as to be indelible, and be signed and dated by the prescriber, issuing it in their usual handwriting with their signature.
- Specify the dose to be taken and, in the case of a prescription containing a controlled drug which is a preparation, the form and, where appropriate, the strength of the preparation, and either the total quantity (in both words and figures) of the preparation or the number (in both words and figures) of dosage units, as appropriate, to be supplied; in any other case, the total quantity (in both words and figures) of the controlled drug to be supplied. If you have any queries in relation to the misuse of drugs, or if you are aware of illicit substances being in the possession of a patient, you must refer to and act on local policy and/or appropriate government health department guidance.

## UNLICENSED MEDICINES

An unlicensed medicine is the term used to refer to a medicine that has no product licence. If an unlicensed medicine is administered to a patient, the manufacturer has no liability for any harm that ensues. The person who prescribes the medicine carries the liability. This may have implications for you in obtaining informed consent.

If a medicine is unlicensed, it should only be administered to a patient against a patient-specific prescription and not against a patient group direction. However, medication which is licensed but used outside its licensed indications may be administered under a patient group direction if such use is exceptional, justified by best practice and the status of the product is clearly described. In addition, you should be satisfied that you have sufficient information to administer the drug safely and, wherever possible, that there is acceptable evidence for the use of that product for the intended indication.

*Source*: NMC, 2002a. This is Crown copyright material which is reproduced with the permission of the Controller of HMSO and the Queen's Printer for Scotland.

# 13 Inter-professional Working and Learning

The focus of this chapter is to encourage the reader to demonstrate an understanding of the role of other health-care professionals by participating in inter-professional working practice. The roles and responsibilities of other health-care professionals are discussed, providing the reader with an understanding of their contribution to the health and wellbeing of the patient. Chapter 7 has already begun to address the importance of working with other health-care professionals and working in a partnership perspective – an inter-agency approach. The promotion of the modernisation of the NHS and the production of key, influencing documents, provided by various governments, has promoted the use of inter-professional working practices.

There is little consensus regarding the term inter-professional working. Several definitions are provided here to help the reader acquire clarity and understanding. It is vital that the nurse understands the terms used if he/she is to engage effectively in inter-professional working and learning. Mutual respect and understanding are common fundamental terms associated with inter-professional working. Being aware of how each professional group perceives the others may enhance understanding and collaboration. Reinforcing and promoting stereotypes, along with harbouring misconceptions, can hinder and harm good working relationships among health-care professionals.

Inter-professional working has much potential to enhance care; it can also produce tensions and concerns within the health-care team. Barriers to effective working relationships associated with inter-professional working and learning are discussed.

To work effectively the nurse must embrace the concept of effective teamworking. Teamworking, like inter-professional working, is defined in many ways and is often used synonymously with group working. This aspect of the chapter considers both teamworking and working as a member of a group.

The latter part of this chapter focuses on inter-professional learning, and it is suggested that learning together will lead to more effective and productive working. Emphasis is placed on the fact that inter-professional learning does not take place in a vacuum. There are many factors that must be taken into consideration, for example the needs and interests of the various stakeholders.

## BACKGROUND AND UNDERLYING PRINCIPLES

The philosophy underpinning inter-professional working lies in the modernisation of the NHS. Chapter 12 commented regarding the 'new NHS' and how it will bring about an overall improvement in the patient experience. The aim of the new NHS is to improve cooperation and partnerships and to enhance communications and working practices across professional and organisational boundaries (Salmon and Jones, 2001). According to Kenny (2002) inter-professional working provides the vehicle whereby existing power structures (i.e. professional elitism) can be replaced with arrangements that are committed to equality and collective responsibility.

The shift from bureaucratic, centralised service provision to more of a focus on patient centredness articulates well with current government policy and the modernisation agenda, a part of which is to enhance inter-professional collaboration (Pollard et al., 2005a; Kenny, 2002; Department of Health, 2000a). Service users (patients) should not become mere recipients of care but should be empowered to become partners in care (Wilby, 2005). The *NHS Plan* (Department of Health, 2000b) claims that problems arise when a system devised in the 1940s tries to operate in the twenty-first century, with old-fashioned demarcations between staff and barriers to services.

It is not only policy development that has required health- and social-care agencies to work together; see for example the NSF for Mental Health (Department of Health, 1999). Glendinning et al. (2003) point out that the Health Act 1999 also imposes a duty on all NHS organisations to work in partnership. The key aim of some legislation, for example the Community Care Act 1990, is to promote closer and collaborative partnerships with service users. Øvretveit et al. (1997) point out that the rationale for improving inter-professional working is to meet the needs of service users more effectively.

Patients often move from one professional group to another depending on their clinical needs. Collaborative arrangements between health-care groups (health-care professionals) are not new: as far back as 1974 the British Medical Association (BMA, 1974) used the term 'primary care team'. Collaborative arrangements, according to Rushmer (2005), have the ability to unite health provision across disciplines (integrated working), across health sectors (intermediate care) and also across agencies (multi-agency working). The aim is to provide the patient with a service that is seamless and joined up (Cabinet Office, 2000). Øvretveit et al. (1997) refer to this as a need for 'coordination-for-continuity'.

## WHAT IS INTER-PROFESSIONAL WORKING?

Cowley et al. (2002) point out that despite the fact that partnership working has been widely recognised for a number of years, in a review of over 52 policy documents there was a lack of consensus in terminology accompanied with a paucity of definitions. Lack of clarity concerning inter-professional working will be reflected in an organisation's philosophy and, as a result, there is a danger that some health-care professionals may dismiss inter-professional working as irrelevant or not needed. It is important to understand what is meant by the term inter-professional working. This is not just the subject of academic debate, it is vital if the nurse is to engage in inter-professional working (and ultimately learning) that he/she understands the concept.

Glenn (1999) suggests that when nurses engage with inter-professional working a forum can occur for them to express themselves and for other health-care professionals to understand and value the role and function of the nurse. Strengthening the professional identity of nursing is seen by Barr (2000) as a prerequisite if nurses are to collaborate effectively with other health-care professionals. Inter-professional working is one way of strengthening nursing's identity.

Lack of clarity and ambiguity can lead to misunderstandings and these misunderstandings, according to Biggs (1997), can multiply. The prefixes 'inter' and 'multi' and the adjectives 'disciplinary' and 'professional' are often used. There are several terms that are used interchangeably, for example, 'multidisciplinary' and 'interdisciplinary' (Wilson and Pirrie, 2000).

There has been much debate about the terminology associated with inter-professional working and many terms exist, for example:

- multiprofessional
- interprofessional
- multidisciplinary
- interdisciplinary
- multi-agency
- inter-agency

Pirrie at al. (1998) state that there is a distinction between 'inter' and 'multi'. This difference is based on three dimensions:

- numerical
- territorial
- epistemological

Pirrie et al. (1998) and Payne (2000) have attempted to summarise the definition quagmire and suggest that evidence gleaned from the literature indicates that 'multi' denotes activities that:

- Bring more than two groups together.
- Focus on complementary procedures and perspectives.
- Provide opportunities to learn about each other.
- Are motivated by a desire to focus on clients' needs.
- Develop participants' understanding of their separate but inter-related roles as members of a team.

They also suggest that the prefix 'inter' is more appropriate when the activity enables team members to:

- Develop a new inter-professional perspective that is more than the sum of the individual parts.
- Integrate procedures and perspectives on behalf of clients.
- Learn from and about each other.
- Reflect critically on their knowledge base.
- Engage in shared reflection on their joint practice.
- Surrender some aspects of their own professional role.
- Share knowledge.
- Develop a common understanding.

Inter-professional therefore relates to relations between different professional groups. A third term also needs to be mentioned: 'inter-agency'. Inter-agency collaboration, according to Biggs (1997), refers to relations that exist between different organisations or agencies. These organisations may be uniprofessional or multiprofessional. Chapter 7 considers inter-agency working in detail and you may note that much of the emphasis there is associated with health- and social-care agencies as well as the voluntary sector. Table 13.1 provides an overview of the three terms.

**Table 13.1** A summary of the three terms often associated with inter-professional collaboration

| Term | Description |
|---|---|
| **Inter-professional** | Relations between different professional groups. Each group will have its own identity and its own professional culture that has been established by professional bodies, e.g. the Health Professions Council (HPC), Nursing and Midwifery Council (NMC) and General Medical Council (GMC). |
| **Inter-agency** | Relations that exist between different organisations and agencies. The agencies may consist of representatives from the health, social and voluntary sector. Each agency is likely to have developed its own culture associated with its policies and procedures. There may be, on occasion, competing funding arrangements. |
| **Multidisciplinary** | This term refers to teams that work in more fluid ways. Members may be from various professional groups but they work towards a focused goal, all aiming to achieve the same outcome. The context is focused, enduring and is often small scale. A shared identity but one with an explicit professional contribution. |

*Source*: Adapted from Biggs, 1997.

Make a list of the different professional groups that you think the nurse might have to collaborate with.

Did you think broad and wide? Compare your list with the following list and the list of professions which are on the Health Professions Register:

- physiotherapists
- paramedics
- radiographers
- occupational therapists
- social workers
- police
- doctors
- probation managers

Each of the groups above has its own unique professional culture and they have all experienced their own unique educational programme preparing them for their practice. These professional groups, therefore, have unique professional identities, yet they are expected to come together to work as a professional group. One common denominator for some of the health-care groups (excluding nursing and medicine) is that they have their own professional regulator – the Health Professions Council (HPC).

Mutual respect, understanding and trust are central components of collaborative working and inter-professional education (Hale, 2003) and are facilitated through open and honest two-way effective communications. This enables the professionals involved in an inter-professional endeavour to develop an understanding of one another's perspectives (Kennison and Fletcher, 2005). Understanding how we perceive other health-care professionals, and being aware of the stereotypes we hold about them, may help us to work more effectively when engaging in inter-professional working.

What do you think are the stereotypical views others hold about nurses? Make a list of them.

Some people have very interesting perceptions, views and clichés about nurses. Did any of the following appear in your list?

- battle axe
- angel
- sex fiend
- all male nurses are gay
- educated
- always on the go
- heavy smoker
- caring
- heavy drinker
- dumb
- killer
- overweight
- all female
- poorly paid

Do you agree with the stereotypes? Do they annoy you at all?

Now think of some of the other health-care professionals that you are required to work with and think about the stereotypes you hold about these other professionals. How do you think they might feel if they think you perceive them in a particular way?

Stereotyping, prejudging and harbouring misperceptions about other health-care professionals can harm good inter-professional working relationships. Working and learning with other health-care professionals may help to address and correct any misconceptions you may have about others.

## THE HEALTH PROFESSIONS COUNCIL

The government aims to improve the quality of services in many ways. Some of these have already been discussed; one other way is to modernise the systems of professional regulation (Whitcombe, 2005). The Health Act 1999 was the Act responsible for replacing the Council for Professions Supplementary to Medicine (CPSM). The move to a smaller and more unified regulative body – the Health Professions Council – was established in 2001 and became operational in 2002.

The HPC maintains a register of health professionals who meet its standards. It also has the power to take action against health professionals who do not meet the standards it has set (HPC, 2004). The aim of the HPC is to protect the health and wellbeing of the people who use the services of the health professionals registered with it. It monitors standards for professional education and conduct. Currently the HPC regulates 13 health professions:

- art therapists
- biomedical scientists
- chiropodists/podiatrists
- dieticians
- occupational therapists
- operating department practitioners
- orthoptists
- orthotists
- paramedics
- physiotherapists
- prosthetists
- radiographers
- speech and language therapists

The HPC has produced standards of proficiency, standards of conduct and standards of performance and ethics (HPC, 2003).

## INTER-PROFESSIONAL WORKING

Many high-profile failures in the health-care system have identified the need for cooperation and collaboration between health and social-care professions (Department of Health, 2002; Laming, 2003). These are the negative consequences that result from a system that has neither cohesive structures for service delivery nor effective inter-professional collaboration (Pollard et al., 2005b). A 'seamless service' is what should occur, however in reality this may not always be the case, as care and collaboration may be fragmented (Miller et al., 2001). Organisational structures and care environments differ across the UK, adding to discoordinated care provision.

Prior to developing inter-professional working it is important to articulate professional identity – nursing's own identity. It is difficult to form collaborative ties, suggests Dombeck (1997), when one is unsure about one's own professional identity. It is possible once this has been achieved to establish a team that is based on an egalitarian and cooperative approach to working together, in partnership with patients (Molyneux, 2001).

Making the change from a uniprofessional approach where traditionally each profession worked in isolation with a rigid hierarchy and a predominant professional (usually medicine) is a challenge. Movement is needed towards a culture that seeks to foster mutual respect as well as shared values (Miller et al., 2001; Molyneux, 2001). Masta (2003) suggests that egalitarian inter-professional relationships have the potential to alter nursing's status and as a result enhance nursing's professionalisation. However, Clarke (1993) states that putting people together in groups that represent various disciplines will not necessarily guarantee the development of a shared understanding. Pirrie et al. (1998), in a study they have undertaken, suggested consolidation of the learning experience, for example inter-professional learning will reduce stereotyping and segregation of professional groups.

An egalitarian relationship with other professions is a key aim associated with inter-professional working. Traditionally nursing has had a very close relationship with medicine and much focus has been on the nurse–doctor relationship. Other relationships with other health-care professionals occur in both health and social care, and they must also be given consideration when proposing an inter-professional working culture.

There are common components between each professional group. However, Biggs (1997) suggests that some concerns arise related to identity and, in particular, the loss of identity as a result of immersing the professions in a wider and less well-defined group. One other concern is the potential problem of one particular professional group (for example nursing) being swamped by another professional group (for example medicine). Pollard et al. (2005a) have demonstrated in their study that hierarchies still persist despite some positive moves towards inter-professional working. They note that junior staff, and in particular student nurses, did not contribute as freely as they might during inter-professional meetings. It was identified that the medical staff initiated or sustained the main leader role.

## INTER-PROFESSIONAL LEARNING

The terms inter-professional learning and inter-professional education are often used interchangeably. Other terms are also used such as transprofessional and interdisciplinary education. Hale (2003) uses the definition of inter-professional education provided by the Centre for the Advancement of Interprofessional Education:

> *An educational activity that uses interactive learning approaches between professionals to cultivate collaborative practice. Multiprofessional education is defined as an education activity where learning is shared passively (e.g. joint lectures).*

Inter-professional learning has become a rapidly developing field as a result of the emphasis on inter-professional practice (Cooper et al., 2004). The United Kingdom Central Council (2001) considered inter-professional education as the ability to enable students from different professional groups to learn from each other with the aim to enhance collaborative practice and improve the effectiveness of care delivery. Inter-professional learning is seen by Young et al. (2003) as learning that takes place when a mix of disciplines congregate in learning groups. The multidisciplinary group is itself the source of material for learning about inter-professional practice.

Promoting and enhancing the concept of inter-professional working may come as a result of inter-professional learning. Indeed, Cooper et al. (2004) suggest that this is the vehicle through which policy goals associated with inter-professional working can be achieved. Barr et al. (1999) consider inter-professional education as a means of:

- Modifying reciprocal attitudes and perceptions.
- Cultivating mutual respect.
- Exploring ways in which collaboration could be made real.

Freeth (2001) makes the observation that education and training are crucial to providing the conditions and skills needed for continued collaboration. However, Laidler (1991) suggests that to be able to cross professional boundaries and feel confident enough to share and defer their professional autonomy, staff from different disciplines need to feel sufficiently confident about their own roles and their own professional identity. Bliss et al. (2000) state that engaging in inter-professional educational activities will facilitate learning in relation to gaining an understanding of one another's roles.

Being able to articulate disciplinary and professional identities is required before inter-professional working can be a success (Dombeck, 1997). Ashworth et al. (2001) see confidence as a key factor in having the ability to influence an individual's capacity to engage with inter-professional working. Freeth et al. (2002) have recognised that education plays a key role in the process of encouraging health-care professionals to address their strong uniprofessional focus, as well as their habitual attitudes and ways of functioning in an inter-professional context.

*Meeting the Challenge* (Department of Health, 2000c) provides a strategy for allied health professions. It also places an emphasis on inter-professional education, suggesting that a change is required in the way health and social-care professionals are educated at both pre-registration and post-registration/graduate levels.

Student nurses in Pollard et al.'s (2005a) study are seen as passive participants when considering inter-professional partnerships. Enhancing inter-professional learning opportunities may be one way of encouraging student nurses to participate in a more active manner. This can only become a reality if students develop assertive skills early on in their nurse education.

Preparation (educational programmes of study) for health-care professionals has been addressed in several seminal documents produced by the government and professional organisations, for example the *NHS Plan* (Department of Health, 2000b). A review declared that providers of education for health-care professionals, for example institutions of higher education, had to develop new common foundation programmes. The aim of these new developments was to enable students (pre-registration) and staff (post-registration) to move between careers and educational pathways more easily. A new type of worker is envisaged, one that is flexible, is more of a teamworker and one who takes on partnership and collaborative activity more easily. A changing workforce programme has already been considered by the Department of Health (2000a). The emphasis of this initiative is on:

- Teamworking across professional and organisational boundaries.
- Flexible working to make the best use of the range of skills and knowledge that staff have.
- Streamlined workforce planning and development that stem from the needs of patients not of professionals.
- Maximising the contribution of all staff to patient care, doing away with barriers that say only doctors or nurses can provide particular types of care.
- Modernising education and training to ensure that staff are equipped with the skills they need to work in a complex, changing NHS.
- Developing new more flexible careers for staff of all professions and non.
- Expanding the workforce to meet future demands.

Inter-professional learning has also been identified by the General Social Care Council (2002) as a key component of pre-registration social work. This requirement is particularly relevant to student nurses who are undertaking the joint social work and registered nurse degree, for example in learning disabilities.

There are various models of learning available when implementing an inter-professional learning approach and some include common learning. This approach, Shaw (1995) suggests, enables students to study topics of common interest whether in single or mixed interdisciplinary groups. Learning takes place in both the classroom and while on clinical placements in the myriad of learning contexts available in the clinical field.

## BARRIERS TO SUCCESSFUL INTER-PROFESSIONAL WORKING AND LEARNING

Barriers to partnership work are evident (Daly, 2004; Glendinning et al., 2003). Some of these are related to structural and organisational changes, for example mergers of Trusts, relocation and withdrawal of services.

Salmon and Jones (2001) point out that one of the key reasons for the modernisation of professional education is the need to develop cooperation and partnerships, with the overarching aim of improving communication and working practices across professional and organisational boundaries. Daly (2004) sees poor communication (written or verbal) between professional groups as a potential threat to effective inter-professional working.

It must also be recognised (Guest et al., 2003) that inter-professional working and learning does not take place in a vacuum. There are several factors to be taken into consideration, such as the needs and interests of the various stakeholders (for example professional organisations), the complex

**Table 13.2** Some potential barriers to inter-professional collaboration and education

- Differences in history and culture.
- Historical inter-professional and intra-professional rivalries.
- Differences in language and jargon.
- Differences in schedules and professional routines (complexities of timetabling).
- Varying levels of preparation, qualifications and status (for example A levels, NVQ).
- Fears of diluted professional identity.
- Differences in accountability, payment and rewards.
- Concerns regarding clinical responsibility and accountability.
- An imbalance between student numbers between different professions.
- Lack of clinical experience.

*Source*: Adapted from Pirrie et al., 1998; Hendrick et al., 1998.

power structures, pay disparities among the integrating groups, gender and socioeconomic differentials. The biggest factor associated with positive outcomes in Young et al.'s (2003) evaluation of multiprofessional programmes was timetabling – various curricula, multisite campuses and uncoordinated clinical placements, which complicated matters and sometimes confused the student. Table 13.2 outlines some barriers to inter-professional collaboration and education.

Daly (2004) makes recommendations that will ensure multiprofessional collaboration. These recommendations may help to overcome some of the barriers to effective inter-professional working and learning. She suggests, for example, regular multiprofessional team meetings to enhance communication and promote team collaboration.

Finally, one question that is yet to be answered is this: does inter-professional learning help to prepare students to manage and perform better in health and social-care settings? There is currently no evidence to support or refute the value of inter-professional learning (Hale, 2003). Zwarenatein et al. (1999), having conducted a systematic review of the literature, determined that at present there is no published evidence to promote inter-professional education as the vehicle to enhance inter-professional collaboration, or that it improves patient outcomes. Freeth et al. (2002) emphasise that more research is needed to evaluate the impact of inter-professional education practice.

## TEAMWORKING

Many government directives or professional edicts frequently require teams to do various things. Often, however, they do not define what they mean by a team. Pollard et al. (2005b) state that what is meant and understood by the term 'team' can vary a great deal. Cook (2004) suggests that the label 'team' is being added to any group of people who work together.

He provides a helpful definition of a team and distinguishes between a group and a team. A group, he proposes, is made up of members who want to create a shared view of goals and develop an efficient and effective organisational structure on which to accomplish those goals. According to Wheelan (1999), a group does not become a team until those shared goals have become established, methods have been developed to accomplish the goals and the goals are in place. Teams, according to Northcott (2003), are different people with different skills all working together towards the same goal(s). Katzenbach and Smith (1993) suggest they are committed to a common purpose with skills that complement each other.

Until the purpose of the team has been decided, it will be unable to function as an effective team (Bliss, 2004). Agreeing on aims, objectives and goals has been identified as a central component of teamworking (Pearson and Spencer, 1997). Clarity is required not only regarding aims, objectives and goals but also about responsibilities within the team. The team must also agree on ways in which it will judge its successes or failures.

Teams may be tight-knit units that are composed of individuals who, on a regular basis, work together; alternatively they may be *ad hoc*, loosely woven entities meeting to address or meet specific demands. Teams, according to Pollard et al. (2005b), can be formally constituted, with a particular structure or objective, or they can be organic entities that occur with no formal recognition. Depending on circumstances, they may be consensual, democratic or hierarchical, or even all of these. Øvretveit et al. (1997) note that there are several permutations associated with team structures and processes. The definition of team is not precise, just as the definitions of light and energy are beyond description and explanation; they cannot be reduced to a simple definition (Adair, 1987). Teams and organisations become more concrete when set within a context.

Team values need to come to terms with individual team members, the priorities of the organisation and the needs of the patient. The RCN (2000) suggests that to function as an effective team, the team members need to agree answers to some questions:

- Who are we? What are our unique qualities, qualifications, interests and enthusiasms?
- What do we do? What exactly are we offering and how does our role differ from that of others?
- How do we do it? Consider the technical, interpersonal and educational skills and our commitment to multidisciplinary and multi-agency working.

There are structural, historical and attitudinal barriers to effective teamworking. In some instances individuals working alone may perform better than a team (Royal Pharmaceutical Society of Great Britain and the British Medical Association, 2000).

Cole (2005) points out that the best teams have the following components:

- clear objectives
- high levels of participation
- a focus on quality
- being supportive of innovations
- using all available opportunities to learn
- regularly reviewing what they are trying to achieve

In some NHS trusts some staff feel poorly supported, and only approximately half of staff say they are encouraged to suggest ideas to improve care provision, with a third of staff suggesting they are not involved in important decisions. In NHS organisations where staff work in formal teams, patient mortality was consistently 5 per cent lower, as opposed to those organisations where staff were not a part of a formal team (West et al., 2002). The need for effective teamworking is evident.

## CONCLUSIONS

A modern NHS is one that provides and delivers care to patients in such a way that it is sensitive and respects their needs and expectations. The NHS provides advice and support to help people manage their own care, quickly and effectively. Care should be streamlined, allowing and facilitating the integration of other services, for example social services.

Inter-professional working and inter-professional education are not the panacea for all ills that befall health and social-care provision; they provide many challenges. Disasters such as the tragedy associated with the death of Victoria Climbié are examples of how lack of collaboration, blurring of roles and responsibilities and poor communication contributed to ineffective child protection.

The modernisation agenda associated with the NHS is seeking fast and radical changes to the way services are provided. However, if inter-professional teamwork is to be a success, then this will require time, as trust building and mutual professional respect are the foundations on which inter-professional working is based. The common goal shared by all who are employed by the NHS is the wellbeing of the patient but, as Daly (2004) suggests, this becomes a singular ideal when each discrete discipline retains its strong and competing dominating identity. Organisations must promote the development of professionalism with independent professional identities and values, and at the same time move towards inter-professional working and collaboration, delivering services to members of the public that they want in response to their needs and expectations.

Nurses are central to inter-professional working. Nurses need to strive to ensure that traditional hierarchies (still evident) are no longer the norm with one profession dominating other(s).

The Centre for the Advancement of Interprofessional Education (1996) has produced a list of principles that underpin effective inter-professional education. This list, reproduced here, aims to summarise some of the key points made in this chapter. Effective inter-professional education:

- Works to improve the quality of care.
- Focuses on the needs of service users and carers.
- Involves service users and carers.
- Promotes inter-professional collaboration.
- Encourages professions to learn with, from and about one another.
- Enhances practice within professions.
- Respects the integrity and contribution of each profession.
- Increases professional satisfaction.

While inter-professional working and learning have their merits, there has been insufficient attention paid to the impact they have on the student experience, and above all patient outcome. More evidence is needed to help guide the way forward. Policies currently formulated must be revisited regularly to determine if they are indeed doing what they say they should be doing.

## REFERENCES

Adair, J. (1987) *Effective Teambuilding: How to Make a Winning Team*. Pan. London.

Ashworth, P., Gerrish, K. and McManus, M. (2001) 'Whither nursing? Discourses underlying the attribution of master's level performance in nursing'. *Journal of Advanced Nursing*. Vol 34, No 5, pp 621–628.

Barr, H. (2000) 'New NHS, new collaboration, new agenda for education'. *Interprofessional Care*. Vol 14, No 1, pp 81–86.

Barr, H., Hammick, M., Koppel, I. and Reeves, S. (1999) 'Evaluating interprofessional education: Two systematic reviews for health and social care'. *British Educational Research*. Vol 24, No 4, pp 533–544.

Biggs, S. (1997) 'Interprofessional collaboration: Problems and prospects' in Øvretveit, J., Mathias, P. and Thompson, T. (eds) *Interprofessional Working for Health and Social Care*. Macmillan. London. Ch 9 pp 186–200.

Bliss, J. (2004) 'Effective team management by district nurses'. *British Journal of Community Nursing*. Vol 9, No 12, pp 524–526.

Bliss, J., Cowley, S. and White, A. (2000) 'Inter-professional working in palliative care in the community: A review of the literature'. *Journal of Interprofessional Care*. Vol 14, pp 281–290.

British Medical Association (1974) *Primary Health Care Teams*. BMA. London.

Cabinet Office (2000) *Wiring It Up: Whitehall's Management of Cross-cutting Policies and Services.* Performance and Innovation Unit. London.

Centre for the Advancement of Interprofessional Education (1996) 'Principles of interprofessional education'. *CAIPE Bulletin*, No 11.1. Centre for the Advancement of Interprofessional Education. London.

Clarke, P.G. (1993) 'A typology of multidisciplinary education. Gerontology education and geriatrics: Are we really doing what we say we are?'. *Journal of Interprofessional Care*. Vol 7, No 3, pp 217–227.

Cole, A. (2005) 'Reaping the benefits of teamwork'. *Nursing Times*. Vol 101, No 1, p 59.

Cook, M. (2004) 'Interprofessional post-qualifying education: Team leadership' in Glenn, S. and Leiba, T. (eds) *Interprofessional Post-Qualifying Education for Nurses Working Together in Health and Social Care*. Palgrave. Basingstoke. Ch 6 pp 79–101.

Cooper, H., Braye, S. and Geyer, R. (2004) 'Complexity and interprofessional education'. *Learning in Health and Social Care*. Vol 3, No 4, pp 179–189.

Cowley, S., Bliss, J., Mathew, A. and McVey, G. (2002) 'Effective interagency and interprofessional working: Facilitators and barriers'. *International Journal of Palliative Nursing*. Vol 8, No 1, pp 30–39.

Daly, G. (2004) 'Understanding the barriers to multiprofessional collaboration'. *Nursing Times*. Vol 100, No 9, pp 78–79.

Department of Health (1999) *National Service Framework for Mental Health*. Department of Health. London.

Department of Health (2000a) *A Health Service of All the Talents: Developing the NHS Workforce*. Department of Health. London.

Department of Health (2000b) *The NHS Plan: A Plan for Investment, A Plan for Reform*. Department of Health. London.

Department of Health (2000c) *Meeting the Challenge: A Strategy for the Allied Health Professions*. Department of Health. London.

Department of Health (2002) *Learning from Bristol: The Department of Health's Response to the Report of the Public Inquiry into the Children's Heart Surgery at the Bristol Royal Infirmary 1984–1995*. The Stationery Office. London.

Dombeck, M. (1997) 'Professional personhood: Training territoriality and tolerance'. *Journal of Interprofessional Care*. Vol 11, pp 9–21.

Freeth, D. (2001) 'Sustaining interprofessional collaboration'. *Journal of Interprofessional Care*. Vol 15, pp 37–46.

Freeth, D., Hammick, M., Koppel, I., Reeves, S. and Barr, H. (2002) *A Critical Review of Evaluations of Interprofessional Education*. Learning and Teaching Support Network, Health Sciences and Practice. London.

General Social Care Council (2002) *Accreditation of Universities to Grant Degrees in Social Work*. GSCC. London.

Glendinning, C., Coleman, A., Shipman, C. and Malbon. G. (2003) 'Progress in partnerships'. *British Medical Journal*. Vol 323, pp 28–31.

Glenn, S. (1999) 'Education for interprofessional collaboration: Teaching about values'. *Nursing Ethics*. Vol 6, No 3, pp 202–213.

Guest, C., Smith, L., Bradshaw, M. and Hardcastle, W. (2003) 'Facilitating interprofessional learning for medical and nursing students in clinical practice'. *Learning in Health and Social Care*. Vol 1, pp 132–138.

Hale, C. (2003) 'Interprofessional education: The way to a success workforce'. *British Journal of Therapy and Rehabilitation*. Vol 10, No 3, pp 122–127.

Health Professions Council (2003) *Standards of Conduct and Ethics: Your Duties as a Registrant*. HPC. London.

Health Professions Council (2004) *Welcome to the Health Professions Council*. HPC. London.

Hendrick, L.A., Wilcock, P.M. and Batalden, P.B. (1998) 'Interprofessional working and continuing medical education'. *British Medical Journal*. Vol 316, pp 771–774.

Katzenbach, J. and Smith, D. (1993) *The Wisdom of Teams*. Harvard Business School Press. Boston.

Kennison, P. and Fletcher, R. (2005) 'Police' in Barrett, G., Sellman, D. and Thomas, J. (eds) *Interprofessional Working in Health and Social Care*. Palgrave. Basingstoke. Ch 10 pp 119–131.

Kenny, G. (2002) 'Interprofessional opportunities and challenges'. *Nursing Standard*. Vol 17, No 6, pp 33–35.

Laidler, P. (1991) 'Adults and how to become one'. *Therapy Weekly*. Vol 17, No 35, p 4.

Laming, Lord (2003) *Inquiry into the Death of Victoria Climbié*. The Stationery Office. London.

Masta, O. (2003) 'Night cover'. *Nursing Standard*. Vol 17, No 49, pp 16–18.

Miller, C., Freeman, M. and Ross, N. (2001) *Interprofessional Practice in Health and Social Care: Challenging the Shared Learning Agenda*. Arnold. London.

Molyneux, J. (2001) 'Interprofessional team working: What makes teams work well'. *Journal of Interprofessional Care*. Vol 15, No 1, pp 29–35.

Northcott, N. (2003) 'Working within a health care team' in Hinchliff, S., Norman, S. and Schober, J. (eds) (4th edn) *Nursing Practice and Health Care*. Arnold. London. Ch 16 pp 371–389.

Øvretveit, J. (1997) 'How to describe interprofessional working' in Øvretveit, J., Mathias, P. and Thompson, T. (eds) *Interprofessional Working for Health and Social Care*. Macmillan. London. Ch 9 pp 9–33.

Øvretveit, J., Mathias, P. and Thompson, T. (eds) (1997) *Interprofessional Working for Health and Social Care*. Macmillan. London.

Payne, M. (2000) *Teamwork in Multiprofessional Care*. Macmillan. Basingstoke.

Pearson, P. and Spencer, J. (1997) *Promoting Teamwork in Primary Care*. Arnold. London.

Pirrie, A., Wilson, V., Elsegood, J., Hall, J., Hamilton, S., Harden. R., Lee, D. and Stead, J. (1998) *Evaluating Multidisciplinary Education in Health Care*. The Scottish Council for Research in Education. Edinburgh.

Pollard, K.C., Ross, K. and Means, R. (2005a) 'Nurse leadership, interprofessionalism and the modernization agenda'. *British Journal of Nursing*. Vol 14, No 6, pp 339–344.

Pollard, K.C., Sellman, D. and Senior, B. (2005b) 'The need for interprofessional working' in Barrett, G., Sellman, D. and Thomas, J. (eds) *Interprofessional Working in Health and Social Care*. Palgrave. Basingstoke. Ch 1 pp 7–17.

Royal College of Nursing (2000) *Children's Community Nursing: Promoting Effective Teamworking for Children and Their Families*. RCN. London.

Royal Pharmaceutical Society of Great Britain and the British Medical Association (2000) *Team Working Primary Health Care: Realising Shared Aims in Patient Care*. Royal Pharmaceutical Society of Great Britain and the British Medical Association. London.

Rushmer, B. (2005) 'Blurred boundaries damage inter-professional working'. *Nurse Researcher*. Vol 12, No 3, pp 74–85.

Salmon, D. and Jones, M. (2001) 'Shaping the interprofessional agenda: A study examining qualified nurses' perception of working with others'. *Nurse Education Today*. Vol 21, No 1, pp 18–25.

Shaw, I. (1995) *Locally Based Shared Learning: Surveys in Two English Counties.* Centre for the Enhancement for Interprofessional Learning. London.

United Kingdom Central Council (2001) *Fitness for Practice and Purpose.* UKCC. London.

West, M., Borrill, C., Dawson, J., Scully, J., Carter, M., Anealy, S., Patterson, M. and Waring, J. (2002) 'The link between management of employees and patient mortality in acute hospitals'. *International Journal of Human Resource Management.* Vol 13, No 8, pp 1299–1310.

Wheelan, S.A. (1999) *Creating Effective Teams: A Guide for Members and Leaders.* Sage. Thousand Oaks.

Whitcombe, S.W. (2005) 'Understanding healthcare professions from sociological perspectives' in Clouston, T.J. and Westcott, L. (eds) *Working in Health and Social Care: An Introduction for Allied Health Professionals.* Churchill Livingstone. Edinburgh. Ch 4 pp 63–73.

Wilby, P.K. (2005) 'Thinking about teamworking and collaboration' in Clouston, T.J. and Westcott, L. (eds) *Working in Health and Social Care: An Introduction for Allied Health Professionals.* Churchill Livingstone. Edinburgh. Ch 5 pp 75–85.

Wilson, V. and Pirrie, A. (2000) *Multidisciplinary Team Working: Beyond Barriers? A Review of the Issues.* The Scottish Council for Research in Education. Edinburgh.

Young, G., Mitchell, F., Sensky, T. and Rhodes, M. (2003) 'Evaluation of the joint universities multiprofessional programme'. *Journal of Inter-professional Care.* Vol 17, p 404.

Zwarenatein, M., Atkins, J., Barr, H., Hammick, K., Koppel, I. and Reeves, S. (1999) 'A systematic review of interprofessional education'. *Journal of Interprofessional Care.* Vol 13, No 4, pp 417–424.

# 14 Competence, Accountability and Delegation

The thrust of this chapter is the delegation of duties to others. The nurse, prior to delegating duties to others, must take into account the role and competence of the person to whom he/she is delegating a duty. The chapter will demonstrate that the nurse is ultimately accountable for his/her actions or omissions, both professionally and from a legal perspective in relation to a duty of care.

This chapter discusses delegation, competence and accountability from various perspectives. It addresses issues concerning those nurses who accept delegated duties and responsibilities from other nurses and other health-care professionals and those who delegate to others. It must be said at the outset, and it will be reiterated throughout this chapter, that accountability can never be delegated.

In everyday life we delegate responsibility to others. In professional practice delegation has the potential to enhance patient care and provide staff with career-development opportunities if it is carried out in an appropriate manner. This chapter addresses some of the issues that impinge on effective delegation.

There are legal ramifications associated with delegation. Delegation may reduce health-care costs, but this must not be the sole reason for delegation of responsibility occurring. Modernisation of the NHS has and will continue to demand role changes within the service of all personnel. Prior to accepting or delegating tasks, the nurse must consider the impact this may have on patient care. The nurse is legally accountable and there are four spheres of accountability: to the patient, to society, to the profession and to the employer. These issues are outlined in this chapter.

There are seven aspects associated with the delegation process that are discussed and elaborated on. It is suggested that the most important aspect is associated with knowing to whom you are delegating and his/her level of competence.

## DELEGATION AND ACCOUNTABILITY

In Chapter 1 accountability was discussed in detail. This chapter considers accountability and its relation to delegation. The code of professional conduct (NMC, 2004a) makes clear the roles and responsibilities of the nurse when delegating care delivery. Section 4 addresses issues associated with cooperation and working with other team members. Section 4.6 specifically considers delegation:

*You may be expected to delegate care delivery to others who are not registered nurses or midwives. Such delegation must not compromise existing care but must be directed to meeting the needs and serving the interests of patients and clients. You remain accountable for the appropriateness of the delegation, for ensuring that the person who does the work is able to do it and that adequate supervision or support is provided.*

When you become a registered nurse your responsibilities will increase, you will be taking on new duties and people will assume more about you, for example they will be aware that you are now deemed a competent nurse. Having undertaken and successfully completed a three-year period of education, you will now be a professional in your own right registered with the NMC. Delegation is essential for developing nursing practice. With time and practice you will become better at delegating appropriately, you will gain more insight and confidence (Lawrence et al., 2003).

Accountability can never be delegated. At no stage during the delegation process can the nurse hand over accountability (Hansten and Jackson, 2004a). Delegation involves the transferring of authority to another competent person to perform a selected task in a particular situation. However, the person delegating that task to the person deemed competent retains accountability for the outcome (National Council of State Boards of Nursing, 1995). The key factor here is the retention of accountability; this makes delegation different from abdication.

Delegation is a management/leadership activity and involves managing your own workload and developing other colleagues (Pearce, 2004). Other colleagues may include, for example, other registered nurses as well as health-care assistants, physiotherapists, occupational therapists and operating department practitioners.

Mullins (2002) defines delegation as the process of entrusting authority and responsibility to others and most cases of delegation occur from the top down. Delegation is more than just giving jobs to others to perform, it encompasses allowing others to develop understanding and confidence (Weightman, 2004).

Cartwright (2002) considers delegation to be the handing down of responsibility for action. He also suggests that it is not enough to just hand down that responsibility, the person delegating must also ensure that there are necessary resources available to carry out the task, as well as providing the person with the authority to delegate. At all times, he states, the delegator still remains accountable for the task and how it is implemented. Delegation plus the encouragement of initiative is empowerment as well as providing a degree of accountability.

Mullins (2002) points out that delegation is founded on three concepts:

- *Authority* – the right to make decisions and take actions.
- *Responsibility* – the obligation to perform certain duties.
- *Accountability* – this cannot be delegated.

**Figure 14.1** The four component parts associated with accountability
*Source*: Bergman, 1981.

Bergman (1981) provides insight into the various levels associated with accountability. Figure 14.1 demonstrates the component parts related to accountability.

Ability, according to Bergman (1981), is associated with the competence to undertake a task or delegated role, having the right knowledge and skills. Responsibility is ensuring that the role or task undertaken is done so in relation to your education and within the framework that you have been asked to work within. Accountability – the ability to act and decide on what needs to be done along with being answerable for decisions made – can only be achieved if you have been given the authority to act. Without authority, accountability will not occur. Therefore, to be accountable you must be able, responsible and have authority invested in you. When these are achieved you can provide care in an autonomous and accountable manner.

Responsibility without the authority to achieve things should be avoided. Frustration is the result of this and does little to enhance motivation. Delegation allows people scope to encourage commitment. This comes about as people are motivated by having something more responsible and complex to do (Mullins, 2002).

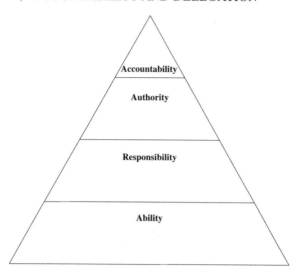

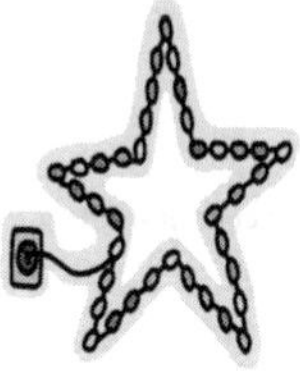

In everyday life (not only when we are at work) we often delegate. Think about some of the things in your everyday life that you delegate to others.

Things we often delegate can include:

- Allowing somebody else to go shopping for you.
- Ordering your shopping from an online shopping service.
- Allowing another person to collect your children from school/nursery.
- Permitting someone else to look after your pets while you are away.
- Taking your child to the childminder/babysitter.
- Ordering food in a restaurant and allowing somebody else to cook it for you to eat.

Hoban (2003) is of the opinion that delegation has a bad name. She considers that delegation tends to be either labelled as a leadership skill needed only by those in charge, or as a way of burdening other colleagues with tasks that you would rather not do yourself. Cohen (2004) discusses the difference between delegation and 'dumping'. There is a difference between delegating a task/activity and abdicating that activity. Belbin (2001) considers delegation not as offloading in relation to the volume of work and the responsibility attached to it, but as the choice of that responsibility.

## SKILL MIX AND DELEGATION

The nature and delivery of health care are changing as a result of policy initiatives and work-force planning developments. As the introduction of skill-mix teams is gaining momentum, the issue of delegation becomes very important and needs to be given much consideration (Forester, 2002). Not only in the UK but universally, policy is being devised to enable more people to access health care and improve the quality of care. Often, however, this is against a backdrop of tight budgetary constraints.

### ROLE CHANGE AND POLICY

Many tasks and roles hitherto associated with and undertaken by doctors, for example, are now becoming a part of the role and function of the nurse. There are many reasons for this. For instance, the reduction of junior doctors' working hours, the result of a European Union Working Time Directive, necessitated a review of skill mix. The introduction of the GMS (General Medical

Services) contract in 1990 (Department of Health and Welsh Office, 1998) heralded new roles within general practices that would impinge on the work of practice nurses in England and Wales.

The Wanless Report (2002) made recommendations that there should be a full exploitation of the potential for a transfer of work from doctors to nurse practitioners in an attempt to ease the burden on medical staff. However, Brown and Grimes (1995) had previously conducted a meta-analysis that concluded that a shift in this direction would introduce a potential shortfall in the supply of nurses, a concern the RCN (2003) also later expressed.

In general practice surgeries some practice nurses are now managing their own clinics, for example asthma and blood-pressure clinics. They are making diagnoses and in certain instances have the power to prescribe treatments. Further developments linked with the changing role of the nurse are associated with those nurses who carry out anaesthetic, endoscopy and surgical work.

While this approach to enhancing patient care should be commended, there are some concerns. There is a lack of clear definition regarding the roles, functions, levels of experience and expertise of the advanced practitioner. The lack of clarity is resulting in confusion not only for those within the health service, but also for the patient (Lankshear et al., 2005).

Health-care practice may be changed either through substitution or complementarity, for example nurses may be replaced by others, such as health-care assistants, or they may replace others, such as doctors. It could be that nurses will complement and enhance the work of others, for example physiotherapists. The RCN (2003) has nevertheless expressed concern about the extra demand that would be placed on nurses, especially during a time when nurses are in short supply.

Forester (2002) considers both skill mix and grade mix. She defines skill mix as:

> *The balance of relevant skills and experience required by staff working in a particular environment with a specific client group. This balance will relate to the nature of the experience and educational background of the staff concerned and the nature of the work.*

Grade mix is defined as:

> *The profile of the mix of grades of staff in a particular working environment. It may not reflect the skills of the staff concerned at all.*

While at first glance it may appear obvious that the differences between the two concepts are about the grade a person has, as opposed to the skills, there are some other differences (see Table 14.1).

There are many examples of good practice associated with skill-mix teams; this is as a result of careful assessment of patient needs. The introduction of skill-mix teams should be viewed as a positive approach to developing the most appropriate methods of providing care to individual patients and patient groups.

**Table 14.1** The essential differences associated with skill mix and grade mix

| Skill mix | Grade mix |
|---|---|
| • What are the needs of the group of patients?<br>• What particular mix of skills is suited to address and meet the needs of the patient?<br>• Which groups of staff have those particular skills to meet the patient's needs?<br>• How best can the team be organised to ensure appropriate allocation of responsibility? | • How much does the service to be provided cost?<br>• How could the proposed service provided by a different mix of grades be carried out more cheaply?<br>• What aspect of work performed by more expensive grades could be carried out by those who are cheaper grades? |

*Source*: Adapted from Forester, 2002.

Most nurses work in variety of teams; this is not a new concept and they may include members from social care, education and the voluntary sectors.

The use and development of skill-mix teams must be based on the following:

- The needs, wishes, wellbeing and interests of the patient must be paramount and will override any other concerns to be considered.
- The use of the skill-mix team must be evidence based.
- All staff that are a part of the skill-mix team must have ownership.
- Any roles and tasks that are to be delegated must be done after a clear assessment of competency to the delegated person/team has been undertaken.
- Ongoing monitoring of performance must occur.
- There has to be an evaluation of the skill-mix team's performance.

The Community Practitioners' and Health Visitors' Association (CPHVA) has noted, however, that there have been incidences where inappropriate delegation of some health-visiting responsibilities has occurred (Forester, 2002). The consequences of inappropriate delegation (not only within the sphere of health visiting) may have implications for the quality of patient care and, as such, the protection of the public. The impact on patient care and patient outcomes associated with delegation – the transfer of work from nurses to others and from others to nurses – needs to be given serious consideration.

Salvage (2003) suggests that there are times when tasks delegated to nurses – for example tasks usually undertaken by a doctor – are delegated because the doctor recognises that the nurse has superior skills and expertise. Often, however, she points out that this may be because the task is routine, unpopular and time consuming.

In developing the role, function and contribution that nurses make to enhance the health of society, this will inevitably result in the need to take on delegated roles. These delegated roles and functions may be situated in unpopular locations, at night, at the weekend and with unpopular patient groups such as the homeless and sex workers (Salvage, 2003). The nurse should not strive to become a mini doctor but a maxi nurse (RCN and Department of Health, 2005).

Prior to taking on these delegated roles and functions, Gibbons (2003) suggests that the nurse consider the following points:

- Is this in the best interest of the patient?
- Do I have the appropriate skills and knowledge?
- Are there the appropriate resources available to support me undertaking this task?
- Will no other element/aspect of patient care suffer if I take on this role?

If the nurse is unable to meet the criteria above, then he/she must refuse to take on the role, seek help and advice from senior colleagues and consult the code of professional conduct.

## DELEGATION: THE LEGAL PERSPECTIVE

Accountability has been addressed in many chapters in this text. Indeed, it could be tentatively suggested that accountability impinges on every aspect of nursing practice and as such should apply to and is associated with every chapter. However, to reiterate, the registered nurse has four explicit lines of accountability:

- to the patient
- to society
- to the profession
- to the employer

When accepting delegated responsibility or when giving delegated responsibility, the nurse must bear in mind the following:

- When working as a team member you are personally accountable for your own actions or omissions – there is no such concept as team negligence. If harm occurs, you are individually accountable.
- You must determine if the person you are delegating to is able to undertake the task. You must provide him/her with adequate resources and supervision. He/she must be deemed competent.
- You must keep up to date your knowledge and skills in order to practise safely and effectively within the scope of the law. You must acknowledge your limitations.
- You must make known and obtain help and supervision from a competent practitioner if you feel an aspect of practice lies beyond your level of competence or outside your area of registration.

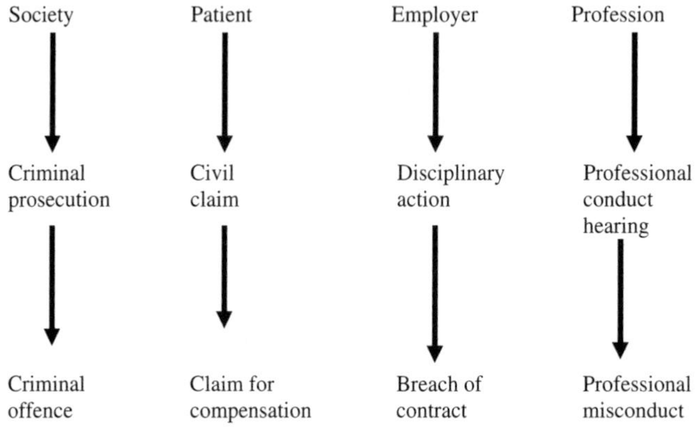


**Figure 14.2** Legal accountability

Figure 14.2 considers the four spheres of accountability.

There are some aspects of health-care-related activity that under statutory provision prohibit delegation. For example:

- The Mental Health Act 1983 provides that only a registered medical practitioner (a doctor) can recommend detention and carry out other statutory functions in relation to a mentally ill patient.
- Only specified registered practitioners (see Chapter 12) can prescribe certain medicines as result of the Medicines Act 1968.
- Dimond (2005a) uses an example from midwifery practice under article 45 of the Nursing and Midwifery Order (2001) – attendance by unqualified persons at childbirth. Section 45 (i) states: 'A person other than a registered midwife or registered medical practitioner shall not attend a woman in child birth.' This section of the order prohibits the delegation of attendance at the birth of a child.

In cases where the law (statute) does not specify that a particular profession carries out a particular activity, then common law (this is also known as judge or case-made law) will apply. The principle underpinning common law in relation to delegation is that provided the activity is carried out to a reasonable degree, which could have been met by the person who has delegated the activity, then delegation is not against the law.

The Bolam Test (see for example *Bolam* v *Friern Barnet HMC* [1957] 2 All ER 118) is a legal test that determines if the reasonable standard of care required is of the same standard that would have been provided by the person delegating the responsibility. In one particular case (*Wilshire* v *Essex Area Health Authority CA* [1986] 3 All ER 801) a junior doctor had failed to provide a reasonable standard of care to a premature infant. The doctor had placed a cannula measuring oxygen levels in a vein instead of an artery. The error resulted in serious harm to the baby. The duty delegated to the doctor was inappropriately delegated. It would similarly be inappropriate, indeed irresponsible, to delegate duties normally carried out by an experienced staff nurse to a junior student nurse.

In determining what to delegate, and to perform the delegated responsibilities to the requisite standard, the delegator has the responsibility to ensure that the person carrying out the activities has the following:

- knowledge
- experience
- education
- competence

From the outset the delegator determines if it is appropriate to delegate the task or duty. Assessment of the competence of the delegatee, for example the health-care assistant, is required. Often this is done by observing and supervising the health-care assistant carrying out the task. The degree of supervision required may reduce over time as the delegatee gains confidence and competence (Dimond, 2005a), but to reiterate, at no time must the delegator delegate accountability.

Having carefully supervised the delegatee and deemed him/her competent, the delegator has acted in a reasonable manner in ensuring that the delegatee is competent, has adequate resources and is appropriately supervised. However, if harm occurs to the patient as a result of negligence caused by the person to whom responsibility has been delegated, according to Dimond (2005a) the delegator is not negligent as he/she had taken all reasonable precautions.

## DELEGATION: SEVEN ASSOCIATED ASPECTS

Hansten and Jackson (2004a) have suggested that there are seven aspects associated with the delegation process. Like the nursing process they are cyclical (see Figure 14.3).

### KNOW YOUR WORLD

Clearly, health-care delivery systems and ways of working are changing and will continue to change. Shortened lengths of stay in hospital, the introduction of critical care pathways, advances in technology, increased consumer involvement and demographic trends are examples of how health and social-care provision is influenced by the modernisation agenda. Porter-O'Grady (2003) notes that one of the biggest areas of change involves the provision of care through others – the delegation of traditional nursing tasks to others.

Increasingly, the nurse is being requested and required to delegate work to care givers such as health-care assistants whom they may know little about. Understanding issues that impinge on your role and your ability to provide quality care – the driving forces leading to the changes above – will help you delegate effectively.

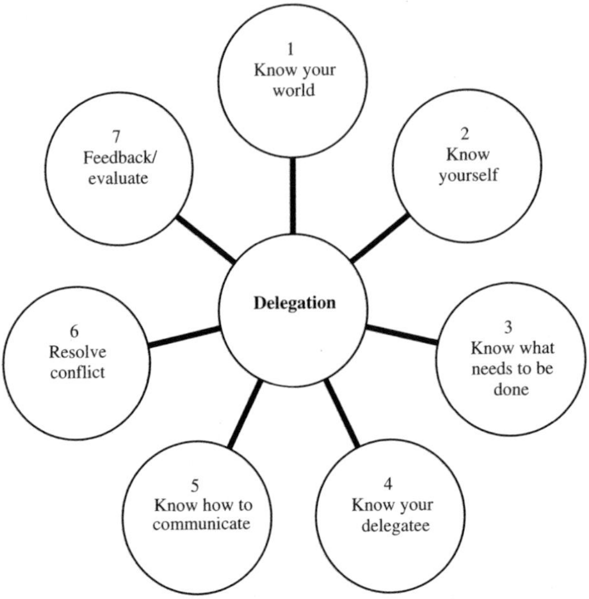


**Figure 14.3** The seven aspects associated with delegation
*Source*: Handsten and Jackson, 2004a.

## KNOW YOURSELF

Knowing your own abilities and limitations is an essential component of effective delegation. Self-analysis and self-understanding are prerequisites, according to Hansten and Jackson (2004b). Being able to recognise your own attributes that may impede effective delegation, such as emotions or beliefs, may enable you to understand your actions.

Take time also to examine your motivation and the reason you are delegating the particular task. Determine that you are delegating for the right reasons (Hoban, 2003).

## KNOW WHAT NEEDS TO BE DONE

Pressure and the amount of work to be done often result in delegation of duties. Working with others in a successful manner necessitates knowledge of the total picture – knowing what needs to be done. The nurse must ensure that that he/she delegates appropriately, effectively and efficiently. Care will need to be prioritised as well as delegating to the right individual based on competence. The key components are an extensive knowledge base and the ability to make sound judgements.

## KNOW YOUR DELEGATEE

Having examined yourself (know yourself) and knowing what needs to be done, it is imperative that you know to whom you are delegating – the delegatee. Perhaps this is the most important aspect of the cycle.

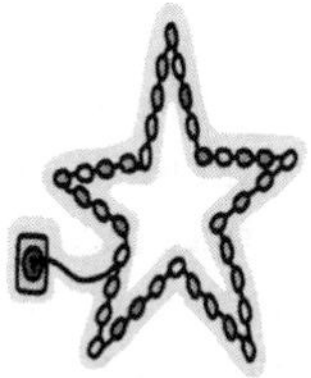

Make a list of those to whom you think you (as registered nurse) may need to delegate.

Here are some of the potential delegatees:

- student nurses (was this first on your list?)
- new staff nurses
- health-care assistants (at various levels)
- speech and language therapists
- physiotherapists
- occupational therapists
- paramedics
- pharmacists
- clerical staff/ward clerks
- volunteers
- social workers
- medical students
- doctors
- phlebotomists

You may think that strictly speaking nurses do not delegate to some of the people listed above. Nurses may not ask some of those people to carry out nursing tasks, but they may ask them to do things for the patient and the nurse acts as coordinator of care. Therefore the same principles associated with safe and effective delegation will apply.

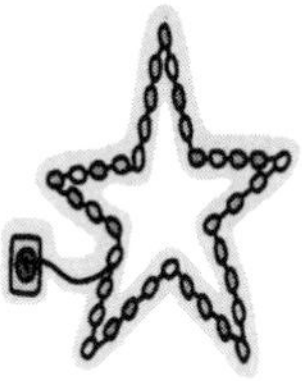

Think about your own family. Who in the family does the cooking and the cleaning? Is that left up to your mother/partner? Is your father/partner responsible for fixing things around the house or on the car? What is your responsibility in the house – do you have any tasks that fall to you to perform?

If this is the case then each person has a role to play and certain things are expected of them – they have their 'job descriptions'. However, family roles and responsibilities are changing. For example, the father may be the only parent and it may be him who is responsible not only for cleaning and cooking, but also for maintaining things around the house. The family analogy used here can also apply to professional practice: the role of the nurse (and it has been said many times in this text) is changing. Families and family roles are becoming more flexible, fluid and dynamic; so too are nurses' roles. Job descriptions for family members may not be written as a job description is written for your work. Job descriptions at work not only have a written element to them but also an unwritten element attached to them.

Before you delegate to others you must have some insight into their roles. Understanding what their role is (as well as your own) will enable you to be clear about what your expectation of the other is. Whatever you delegate must fall within the remit of the job description of the delegatee; to do otherwise would be inappropriate and potentially dangerous.

Assessing the competency of the person to whom you are delegating is an important activity. The Nursing and Midwifery Council is required by law (Nursing and Midwifery Order 2001) to establish standards of proficiency that must be met by applicants to different parts of the professional register. These standards are mandatory and in accordance with statutory legislation and are seen as necessary to provide safe and effective practice. The standards of proficiency for nursing are the overarching principles of being able to practise as a nurse (NMC, 2004b). The standards of proficiency for nursing can be found in Appendix 14.1. You may note that one of the proficiencies is:

*Delegate duties to others, as appropriate, ensuring that they are supervised and monitored.*

A result of this requirement is that the NMC has standardised all educational programmes leading to registration and has produced standards of proficiency for pre-registration nursing education (NMC, 2004b). The NMC has:

- Defined competence.
- Set standards of proficiency.
- Evaluated nurses (through devolved responsibility to institutions of higher education).
- Implemented a system that manages those who fall below the level of competency expected after registration.

Every nurse who appears on the NMC's register will therefore be expected to be able to perform to a particular standard on registration, and at that point he/she is deemed competent. This provides reassurance to the public that the nurse has met the requisite standards of proficiency.

Health-care assistants' standards of competence may be found in their job descriptions or associated with their programme of study, for example SNVQ or NVQ. Currently there is no regulation for health-care assistants in the UK (Salvage, 2003); however this may change in the near future (Dimond, 2005a). Specific behaviours that might be expected of health-care assistants may also be cited explicitly in their job description, for example:

- Reporting and advising the registered nurse of any change in the patient's condition.
- Collecting of urine, sputum and stool specimens.
- Testing of urine and stool specimens.
- Taking vital signs.
- Providing oral hygiene.

In some trusts health-care assistants may be deemed competent to administer enemata, perform venepuncture or apply dressings, and in others this may not be allowed. The lack of consistency provides a challenge for the nurse when considering the delegation of some tasks. It is important, therefore, to know whom you are delegating to. You must fully understand the job description and other organisational policies associated with the role of the people you may delegate to; you need to match the job description to the delegated activity. You should never allow a delegatee to perform beyond their role and level of competence.

While much of the above discussion centres on the 'official' role expectations of personnel, there are, as has been suggested, some unofficial expectations. These 'grey areas' can arise when you (or the delegatee) may have inappropriate expectations of the delegatee. Understanding the job description of the delegatee and encouraging effective, honest, open two-way communication can result in better clarification of role expectations, reduction in conflict and improvement in patient care. The expectations of all parties concerned should be openly expressed in a non-threatening manner.

Table 14.2 summarises some of the important points you need to consider in an attempt to know yourself and the delegatee better.

## KNOW HOW TO COMMUNICATE

Open, honest and effective two-way communication is vital if delegation is to work efficiently, as already discussed. Washburn (1991) suggests that there are four Cs associated with effective communication – it must be:

- **C**lear
- **C**oncise
- **C**orrect
- **C**omplete

**Table 14.2** Some points to consider when getting to know the delegatee

- Know your job description and the job description of the delegatee.
- Make sure the person is interested in the task and has the necessary skills and ability to achieve it.
- Know the policies and procedures in place in your organisation that may impinge on the delegation process.
- Be constantly aware of the concepts of competency and accountability.
- Know your own strengths and weaknesses and the strengths and weaknesses of the delegatee.
- Know how to motivate and support others.
- Continually supervise, monitor and provide feedback to the delegatee.
- Be realistic.
- You cannot control every action of those to whom you delegate.
- Remember that delegatees are also responsible for their actions or omissions.
- Be aware of the delegatee's workload.

*Source*: Adapted from Hansten and Jackson, 2004c; Pearce, 2004; Hoban, 2003.

When the nurse delegates to another he/she is entrusting another person to act in his/her place for that particular task (O'Neill, 2004). It is important for this reason that the nurse communicates effectively. The person you are delegating to is not you, and you must be aware that he/she may not perform the task to your standards. Therefore you must make every effort to ensure that he/she knows exactly what is expected of them.

It may seem obvious, but you must know what it is you are delegating. If you cannot explain (communicate effectively) to the delegatee what it is you are delegating then the task is not to be delegated. Ensure that you are specific about the task to be delegated, that you are able to measure and determine if the task has been completed, be realistic in your expectations and apply a time element to the task being delegated.

At all times during the delegation process allow the delegatee the opportunity to raise any concerns or questions he/she may have (Hoban, 2003). Listen to any concerns and provide appropriate responses. You may also need to inform other team members of what has been delegated and to whom (Pearce, 2004). However, Mullins (2002) notes that the more specific the instructions and terms of reference, the less stimulating the task is and as a result of this little learning will occur. The criterion for assessing if delegation has been successful, according to O'Neill (2004), is the completion of the task.

## RESOLVING CONFLICT

Conflict is inevitable and the way it is managed will determine the outcome of delegation, the ability to move on and enhance nursing practice and the ability to continue to delegate appropriately. Even prior to delegating conflict may occur: for example the delegatee may be unable or unwilling to accept the delegated task or there may be a shortage of staff, meaning no one else is available to delegate to (Boswell, 2005). Attempt to resolve conflict prior to delegating or as soon as there is evidence of it arising.

### GIVING FEEDBACK AND EVALUATING

Providing feedback and evaluating processes constitute the final stage of the seven-step approach. This also has the ability to feed into the first stage, 'knowing your world', and starting the cycle over again when the next occasion to delegate arises. Feedback, when given appropriately, can have positive repercussions, can enhance working relationships and can encourage reflection and improve self-awareness (Boswell, 2005). The delegatee should be given the opportunity to self-assess his/her performance, highlighting any difficulties that may have occurred. The outcome of evaluation may provide you with a chance to develop training needs and to enhance and improve your own delegating skills.

Providing the delegatee with feedback and evaluating outcomes – be it a thank-you or a more in-depth discussion – means that you have fulfilled your obligations in association with the cycle. You have monitored, evaluated and followed up on your delegated activity. Feedback and evaluation do not occur as one-off activities, they are continuous activities that enable you to intervene should the need arise. Offering feedback can also be seen as offering support and supervision. Robbins (2005) suggests that providing praise and encouragement when difficulties are being encountered may help ease the situation and restore self-confidence.

## FACTORS ASSOCIATED WITH DELEGATION

There are many influencing factors that need to be considered regarding delegation: delegation from doctors to nurses, between nurses and other health-care professionals. The attitude of the person delegating responsibility will facilitate or inhibit the level of task and role sharing (Richardson et al., 2000). Some tasks they found, such as ear syringing and dressings, were easily delegated to the nurse by the general practitioner. However, there are other tasks that the GP was more reluctant to delegate. Reasons for this centred on:

- fear of incompetence
- loss of independence
- creation of more work
- loss of doctor–patient relationship

Attitudes towards delegation are changing and some areas where this is occurring have been identified, for example the endoscopy nurse practitioner, the emergency nurse practitioner.

Effective delegation is delegating with trust – Brown (1997) sees trust as the key word when delegating – with only the minimum of controls. The outcome will depend on the blend between trust and control, the difficulty of the task and the risks associated with it. The delegatee's skills, experience and willingness to take on the task and finally the nurse's skills, experience, willingness to delegate the task and ability to provide constructive feedback will have ramifications for the outcome of delegated actions.

Some of the barriers to effective delegation have already been mentioned, for example lack of confidence, loss of power and loss of authority. Delegation brings with it a degree of risk. The nurse must balance the risks and benefits to the patient before delegating – always acting in the patient's best interests.

Lack of experience, both of the delegator (staff nurse for example) and delegatee (for example student nurse), is a factor that needs consideration. Often when delegating to student nurses the staff nurse needs to consider the level of the student's education, skill acquisition and experience. Using delegation as a form of coaching can help both student and staff nurse to enhance and increase experience and expertise – it is a two-way learning process. Step by step the staff nurse can develop the student's skills and levels of competence as well as his/her own.

## CONCLUSIONS

The role and function of the nurse will continue to expand. This is primarily in response to the government's attempts to modernise the NHS. One result of this is a change in the skill mix. Ongoing evaluation is required to determine if the expanding roles undertaken by the nurse and the delegation of roles and duties previously held by the nurse to others are effective.

Effective delegation is the allocation of tasks and responsibilities to those staff who are best suited to do them. This then provides them with the freedom to perform the activity safely and in the most appropriate and effective manner, in the patient's best interests.

Effective delegation is not easy: it is concerned with trusting other people and having confidence in them. The nurse faces challenges when he/she delegates. A balance must be achieved between delegating too much or too little and between over-supervision and under-supervision (Pearce, 2004). Delegation is a useful tool in career development; it can also enhance individual skill development.

The NMC is yet to decide what duties, responsibilities or tasks the registered nurse can delegate. Dimond (2005b) suggests that it would be useful if the NMC would identify principles that would apply to the delegation of activities, as well as suggesting the educational and training requirements for delegation.

There is evidence that nurses can substitute effectively for doctors in some areas, such as arthritis, diabetes mellitus and Parkinson's disease (Hewitt et al., 2003). This evidence, applied in an appropriate manner, has the potential to enhance patient care. This should be the primary aim of delegating responsibility to others.

When a task has been delegated the nurse cannot just withdraw from it. The nurse remains accountable for what the delegatee does or does not do.

## REFERENCES


Belbin, R.M. (2001) *Team Roles at Work*. Heinemann. Oxford.

Bergman, R. (1981) 'Accountability – Definition and dimensions'. *International Nursing Review*. Vol 28, No 2, pp 53–59.

Boswell, A. (2005) 'How effective delegation can build better teams'. *Nursing Times*. Vol 101, No 20, pp 60–61.

Brown, C. (1997) *Essential Delegation Skills*. Gower. Aldershot.

Brown, S.A. and Grimes, D.E. (1995) 'A meta-analysis of nurse practitioners and nurse midwives in primary care'. *Nursing Research*. Vol 44, No 6, pp 332–339.

Cartwright, R. (2002) *Mastering Team Leadership*. Palgrave. Basingstoke.

Cohen, S. (2004) 'Delegating vs. dumping: Teach the difference'. *Nursing Management*. Vol 35, No 10, pp 14–18.

Department of Health and Welsh Office (1998) *General Practice in the NHS: A New Contract*. HMSO. London.

Dimond, B. (2005a) 'Legal liability of the midwifery delegator'. *British Journal of Midwifery*. Vol 13, No 1, p 41.

Dimond, B. (2005b) 'Is the delegation of midwifery tasks ever legal?'. *British Journal of Midwifery*. Vol 13, No 1, p 42.

Forester, S. (2002) *Professional Briefing: Delegation and Professional Accountability*. Community Practitioner's and Health Visitor's Association. London.

Gibbons, P. (2003) 'Ethical dimensions of practice' in Hinchliff, S., Norman, S. and Schober, J. (eds) (4th edn) *Nursing Practice and Health Care*. Arnold. London. Ch 5 pp 77–97.

Hansten, R.I. and Jackson, M. (2004a) 'The overall process of delegation' in Hansten, R.I. and Jackson, M. (eds) (3rd edn) *Clinical Delegation Skills: A Handbook for Professional Practice*. Jones and Bartlett. Boston. Ch 1 pp 1–9.

Hansten, R.I. and Jackson, M. (2004b) 'Know yourself' in Hansten, R.I. and Jackson, M. (eds) (3rd edn) *Clinical Delegation Skills: A Handbook for Professional Practice*. Jones and Bartlett. Boston. Ch 5 pp 113–146.

Hansten, R.I. and Jackson, M. (2004c) 'Know your delegate' in Hansten, R.I. and Jackson, M. (eds) (3rd edn) *Clinical Delegation Skills: A Handbook for Professional Practice*. Jones and Bartlett. Boston. Ch 7 pp 193–234.

Hewitt, C., Lankshear, A., Maynard, A., Sheldon, T. and Smith, K. (2003) *Health Service Workforce and Health Outcomes: A Scoping Exercise*. University of York. York.

Hoban, V. (2003) 'How to . . . enhance your delegation skills'. *Nursing Times*. Vol 99, No 13, pp 80–81.

Lankshear, A., Sheldon, T., Maynard, A. and Smith, K. (2005) *Health Policy Matters: Helping Decision Makers Put Health Policy into Practice*. University of York. York.

Lawrence, C., Gibson, F. and Zur, J. (2003) 'Care delivery: The needs of children' in Hinchliff, S., Norman, S. and Schober, J. (eds) (4th edn) *Nursing Practice and Health Care*. Arnold. London. Ch 8 pp 177–202.

Mullins, L. (2002) (6th edn) *Management and Organisational Behaviour.* Prentice Hall. Harlow.

National Council of State Boards of Nursing (1995) *Delegation: Concepts and Decision-Making Process.* National Council of State Boards of Nursing. Chicago.

Nursing and Midwifery Council (2004a) *The NMC Code of Professional Conduct: Standards for Conduct, Performance and Ethics.* NMC. London.

Nursing and Midwifery Council (2004b) *Standards of Proficiency for Pre Registration Nursing Education.* NMC. London.

Nursing and Midwifery Order (2001) Statutory Instrument 2002 No 253.

O'Neill, L. (2004) 'Know how to communicate' in Hansten, R.I. and Jackson, M. (eds) (3rd edn) *Clinical Delegation Skills: A Handbook for Professional Practice.* Jones and Bartlett. Boston. Ch 8 pp 235–254.

Pearce, C. (2004) 'Honing the art of effective delegation'. *Nursing Times.* Vol 100, No 29, pp 46–47.

Porter-O'Grady, T. (2003) 'A different age for leadership, Part 1'. *Journal of Nursing Administration.* Vol 33, No 2, pp 115–110.

Richardson, A., Carley, J., Jenkins-Clarke, S. and Richards, D.A. (2000) 'Skill mix between nurses and doctors working in primary care – delegation or allocation: A review of the literature'. *International Journal of Nursing Studies.* Vol 37, pp 185–197.

Robbins, F. (2005) 'Managing the performance of staff teams and individuals'. *Nursing and Residential Care.* Vol 7, No 4, pp 148–150.

Royal College of Nursing (2003) *More Nurses, Working Differently? A Review of the UK Nursing Labour Market for 2002–2003.* RCN. London.

Royal College of Nursing and Department of Health (2005) *Maxi Nurses: Working in Advanced and Extended Roles Promoting and Developing Patient Centred Health Care.* RCN. London.

Salvage, J. (2003) 'Nursing today and tomorrow' in Hinchliff, S., Norman, S. and Schober, J. (eds) (4th edn) *Nursing Practice and Health Care.* Arnold. London. Ch 1 pp 1–24.

Wanless, D. (2002) *Securing Our Future Health: Taking a Long Term View.* HM Treasury Public Enquiry Unit. London.

Washburn, M.J. (1991) 'Delegation: The art of getting things through others'. *AZ Nurse.* January, p 1.

Weightman, J. (2004) (2nd edn) *Managing People.* The Charted Institute of Personnel and Development. London.

## APPENDIX 14.1 THE STANDARDS OF PROFICIENCY FOR NURSING

- Manage oneself, one's practice, and that of others, in accordance with *The NMC code of professional conduct: standards for conduct, performance and ethics* (the Code), recognising one's own abilities and limitations.
- Practise in accordance with an ethical and legal framework which ensures the primacy of patient and client interest and well-being and respects confidentiality.

- Practise in a fair and anti-discriminatory way, acknowledging the differences in beliefs and cultural practices of individuals or groups.
- Engage in, develop and disengage from therapeutic relationships through the use of appropriate communication and interpersonal skills.
- Create and utilise opportunities to promote the health and wellbeing of patients, clients and groups.
- Undertake and document a comprehensive, systematic and accurate nursing assessment of the physical, psychological, social and spiritual needs of patients, clients and communities.
- Formulate and document a plan of nursing care, where possible in partnership with patients, clients, their carers and family and friends, within a framework of informed consent.
- Based on the best available evidence, apply knowledge and an appropriate repertoire of skills indicative of safe nursing practice.
- Provide a rationale for the nursing care delivered which takes account of social, cultural, spiritual, legal, political and economic influences.
- Evaluate and document the outcomes of nursing and other interventions.
- Demonstrate sound clinical judgement across a range of differing professional and care delivery contexts.
- Contribute to public protection by creating and maintaining a safe environment of care through the use of quality assurance and risk management strategies.
- Demonstrate knowledge of effective inter-professional working practices which respect and utilize the contributions of members of the health- and social-care team.
- Delegate duties to others, as appropriate, ensuring that they are supervised and monitored.
- Demonstrate key skills.
- Demonstrate a commitment to the need for continuing professional development and personal supervision activities in order to enhance knowledge, skills, values and attitudes needed for safe and effective nursing practice.
- Enhance the professional development and safe practice of others through peer support, leadership, supervision and teaching.

*Source*: NMC, 2004b. This is Crown copyright material which is reproduced with the permission of the Controller of HMSO and the Queen's Printer for Scotland.

# 15 Key Skills

Key skills that underpin the practice of all nurses, demonstrating proficiency at literacy, numeracy and problem solving are vital components of safe and effective practice (Lawrence et al., 2003). Failure to articulate clearly using words and numbers can impinge on the quality of care. The nurse is not only required to calculate in order to ensure drug doses are safe, but also to communicate coherently and document accurately.

The key skills concerned in this chapter are:

- skills associated with literacy
- skills required for numeracy
- computer skills

The above issues are addressed and related to the need to develop these skills in order to record, enter, store, retrieve and organise data essential for care delivery. One aspect of the chapter will provide you with study skills guidance. In this section you will be offered points and tips to consider using when writing essays and preparing for assignments. These proficiencies may be required during your programme of study and beyond.

Prior to entering nurse education, educational institutions are required by the NMC (NMC, 2004c) to ensure that all applicants provide evidence of literacy and numeracy. This is to enable the candidates to cope with the demands of pre-registration nursing programmes and to ensure that the interests of the public are served. If candidates are applying to an educational institution in Wales, they must, where required, be able to demonstrate proficiency in the use of the Welsh language.

Computer skills and the use of information technology will be addressed briefly in this chapter. You are encouraged to seek support while on clinical placement and also when attending theory sessions to develop and enhance your skills in these domains. It is not the aim of this chapter to provide the reader with in-depth information regarding key skills, merely to emphasise the importance of becoming proficient in them.

## NUMERACY

Woodrow (1998) suggests that people do not become nurses to practise mathematics. However, all nurses need to have an understanding of calculation in order to perform their job effectively and, above all, safely. It is important, therefore, that nurses are able to carry out accurate drug calculations and other arithmetically based activities to perform within the code of professional conduct (NMC, 2004a). In doing patients no harm and acting in their best interests, drug calculations are an essential skill (Wright, 2005; NMC, 2004b). More often than not the use of calculation is predominantly, but not exclusively, associated with drug administration.

Hutton (2005) points out that the nurse should apply common-sense rules to drug calculations, for example knowing what a sensible answer should be. This will come with experience. The nurse should never, however, make assumptions. He/she should never assume that the prescription is correct and if in doubt referral to recommended dose ranges published in drug formularies is required.

It has been demonstrated that the nurse's ability to calculate accurately is flawed. Trim (2004) points out that over the last decade discrepancies associated with the nurse's ability to calculate correctly have been highlighted (see for example Bindler and Bayne, 1991; Blais and Bath, 1992; Segatore et al., 1993; Arnold, 1998). Errors associated with incorrect calculations occur in all branches and within all areas of nursing and this can threaten the lives and wellbeing of patients (Gray and Jackson, 2004; Weeks et al., 2000).

In a study undertaken by Taxis and Barber (2003) associated with intravenous medication errors, it was determined that out of 1042 intravenous medications, 49 per cent of errors were linked with the preparation and administration of the drugs. There are many reasons why drug errors may occur. Gray and Jackson (2004) posit that this may be because of the increase in technology and the vast range of drugs available. Hall (2000), when considering neonatal drug calculations, states that medicines are not usually manufactured with the neonate in mind, and as such this makes the administration and calculation of medicines for neonates potentially difficult. On a similar note, Woodrow (1998) considers the difficulties faced by paediatric nurses, as paediatric patients have less physiological reserve than adults and as a result are less able to compensate for approximations or mistakes. Weeks et al. (2000) suggest that the mathematics nurses are required to deal with, such as calculating drug doses, are becoming more critical and complex.

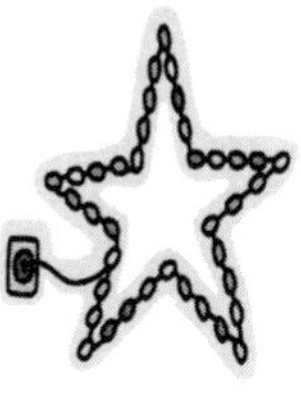

What other areas (apart from the administration of medicines) associated with the role of the nurse do you think require the use of calculations and demonstrate numeracy?

The following is a possible list:

- Nurse educationalists/mentors when calculating final grades for theoretical and practice assessments.
- When working out blood results, for example a nurse working in a renal unit and caring for patients who are undergoing renal dialysis.
- When a charge nurse needs to calculate the number of staff to safely staff a ward or unit.
- When working in accident and emergency units/burns units and calculating the percentages of burns a patient has suffered (see Chapter 6 and the rule of nines).
- When working out the body mass index (BMI).
- When dealing with a patient's money after admission to a ward or hospital department, e.g. an acute psychiatric admissions ward.

The government's publication *Building a Safer NHS for Patients* (Department of Health, 2004) focuses on the importance of safe medicines administration. The most common incidents reported by the National Audit Office (2005) were falls, followed by medication errors. Chapter 12 of this text has also highlighted the importance of safe drug administration.

The problems faced by nurses regarding computation are not exclusive to the UK. Problems are evident in the Unites States (Polifroni et al., 2003), Sweden (Kapborg, 1994), Canada (Segatore et al., 1993) and Japan (Kawamura, 2001). The reasons why problems associated with medication error occur are often related to the poor skills and competence levels of the nurses who make the calculations (Wright, 2004).

For student nurses and all health-care professionals, learning how to calculate drug dosages is an important skill (Wright, 2005). Kapborg (1994) states that numerous research studies have demonstrated that both student nurses and qualified nurses are unable to calculate all drug doses presented to them in a maths test, with an error rate of approximately 1 in 10 calculations. Improving the drug-calculation skills of nurses is one way in which drug errors, the harm caused to patients (iatrogenic complications) and the potential ensuing litigation may be reduced.

Weeks et al. (2000) acknowledge that it is essential that continued efforts are made for student nurses in theoretical and clinical domains in order to promote and develop this essential skill. Woodrow (1998) suggests that in spite of the increasing numbers and complexity of calculations that nurses are making on a daily basis, there is little preparation or support for the development of mathematical skills. Wilson (2003) concludes that poor mathematical skills are the primary reason why nurses sometimes fail to calculate correctly.

To reduce the numbers of medication errors caused by drug dose or volume errors, Trim (2004) suggests that the nurse must be familiar with the various formulae available. Calculators may be used in the clinical area to help the nurse; however, Preston (2004) states that mistakes with calculators do occur.

This chapter cannot address every mathematical problem that the nurse may face. It provides a basic introduction to simple mathematical calculations and their application to practice. This section of the chapter is not intended as a remedial course for those with numeracy problems. You are strongly advised to hone your numeracy skills whenever the opportunity arises; there are several resources available to you, both human and material. At every stage of the calculation process, should you feel unsure or in doubt, you must seek help, advice and support.

The following points may help you in the clinical area to ensure safe practice:

- Remember at all stages that the patient's best interests come first.
- Take your time and if possible work out calculations in a quiet area.
- If the answer looks unusual, recheck and ask a colleague to examine what you have done.
- Use a calculator and other aids if you need to.
- If you are still unsure do not give the drug, seek help.

In the UK the predominant system of measurement in health care is the metric system, SI. Le Système International d'Unités (SI) came into operation in the 1960s and has been widely adopted and recognised by nearly all countries. Table 15.1 outlines common decimal weights.

**Note:** Milligrams and millilitres are plural, as are metres, centimetres and millimetres. However, the appropriate abbreviations are mg ***not*** mgs and ml ***not*** mls, m ***not*** ms, cm ***not*** cms and mm ***not*** mms.

Place value is associated with numbers and each number from 0 to 9 is written in a column, for example:

- units
- tens

**Table 15.1** Common decimal weights, volumes and lengths

| | |
|---|---|
| **Weights** | |
| 1 gram (g) | = 1000 milligrams (mg) |
| 1 mg | = 1000 micrograms (mcg) (never use ug, this may be mistaken for mg) |
| 1 mcg | = 1000 nanograms (ng) (always write nanograms in full, ng can easily be mistaken for mg) |
| **Volumes** | |
| 1 litre (l) | = 1000 millilitres (ml) |
| **Lengths** | |
| 1 metre | = 100 centimetres (cm) |
| 1 cm | = 10 millimetres (mm) |

**Table 15.2** Numbers in words and figures

| Numbers in words | Numbers in figures | | | |
|---|---|---|---|---|
| | Thousands | Hundreds | Tens | Units |
| Two hundred and fifty eight | – | 2 | 5 | 8 |
| Six thousand four hundred | 6 | 4 | 0 | 0 |
| Eighty nine | – | – | 8 | 9 |
| Twenty one | – | – | 2 | 1 |

**Table 15.3** Numbers and the decimal point

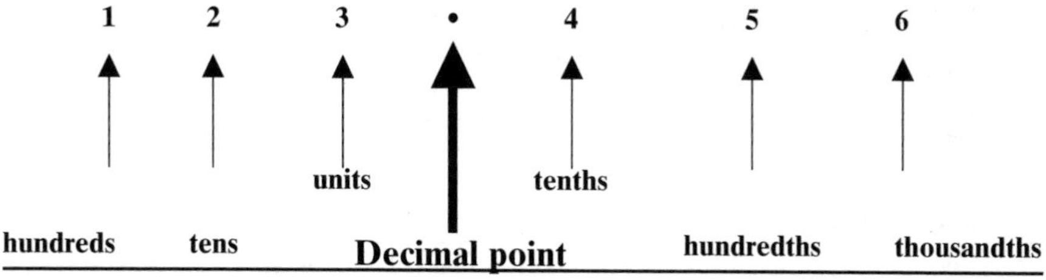


- hundreds
- thousands

Table 15.2 demonstrates numbers written and in figures.

Numbers that are smaller than one unit are decimals, for example tenths, hundredths and thousandths. These are separated by the decimal point; see Table 15.3.

## ADDING AND SUBTRACTING DECIMALS

You will be required to use addition and subtraction nearly every day in your work, for example when calculating a patient's fluid balance. In most cases of fluid balance decimal points are not required; you would round up or down to the nearest whole number. However, in the acutely ill or the neonate, for example, exact amounts may be required.

In Figure 15.1 calculate the amount of fluid the child has had via the intravenous route for 24 hours. Then calculate the amount of fluid aspirated from the nasogastric tube and urine via the urinary catheter. Total the input and output values, subtracting input from output, and arrive at the child's fluid balance. Is it negative or positive?

Numbers that are left of the decimal point are greater than one. Those numbers situated right of the decimal point are less than one. In the following example note the position of the decimal point:

| | | | | | |
|---|---|---|---|---|---|
| **Anytown Hospital** | | | | | |
| **Fluid Balance Chart** | | | | | |
| Name..................................................................................................... | | | | | |
| Ward..................................................................................................... | | | | | |
| Hospital Number..................................................................................................... | | | | | |
| DoB..................................................................................................... | | | | | |

| Time | Input (in ml) | | Output (in ml) | | |
|---|---|---|---|---|---|
| | **Intravenous** | **Oral/other** | **Urine** | **Other** | **Comments** |
| **0000** | 2.60 | NBM | 20 | | |
| **0100** | 2.65 | | 10 | 1.20 | Nasogastric |
| **0200** | 2.75 | | 10 | | |
| **0300** | 3.84 | | 8.2 | | |
| **0400** | 8.70 | | 2.6 | | |
| **0500** | 6.00 | | 8.0 | 1.80 | Nasogastric |
| **0600** | 6.00 | | 12.2 | | |
| **0700** | 9.90 | | 10.2 | | |
| **0800** | 3.65 | | 10 | | |
| **0900** | 7.75 | | 14 | 1.10 | Nasogastric |
| **1000** | 12.00 | | 13 | | |
| **1100** | 12.75 | | 14.7 | | |
| **1200** | 20.00 | | 12.4 | | |
| **1300** | 21.20 | | 20 | 1.20 | Nasogastric |
| **1400** | 22.00 | | 32 | | |
| **1500** | 75.00 | | 36 | | |
| **1600** | 75.00 | | 26 | | |
| **1700** | 15.00 | | 28 | 1.75 | Nasogastric |
| **1800** | 0.75 | | 23 | | |
| **1900** | 0.75 | | 22 | | |
| **2000** | 1.75 | | 18 | | |
| **2100** | 10.75 | | 12.8 | 1.80 | Nasogastric |
| **2200** | 20.75 | | 14.6 | | |
| **2300** | 21.75 | ▼ | 12.4 | | |
| **Total** | | Nil | | | |

**Figure 15.1** A neonate's fluid balance chart

- 1.60 is equal to one plus a fraction of one (6/10).
- 0.75 is equal to a fraction of one (75/100).

## MULTIPLYING DECIMALS

Often drug calculations require you to multiply and divide. Multiplying a decimal is done in exactly the same way as you multiply whole numbers; however, you have to consider the decimal point. Always remember to put the decimal point in the correct place when you arrive at your answer.

When multiplying, you have to use the 'power of ten' rule:

- $\times$ 10 move the decimal point 1 place to the right.
- $\times$ 100 move the decimal point 2 places to the right.
- $\times$ 1000 move the decimal point 3 places to the right.

Here is an example:

$$6.178 \times 100 = 617.8$$

Try this one next:

$$0.0345 \times 10 = 0.345$$

Division also has 'power of ten' rules. In multiplication you move the decimal point to the right, in division it is to the left.

- $\div$ 10 move the decimal point 1 place to the left.
- $\div$ 100 move the decimal point 2 places to the left.
- $\div$ 1000 move the decimal point 3 places to the left.

For example, if dividing 35.42 by 10, 100 and 1000:

- $\div$ 35.42 by 10 = 3.542.
- $\div$ 35.42 by 100 = 0.3542.
- $\div$ 35.42 by 1000 = 0.03542.

Table 15.4 shows multiplication and division of decimals.

## CONVERTING FROM ONE UNIT TO ANOTHER

In some instances you will be required to convert from one unit to another, for example from grams to milligrams or from milligrams to micrograms. It is often safer to work in whole numbers, for example 275 mcg as opposed to 0.275 mg. Fewer mistakes are made when working this way. When being able

**Table 15.4** Movement of the decimal point in multiplication and division

| Multiplying by | Number of zeros | Movement of the decimal point to the right |
|---|---|---|
| 10 | 1 | 1 place |
| 100 | 2 | 2 places |
| 1 000 | 3 | 3 places |
| 10 000 | 4 | 4 places |
| **Dividing by** | **Number of zeros** | **Movement of the decimal point to the left** |
| 10 | 1 | 1 place |
| 100 | 2 | 2 places |
| 1 000 | 3 | 3 places |
| 10 000 | 4 | 4 places |

to convert from one unit to another is required, you need either to multiply or divide. When converting from a larger unit (grams) to a smaller unit (milligrams), multiply by 1000. When converting from a smaller unit (milligrams) to a larger unit (grams), divide by 1000.

Converting 4 g to milligrams, for example (a larger unit to a smaller unit), requires you to multiply by 1000 (1 g = 1000 mg). 4 g is equal to 4000 mg. If you were required to convert 10 kg to grams (recall 1 kg = 1000 g): 10 × 1000 = 10 000 g.

The above are being converted from a larger unit to a smaller unit. Consider now how you would convert from a smaller unit to larger unit, 3300 mg to grams. You need to divide: 3300 ÷ 1000 = 3.3 g.

Converting g to mcg requires you to do this using two steps: convert g to mg then convert mg to mcg.

For example, convert 3.5 g to mcg:

- 3.5 × 1000 = 3500 mg
- 3500 mg × 1000 = 3 500 000 mcg

The above examples are easier than some real-life challenges you may encounter when working in the clinical field. You must refer to other sources for more detailed explanations of the above, as well as following the examples that are provided to you.

All calculations can be written as equations and this will now be demonstrated. There are several formulae that can be used to calculate drug dosages (Taylor et al., 2005). Formulae consist of ratios to set proportions, and can be used to calculate dosages for solid and liquid preparations. The standard formula for calculating drug dosage is related to the form of medication the patient is to receive (see Table 15.5).

The formula that apples to all of the above is:

$$\text{Volume required} = \frac{\text{Strength required}}{\text{Stock strength}}$$

For example, a patient has been prescribed 75 mg of pethidine intra-muscular injection. The stock you have comes in ampoules of 100 mg in 2 ml.

$$\text{Volume required} = \frac{\text{Strength required (75mg)}}{\text{Stock strength (100 mg)}}$$

$$\frac{75}{100} \times 2\,\text{ml} = \frac{75}{100} \times \frac{2}{1} = 0.75\ \text{ml.}$$

**Table 15.5** Some forms of medicines

| | |
|---|---|
| How much how/many tablets | Solid medication, for example tablets or capsules |
| How much how/many millilitres | Injections |

As another example, a patient is prescribed 225 mg of ranitidine orally. The medication comes in 150 mg tablets.

$$\text{Volume required} = \frac{\text{Strength required (225mg)}}{\text{Stock strength (150 mg)}}$$

$$\frac{225}{150} \times 1 = 1.5 \text{ (or one and a half tablets).}$$

However, you should always avoid halving tablets.

## PRESENTING NUMBERS, CHARTS AND GRAPHS

Using information presented in graphs and charts is a requirement of the twenty-first-century nurse. Much data relating to the care of the patient is presented in graph format. The data provides a means of communication (Bigwood and Spore, 2003). It is important therefore that you develop your skills when dealing with information that is presented in graph, table or chart format. Some data presented is not user friendly and may only serve to confuse; however if it is used appropriately it can communicate numerical data in an easier manner and save time.

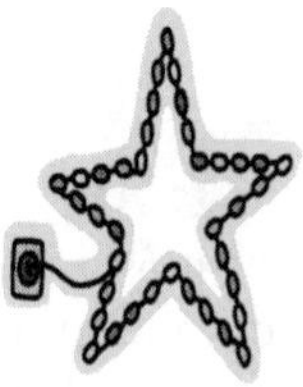

Make a list of data and how it might be presented to nurses in order to help them care for their patients more effectively.

Table 15.6 outlines some methods of data presentation.

### GRAPHS

There are several types of graph that allow the presentation of numerical trends and relationships (Bigwood and Spore, 2003). For example:

- line graphs
- pie charts
- bar charts
- pictographs
- scattergrams

**Table 15.6** Methods of presenting data and providing information

| Type of data | Format |
|---|---|
| Outcomes of research studies | Often presented in:<br>• table format<br>• graph<br>• chart |
| Blood results | Can be presented in many ways and an accumulative account of patients' results can be provided in linear format |
| Percentile charts | Graph format detailing height and weight ratio |
| Information about a patient's current health status | This type of information is often presented in graph format and is related to various aspects of patient care:<br>• observation charts, e.g. blood pressure, temperature and respiration |
| Epidemiological information | This type of data comes in many forms and allows you to determine the health of the nation or a population. It allows the measurement of trends and occurrences related to specific illnesses, diseases or particular social issues, for example the number of teenage pregnancies |

### Line Graphs

Line graphs can be used to show how something changes over time, for example a patient's blood glucose. Line graphs have points that are joined together, this allows the reader to see at a glance any variations or fluctuations in the patient's condition (see Figure 15.2).

### Pie Chart

These charts can be simple or very complex. The data contained within the chart can be percentages of a whole, showing parts of the whole in a circle. Pie charts display categorical data and each segment of the chart represents a particular category. They cannot show a change over time as line graphs can (see Figure 15.3).

### Bar Charts

Bar charts also represent categorical data. They utilise a number of rectangular shapes that represent a particular category. The length of each rectangle is proportional to the number of cases in the category it represents (see Figure 15.4).

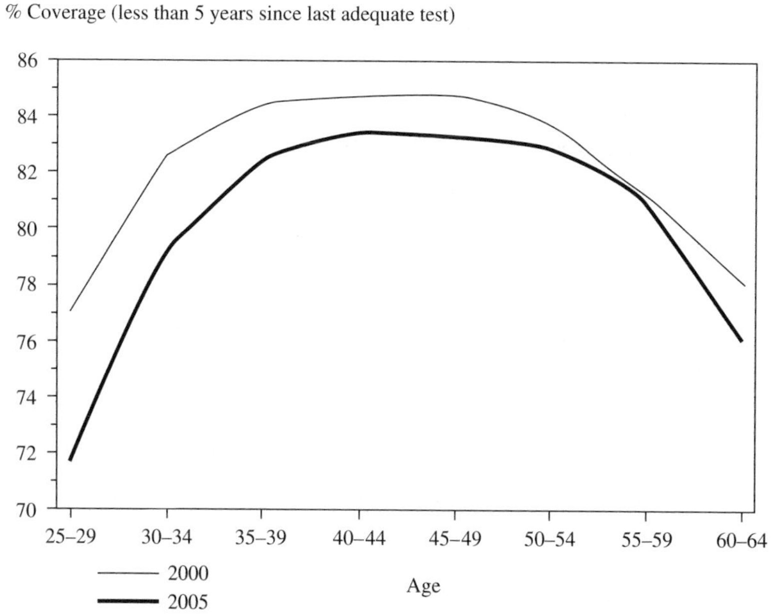


**Figure 15.2** A line graph demonstrating cervical screening by age in England
*Source*: National Statistics, 2005.

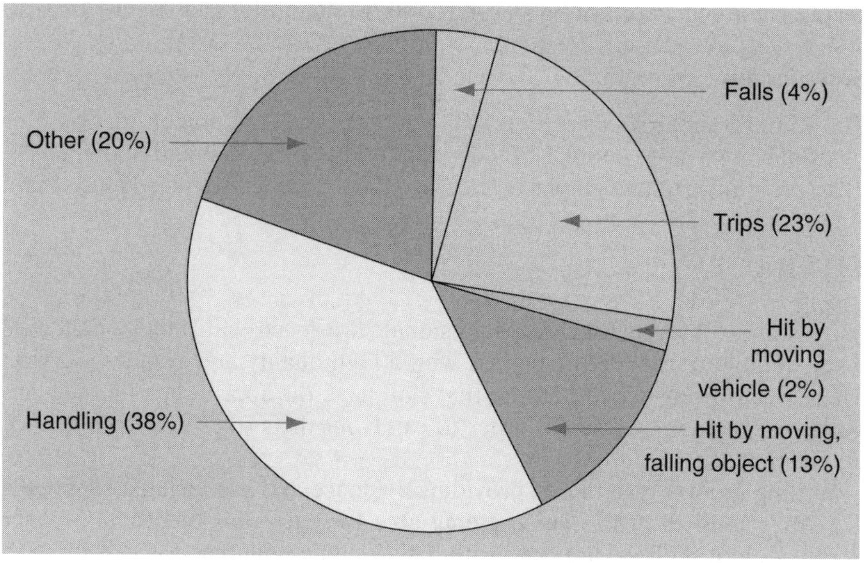


**Figure 15.3** A pie chart demonstrating kinds of accident causation over three-day injury 2001/2
*Source*: Health and Safety Executive, 2004.

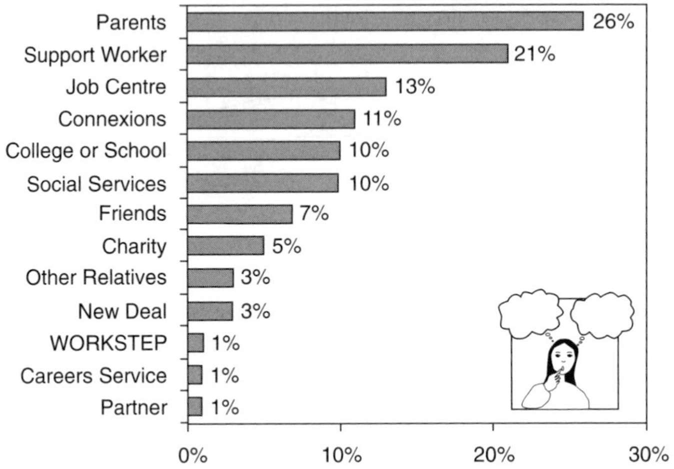


**Figure 15.4** An example of a bar chart: who people would turn to for help finding a job
*Source*: Health and Social Care Information Centre, 2005.

### Pictographs

This type of graph provides the reader with an opportunity to view statistical data with pictures or symbols in a more inviting manner than other types of graph. The pictures or symbols used represent quantities (see Figure 15.5).

### Scattergrams

The scattergram provides readers with a visual representation of relationships by displaying a large number of individual points (Bigwood and Spore, 2003). They are similar to line graphs as they also have $x$ and $y$ axes (see Figure 15.6).

## LITERACY

Nurses and other health-care professionals are faced with many challenges when aiming to provide the patient with a high-quality and seamless service. There is a growing need to ensure that staff have the appropriate literacy, language and numeracy skills in order to carry out their roles with competence and confidence.

Writing reports, statements, providing evidence and producing assignments are key requisites of the nurse. Being able to write competently and confidently are not skills we are born with. This is something that you can strive to acquire; you can become proficient through practice, determination and commitment. The importance of record keeping, writing records and documentation has been discussed elsewhere in the text (see for example Chapter 2). This

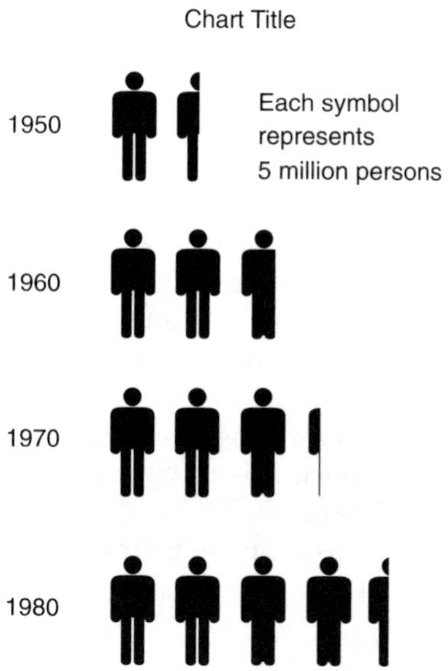


**Figure 15.5** A pictograph

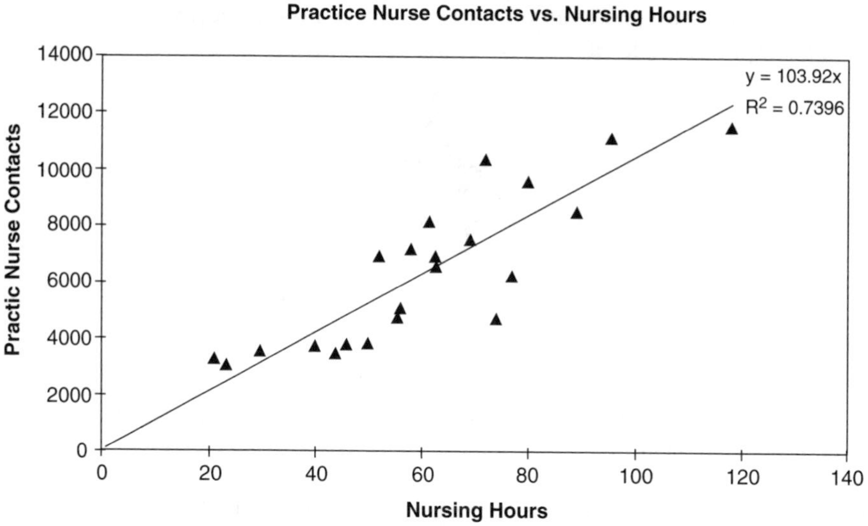


**Figure 15.6** A scattergram
*Source*: Centre for Innovations in Primary Care, 1997.

section of the chapter will provide you with brief guidelines on writing as an aspect of your work as a professional and also as a student (pre-registration or post-registration), for example statement and academic writing. It is not the intention to teach the rules associated with grammar, punctuation or syntax.

The key aim is to encourage you to develop those skills you already possess. As with the previous section of this chapter, you are advised to seek further support (both material and human) about any aspect of report writing, statement production or course assignment work that is required of you and you need help with.

Eborall (2004) points out that poor record keeping and reporting standards, not understanding written information and instructions, along with a poor understanding of numbers and poor oral communication skills, lead to poor handover at the end of each turn of duty. Further outcomes are associated with poor-quality records and paperwork, the risk of errors and accidents and lower standards of care for patients.

There are various types of writing styles and whatever type is chosen should reflect the purpose for which it is to be used. For example, a postcard to a friend would be very different to a set of instructions given to a patient to manage his/her medications at home after discharge. Instructions given to a patient should be factual.

## FACTUAL WRITING

The purpose of using a factual type of writing may be to inform the patient or another health-care professional – to give instruction. Table 15.7 provides you with a simple example of factual writing.

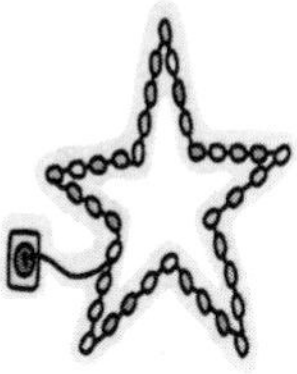

Can you think of any other examples of instructional writing that you may have come across? The following are some examples:

- Instructions provided at the cash till (ATM).
- Instructions given to you in patient information leaflets, explaining how to take your medications.
- Recipes.
- Instructions that accompany flat-pack, self-assembly furniture.
- Information on how to repair a flat tyre.

The common element in all aspects of factual writing (or what should be the common element) is the attention to detail and the provision of fact. Step-by-step guidance is needed in order to proceed safely. If these important components are not present, then this could result in calamity or failure to achieve the desired goal/outcome, such as the baking of a cake. The detail needs to be precise, clear and written in a language the reader will understand.

**Table 15.7** A simple example of factual writing: making a cup of coffee

| | |
|---|---|
| 1 | Fill the kettle with water and allow the kettle to boil. |
| 2 | Take your cup or mug and put the required amount of instant coffee into the cup. |
| 3 | Once the kettle has boiled pour the boiling water into the cup or mug with the instant coffee in it. |
| 4 | Add sugar and milk to taste. |

Report writing is an example of factual writing, for instance the writing of minutes for a formal meeting. The finished minutes should be a true reflection of what actually occurred or what was said during the meeting. There is no place here for the person recording the minutes to add any personal opinions or subjective comments. Factual writing is a key element when you are asked to provide a statement or a report. The information provided in the statement may be used as part of a fact-finding exercise. It is important not to confuse fact with opinion; opinions should always be prefaced with 'I think' or 'I believe'.

You may be asked to write a statement for several reasons, for example in response to an investigation, and as such the content of your statement may need to be disseminated to other parties. Table 15.8 provides you with some pointers that you may find useful if you are asked to write a statement. You must always seek advice and support from your line manager or a member of staff at your educational institution.

You should always seek advice and support before, during and after you have written the statement, bearing in mind that the person you seek advice from cannot write the statement for you. You are strongly advised to ensure that you keep a copy of the statement (Holburn et al., 2000). If you are requested to attend a hearing or formal discussion of any issue(s) arising out of your statement, you may be allowed to take a friend, colleague, member of staff from your educational institution or a trade union representative to accompany you. A summary of issues associated with statement writing can be found in Table 15.9.

## ACADEMIC WRITING

Academic writing will include essay writing, but it is not solely concerned with essay writing. There are many reasons why you may be required to write an essay, for example, you may have been asked to write an essay as part of your entry to determine your suitability for nurse education. Good essay writing demonstrates that you have the ability to communicate clearly using the written word, as well as following the rules of grammar and syntax, taking into account your audience. All formal programmes of nurse education (pre-registration or post-registration) will have essay writing as part of their assessment process.

**Table 15.8** How to write and what to include in a statement

***How to write a statement***

- Write your notes as soon after the event as possible, you will need your notes to construct your statement.
- Be honest.
- Write in the first person singular (e.g. 'I saw . . .').
- Use plain, clear and jargon-free language.
- Be precise and concise.
- Provide the details chronologically.
- Include all details.
- Only provide fact, not opinion.
- Detail and document only what you have seen, and not what you think may have occurred.
- Clearly handwrite or wordprocess your statement.

***What to include in a statement***

- A heading explaining what the statement is about (for example 'Statement regarding the treatment to patient X').
- Page numbers if there are more than one page.
- A brief introduction of who you are, grade, qualifications and what your job is.
- Date, time and place the incident occurred.
- Those others who were also involved, who they are and what their job is.
- Background information (such as the environment, particular circumstances. Occurrence – is this a one-off incident? Was it night or day?).
- What you saw happen, not what you think happened or should have happened but what you saw happen.
- What you did – what action you took.
- What were the outcomes of the action you took.
- Any information given to you by a third party (e.g. Charge Nurse Patel informed me that . . .).
- Any relevant local factors (e.g. was there any relevant equipment available/ unavailable).
- Your contact details.
- You may be required to conclude your statement with the following: 'The contents of this statement are true to the best of my beliefs and knowledge.'
- The date and time you wrote the statement.
- Your signature.

*Source*: Adapted from Robinson, 2004; Holburn et al., 2000.

The following aspect of the chapter provides you with tips and hints. However, this will never replace the advice, guidance and support offered to you by those who have asked you to write the essay. There are many other texts that you may wish to use to help you produce essays and other types of assignments required for your nursing programme.

There is no single 'best' way to write an essay; each individual will differ. However, there are some generalisations and fundamental principles that may help you. To produce a good essay you must take time to plan and to devise the way in which you wish to tackle the question set. Essay writing is a skill:

**Table 15.9** Some key issues associated with statement writing

**The statement should not:**

- Be written in haste.
- Be written under duress.
- Be brief or dismissive.
- Seek to blame others.
- Include statements beyond your recollection or knowledge.
- Comment on the aftermath.
- Comment on what you would have done according to normal practice.
- Be made up if you cannot recall events. If you cannot be sure of a certain aspect or recall the matter in question, say so.
- Include ambiguous statements.
- Speculate on what others were doing or thinking.
- Express opinions on the care given or actions taken by others.
- Include speculation or conjecture.
- Be hostile, rude or defensive.
- Be derogatory or defamatory.
- Be subjective.
- Include abbreviations or jargon.
- Be drawn up in collusion with other witnesses.
- Be signed until you are happy with it.

*Source*: Adapted from Robinson, 2004.

you can work on your essay-writing skill and develop your ability to produce cogent arguments, provide facts or inform others.

Planning ahead and managing your time effectively are skills that will underpin all of your academic endeavours (as well as your clinical work). Good essay writing depends on preparation (Masterson, 2001). This may be related to your time at the university or/and your time at home. Think about reorganising your everyday jobs at home and put your skills of delegation to use. Ensure that your diary or personal planner has all of the important dates in it, for example dates of submission for your course work. It is helpful if you work backwards from the deadline set, in order to organise your time ahead. You are advised to do this at the beginning of term, as you may find time can become limited with other competing activities. Do not forget that you must also ensure that you plan time out for yourself; never forget there may be unexpected events that can occur.

Devise an action plan. You may wish to include the following in your action plan:

- Assignment remit.
- Question breakdown.
- Data gathering/researching the topic.
- Writing up the first draft.
- Proofreading first draft.
- Amendments.

• Final proofreading.
• Submission.

## THE ASSIGNMENT QUESTION

When you receive the assignment question read it – it sounds obvious, but read it, analyse the question that has been set. What exactly have you been asked to do? Assignment questions contain direction words, verbs that will give directions to you, telling you how to answer the question. In the question set, underline the verbs that direct you, words that have a specific focus (see Table 15.10).

Brainstorming your ideas may help. Some people find it helpful to use spider diagrams to consider as much of the topic area as possible. Buzan (2001) recommends the use of a mind map. However, remember that not all of the approaches or suggestions here will suit all people. Find your own approach, whatever that may be, so long as you feel comfortable with it.

Planning the way you structure your response is very important. You will have a word limit that you will have to adhere to and your planning will need to take this into account. Decide on how many words you intend to allocate to each section; clearly the body of the text will require the largest number of words. You may wish to write a draft first and then review this.

There are three key components associated with a logically presented essay:

• introduction
• main part or body
• conclusion

**Table 15.10** Some key verbs that are used to direct your essay

| | |
|---|---|
| **Account for** | Give reasons for |
| **Analyse** | Consider each aspect/issue and discuss |
| **Assess** | Give reasons for what you think is important |
| **Compare** | Show ways in which two things (or more) are alike or similar |
| **Contrast** | Highlight the differences between two things |
| **Criticise/critically evaluate** | Give your judgement, support your judgement |
| **Define** | Provide the exact meaning |
| **Discuss** | Look at all aspects of the issue, investigate and consider the pros and cons |
| **Evaluate** | Give reasons why you think something is important |
| **Explain** | Clearly state why something happens/occurs |
| **Identify** | Make known, describe and highlight |
| **Illustrate** | Provide examples, e.g. figures, graphs, tables, data |
| **Outline** | State what are the main, key/salient points. What are the key issues? |
| **Review** | Go over, re-examine, briefly comment on the issue |

### Introduction

The introduction should tell the reader what you are writing about – the topic. It should also point out the direction in which the essay is going to go. This aspect should be seen as the signpost. In a nutshell, tell the reader what he/she is to expect.

### Main Part or Body

The paragraphs comprising the main body are the paragraphs that should inform the reader of the key/salient points. You will be guided in this section by the verbs used in the assignment remit or title, such as 'discuss' and 'evaluate'. Summarising and paraphrasing will be required. Remain focused on this section of the essay – it is easy to become diverted.

If you are asked to refer to or include examples of clinical practice, be sure to do that but also make certain that you do not breach any aspect of confidentiality. You should ensure you are fully conversant with the rules regarding confidentiality; take into account also the issues regarding confidentiality discussed in the code of professional conduct (NMC, 2004a). Adhere strictly to your educational institution's rules regarding referencing and be aware of what may constitute plagiarism, cheating and collusion.

The concluding sentence or paragraph of the main body should aim to tie all the content of this section together. This section is concerned with 'telling' the reader.

### Conclusion

The main key/salient points of the essay should be provided in summary format. This section brings it all together and recaps. Briefly review the key content with an overall comment related to the topic in question. If appropriate, in the conclusion you may recommend or make suggestions – but only if appropriate. You should not introduce any new ideas at this point. Say what you have already said, 'saying it again' (briefly).

In summary, as a basic rule of thumb, an essay with three parts, an introduction, a body and a conclusion, should aim to:

- Say what you are going to say.
- Say it.
- Say it again.

Prior to submitting your essay or assignment you should always proofread it yourself and also have someone else proofread it for you if possible. Pay attention to the finishing touches. Leave a day or so prior to embarking on proofreading: you may notice things after you have not been working on your essay for a day or two. The aim here is to look at the overall structural coherence and institutional requirements:

- Have you addressed the question set?
- Is there a logical flow – do ideas follow on from idea to idea?
- Consider spelling, syntax and grammar.
- Have you referenced and supported your work using other literature as required and in line with your educational institution's requirements?
- Have you completed the appropriate cover sheet (if required)?
- Does the submission comply with all of the requirements of your educational institution?

Figure 15.7 provides an overview of some of the steps associated with the essay-writing process.

Always ensure that you keep a copy of the assignment in the form of hard copy (photocopy for example) or on a disk. Store copies away carefully, as they may come in handy when you are revising or referring to previous aspects of your programme of study.

If at any stage of the process you are unsure what is required, make an appointment or seek support from the person who set you the assignment. Always attend tutorials if they are being offered to you.

When it comes to the submission of your piece of work, plan in advance for this. If you are required to wordprocess your work then ensure you allow time for printing. Remember, if you are printing off your work at the university there will be other students who also have to submit wordprocessed assignments at the same time as you and they will need to use printers, so expect queues and plan for this. Beware that your printing may be delayed due to pressure on networked equipment.

Always submit work on time. Check out the required submission date as well as the time, and if in any doubt check it out. Some institutions are very strict about this and you run the risk of being penalised if you fail to submit work when required, even if you are late by a few minutes.

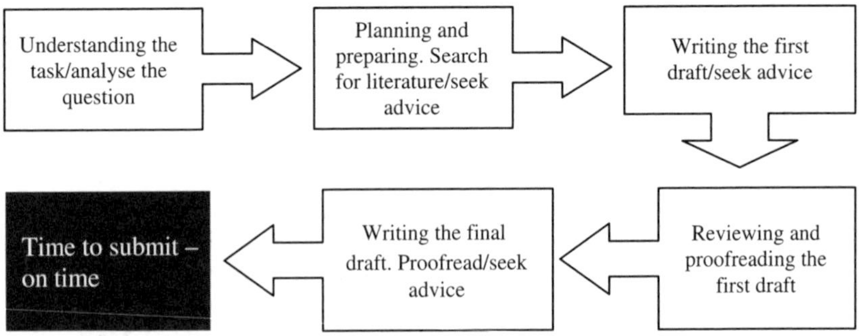


**Figure 15.7** Steps associated with the essay-writing process

**Key Points**

1. Take time to plan and seek out a place that you feel comfortable in when writing your essay.
2. When planning time to write the essay, also plan to give yourself treats and allow yourself 'time out'.
3. Organise yourself.
4. Use a good record-keeping system so that you have all the information you have gathered in the planning stage to write your essay close to hand and in order.
5. Seek help, attend tutorials and ask for clarification.
6. Know the word limit, referencing requirements and submission dates.
7. Proofread prior to submission.
8. Submit on time and plan for submission.
9. Keep copies of your work.
10. Again, if in any doubt at all ask.

In some educational institutions all academic work produced by students for assessment may need to be wordprocessed. Some institutions require students to submit their work online (via the Internet). In order to do this competently you will need to be computer literate and be able to demonstrate a degree of proficiency in computer skills.

## COMPUTER SKILLS

Computer skills are not only required for carrying out academic work. In all aspects of heath-care provision computer skills and the use of information technology are prerequisites, in the hospital and community setting. Offredy in this text (Chapter 8) has already introduced the idea of using information technology when engaging in evidence-based practice. Anthony (2001) points out that a research-aware clinical nurse who wishes to ensure that clinical practice is evidence based will need to make use of some of the common information technology applications that are available.

Many organisations, including educational institutions and NHS Trusts, offer information technology training. You should make use of these facilities and develop your understanding of the basic aspects associated with information technology, and then strive to go on and develop your skills over time. Computer-based information technology workshops and drop-in sessions organised by learning resource centres (or their equivalent) may be available to you.

The NHS has provided guidance regarding the way forward, in the guise of a national strategy. The national strategy (NHS Executive, 1999) aims to equip all staff with the knowledge, skills and expertise required to make better use of information and information technology. Effective information management benefits the patient and as a result, it is hoped, the patient will receive high-quality care.

Clinical information technology is not new and the development of information technology in relation to clinical practice closely follows developments in medicine. Nurses, as is the case with all other health-care professionals, must keep up to date with contemporary practices. There are several ways of doing this, but it could be suggested that the most common way is to access the Internet to retrieve data. In order to do this effectively a basic understanding of information technology is required.

The European Computer Driving Licence (ECDL), an internationally recognised qualification, is available for all NHS staff to acquire. Most higher education institutions also provide access for their students to undertake this qualification. The ECDL addresses competencies in seven key areas:

- Basic concepts of IT.
- Using a computer and managing files.
- Wordprocessing.
- Spreadsheets.
- Databases.
- Presentations.
- Information and communication.

The key aim of the ECDL is to provide an understanding of the concepts associated with information technology. It is important that nurses have access to information technology and also have the skills to use it effectively. The ECDL is one way of becoming a proficient, information-literate practitioner.

## CONCLUSIONS

Nurses need many skills and the skills associated with numeracy, literacy and computers are just as important as all the other key skills. On a daily basis nurses undertake activities associated with numeracy and literacy, and in some instances the patient's life may depend on the nurse's proficiency. It is crucial therefore that the nurse develop his/her skills of computation, problem solving and documentation. Calculating and documenting, like most things, become better and easier with practice. There is an increase in the use of information technology in all aspects of health care. The nurse must also become proficient when using this key skill, just as he/she strives to develop numeracy and literacy skills.

The mathematical skills of nurses have been shown to be poor on several occasions and over many years. It is vital that nurses possess the knowledge and skills required to perform computations and the more complex problem-solving skills involving formulae. These skills are central in ensuring that the patient is safe. Nurses need mathematical skills for several activities, for example to calculate drug dosages safely as well as using formulae to record, enter, store, retrieve and organise data essential for care delivery.

Implementing various strategies to improve confidence and skills may help to address deficiencies. Support must be offered to those who need it in a sensitive and stigma-free context. The support offered can be provided in many forms. The acquisition of the ECDL is one way of demonstrating proficiency associated with information technology.

## REFERENCES

Anthony, D. (2001) 'Using information technology' in Maslin-Prothero, S. (ed.) (3rd edn) *Bailliere's Study Skills for Nurses and Midwives*. Elsevier. London. Ch 4 pp 82–112.

Arnold, G. (1998) 'Refinements in the dimensional analysis of dose calculation problem-solving'. *Nurse Education*. Vol 23, pp 22–6.

Bigwood, S. and Spore, M. (2003) '*Presenting Numbers, Tables and Charts*. Oxford University Press. Oxford.

Bindler, R. and Bayne, T. (1991) 'Medication calculation ability of registered nurses'. *Image Journal of Nursing Scholarship*. Vol 23, No 4, pp 221–224.

Blais, K. and Bath, J.B. (1992) 'Drug calculation errors of baccalaureate nursing students'. *Nurse Education*. Vol 17, pp 12–15.

Buzan, T. (2001) *How to Mind Map: The Ultimate Thinking Tool That Will Change Your Life*. Thorsons-HarperCollins. London.

Centre for Innovations in Primary Care (1997) *How Does Our Nursing and Administrative Staff Provision Compare with Other Practices in PDC*. Centre for Innovations in Primary Care. Sheffield.

Department of Health (2004) *Building a Safer NHS for Patients: Improving Medication Safety*. Department of Health. London.

Eborall, C. (2004) *Basic Skills in Social Care*. Training Organisation for the Personal Social Services. Leeds.

Gray, J. and Jackson, C. (2004) 'The development of an online quiz for drug calculations'. *Nursing Times*. Vol 100, No 4, pp 40–41.

Hall, C. (2000) 'Medication in the newborn' in Boxwell, G. (ed.) *Neonatal Intensive Care Nursing*. Routledge. London. Ch 19 pp 430–442.

Health and Safety Executive (2004) *Getting to Grips with Manual Handling: A Short Guide*. HSE. London.

Health and Social Care Information Centre (2005) *Adults with Learning Disabilities in England 2003/4*. Health and Social Care Information Centre.

Holburn, C.J., Bond, C., Solon, M. and Burn, S. (2000) *Healthcare Professionals as Witnesses to the Court*. Greenwich Medical Media. London.

Hutton, M. (2005) *Calculation Skills: Paediatric Dosages*. RCN Publishing Company. London.

Kapborg, I. (1994) 'Calculation and administration of drug dosage by Swedish nurses, student nurses and physicians'. *International Journal for Quality in Health Care*. Vol 6, No 4, pp 389–395.

Kawamura, H. ( 2001) 'The approaches to factors which cause medication errors from the analysis of many near miss cases related to intravenous medication which nurses experienced'. *Japanese Journal of Cancer and Chemotherapy*. Vol 28, No 3, pp 304–309.

Lawrence, C., Gibson, F. and Zur, J. (2003) 'Care delivery: The needs of children' in Hinchliff, S., Norman, S. and Schober, J. (eds) (4th edn) *Nursing Practice and Health Care*. Arnold. London. Ch 8 pp 177–202.

Masterson, A. (2001) 'Writing skills and developing an argument' in Maslin-Prothero, S. (ed.) (3rd edn) *Bailliere's Study Skills for Nurses and Midwives*. Elsevier. London. Ch 9 pp 185–208.

National Audit Office (2005) *A Safer Place for Patients: Learning to Improve Patient Safety*. TSO. London.

NHS Executive (1999) *Working Together with Health Information: A Partnership Strategy for Education, Training and Development*. NHSE. London.

National Statistics (2005) *Cervical Screening Project: England 2004–05*. National Statistics. London.

Nursing and Midwifery Council (2004a) *The NMC Code of Professional Conduct: Standards for Conduct, Performance and Ethics*. NMC. London.

Nursing and Midwifery Council (2004b) *Guidelines for the Administration of Medicines*. NMC. London.

Nursing and Midwifery Council (2004c) *Standards of Proficiency for Pre-registration Nursing Education*. NMC. London.

Polifroni, C., McNulty, J. and Allchin, L. (2003) 'Medication errors: More basic than a system issue'. *Journal of Continuing Education*. Vol 42, No 10, pp 455–458.

Preston, R.M. (2004) 'Drug errors and patient safety: The need for a change in practice'. *British Journal of Nursing*. Vol 13, No 2, pp 72–78.

Robinson, S. (2004) 'Healthcare professionals in court – professional and expert witnesses' in Payne-James, J., Dean, P. and Wall, I. (eds) (2nd edn) *Medicolegal Essentials in Healthcare*. Greenwich Medical Media. London. Ch 20 pp 233–240.

Segatore, M., Edge, D. and Miller, M. (1993) 'Poslogy errors by sophomore nursing students'. *Nursing Outlook*. Vol 41, pp 160–165.

Taxis, K. and Barber, N. (2003) 'Ethnographic study of incidence and severity of intravenous drug errors'. *British Medical Journal*. Vol 326, p 684.

Taylor, C., Lillis, C. and LeMone, P. (2005) (5th edn) *Fundamentals of Nursing: The Art and Science of Nursing Care*. Lippincott. Philadelphia.

Trim, J. (2004) 'Clinical skills: A practical guide to working out drug calculations'. *British Journal of Nursing*. Vol 13, No 10, pp 602–606.

Weeks, K.W., Lyne, P. and Torrance, C. (2000) 'Written drug dosage errors made by students: The threat to clinical effectiveness and the need for a new approach'. *Clinical Effectiveness in Nursing*. Vol 4, pp 20–29.

Wilson, A. (2003) 'Nurses' maths: Researching a practical approach'. *Nursing Standard*. Vol 17, No 47, pp 33–36.

Woodrow, P. (1998) 'Numeracy skills'. *Nursing Standard*. Vol 10, No 6, pp 26–30.

Wright, K. (2004) 'An investigation to find strategies to improve student nurses' maths skills'. *British Journal of Nursing*. Vol 13, No 21, pp 1280–1284.

Wright, K. (2005) 'An exploration into the most effective way to teach drug calculation skills to nursing students'. *Nurse Education Today*. Vol 25, pp 430–436.

# IV Personal and Professional Development

# 16 Continuing Professional Development

After engaging in three years' nurse education and successful registration with the Nursing and Midwifery Council, you will have fulfilled the NMC's registration requirements and, as such, be entitled to practise your profession. In order to be cognisant of your own professional development, there will be a need for reflective practice and a commitment to the concept of lifelong learning.

Continuing professional development is a requirement for all registered nurses, midwives and community public health nurses. It is one of the two standards associated with PREP (post-registration education and practice). PREP is a legal requirement that must be met by all those who are on the professional register and who wish to have their registration renewed (Nursing and Midwifery Order, 2001). Renewal is required every three years. An outline of the process as required by the NMC will be considered in this chapter.

Reflective practice is introduced and lifelong learning strategies through the development of a personal development plan are discussed. Three reflective models are briefly outlined. The nurse must demonstrate an ability to commit to the need for continuing professional development. Closely related to reflective practice is clinical supervision. Clinical supervision, what it is and what it is not are described. Reflective practice, clinical supervision and the ability to demonstrate continued professional development are all associated with the concept of lifelong learning.

The way in which the nurse provides evidence of continuing professional development is a personal matter. However, he/she must be aware that the NMC, as a part of its audit arrangements, may request and require a nurse to provide evidence of how he/she has maintained his/her professional development. Often the nurse chooses to use a professional portfolio to do this – again, there are no set requirements for how this should look, neither are there any stipulations associated with the content of the portfolio. Advice is provided in this chapter that may help you to devise and develop your own portfolio.

## POST-REGISTRATION EDUCATION AND PRACTICE (PREP)

PREP is a set of standards and guidance produced by the NMC (2004a) designed to enhance patient care. PREP can help the nurse keep up to date and be aware of new developments that are occurring in practice. Nursing practice occurs in an environment that is ever changing (Driscoll and Teh, 2001). PREP has the ability to encourage the nurse to think and reflect, demonstrating to the patient that you are a knowledgeable, up-to-date practitioner who is capable of continuous professional development.

Continuing professional development, although not a guarantee of competence, is a key component of clinical governance and affects all health-care professionals. Continuing professional development is defined as:

> *A process of lifelong learning for all individuals which meets the needs of patients and delivers health outcomes and health care priorities of the NHS which enables professionals to expand and fulfil their potential.* (HSC, 1999/194)

Figure 16.1 provides a useful model of continuing professional development as described in the Department of Health's publication *A First Class Service* (Department of Health, 1998). Although that publication is focused on

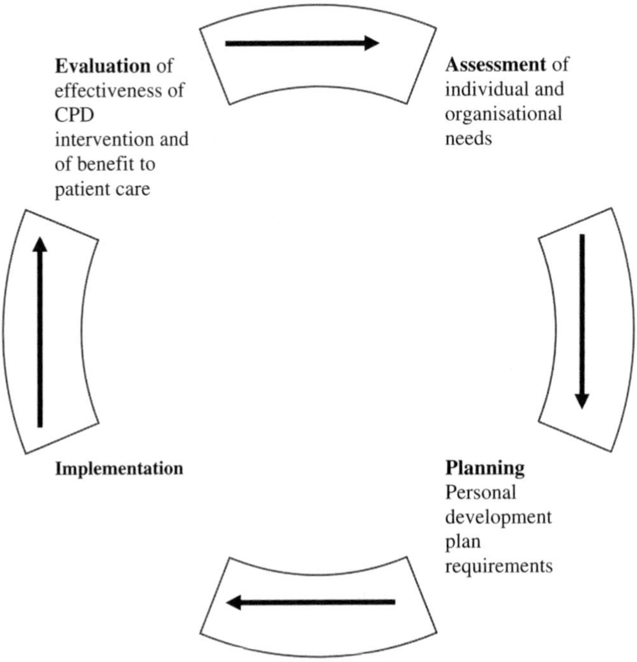


**Figure 16.1** A continuing professional development model
*Source*: Department of Health, 1998.

England, the principles of continuing professional development apply across all four countries in the UK.

## THE NMC AND PREP

You may recall that the role of the NMC is to protect the public. This is done through several mechanisms, one of which is to maintain the professional register. As already discussed, registration allows you to practise legally as a registered nurse in the UK. Every three years you are legally required to renew your registration (and pay a fee for this).

One aspect of this renewal process is that you are required to sign a notification of practice form, accompanied by the registration fee. The notification of practice form requires that you make a declaration relating to the details on the form. This declaration in effect states that the information you have provided is a true and accurate statement of your current practice and continuing professional development status. You also declare that your health and character are sufficiently good to enable you to continue to practise safely and effectively. There is a second section of the form concerned with 'Police cautions and convictions declaration'.

PREP requirements will now be discussed.

## PREP REQUIREMENTS

You must demonstrate the ability to meet PREP requirements. These are legal requirements and you will not be able to register unless you meet them. Since 1995 those wanting to re-register have had to provide evidence that they meet the legal PREP requirements. PREP requirements also feature as an important activity with other health-care professionals, for example physiotherapists (Chartered Society of Physiotherapists, 2005). The Health Professions Council (HPC, 2005) has produced five standards for continuing professional development (see Table 16.1).

**Table 16.1** The five continuing professional development standards produced by the HPC

| **Registrants must:** |
|---|
| 1 Maintain continuous, up-to-date and accurate records of their CPD. |
| 2 Demonstrate that their CPD activities are a mixture of learning and activities relevant to current or future practice. |
| 3 Seek to ensure that their CPD has contributed to the quality of their practice and service delivery. |
| 4 Seek to ensure that their CPD benefits the service user. |
| 5 Present a written profile containing evidence of their CPD on request. |

*Source*: HPC, 2005.

**Table 16.2** The two standards that must be met in order for registration be renewed

| PREP standard | PREP requirements |
|---|---|
| **Practice standard** | You are required to have worked in some capacity by virtue of your nursing or midwifery qualification during the previous five years for a minimum of 100 days (750 hours), or have successfully undertaken an approved return-to-practice course. |
| **CPD standard** | You must have undertaken and recorded your continuing professional development over the three years prior to the renewal of your registration. All registered nurses and midwives must declare on their notice-to-practice form that they have met this requirement when they renew their registration. |

*Source*: NMC, 2004a.

For nurses there are two standards associated with PREP, the PREP 'practice' standards and the PREP 'continuing professional development' standards (see Table 16.2).

## THE PRACTICE STANDARD

This standard aims to ensure that the public are being protected by requiring that the nurse has undertaken a minimum amount of 100 days' practice (750 hours) in some capacity by virtue of his/her nursing qualification. The 100 days (750 hours) must have occurred within the last five years prior to renewal of registration. Failure to meet this requirement means that the person wishing to renew registration must undertake an approved return-to-practice programme of study.

### Return-to-Practice Courses

These courses are run in association with approved or accredited institutions, such as a university or other education institution. The programmes often adopt a flexible approach, fitting in with family life and other commitments. Both theoretical and practice experience is provided. The aims are to:

- Develop competence.
- Develop and enhance confidence.
- Update skills and knowledge.
- Regain registration.
- Return to work.

Outcomes have been set by the NMC against which return-to-practice courses are validated. The programme must not be less than five days in length. The programme takes into account the needs of the student and previous levels of knowledge and experience.

The PREP practice standard can be met regardless of whether the individual is in paid work, for example employed by an NHS Trust, working independently or working with a nursing agency; unpaid work, for example working for a voluntary organisation; or not working, for example the person may be taking a career break, have been on maternity leave or have retired. Whether the person is in part-time or full-time employment is irrelevant.

## THE CONTINUING PROFESSIONAL DEVELOPMENT STANDARD

This element of PREP is referred to as continuing professional development and is also a condition for re-registration with which the nurse must comply. The nurse is committed to undertaking continuing professional development. The NMC (NMC, 2004a) has decreed that there are three aspects associated with this standard. The nurse must:

- Undertake at least five days or 35 hours of learning activity relevant to his/her practice during the three years prior to renewal of registration.
- Maintain a personal professional portfolio of learning activity.
- Comply with any request from the NMC to audit how those requirements have been met.

The way in which this standard is met is up to the nurse. The person who is required to demonstrate continuing professional development activities is the best person to decide what learning activities are needed to comply with the standard.

What is essential is that you document your learning activities. This is best done in your personal professional portfolio (on which there is more in the next section). There must be evidence that the learning activity you have undertaken has informed and influenced your practice. The important issues associated with the continuing professional development standard are outlined in Table 16.3.

You may be asked to demonstrate to the NMC how you have met the continuing professional development standard. You must be able to provide documentation regarding your learning activities that you have completed within

**Table 16.3** Important things to remember in relation to the continuing professional development standard

- It does not have to cost you any money.
- There is no such thing as approved PREP (CPD) learning activity.
- You do not need to collect points or certificates of attendance.
- There is no approved format for the personal professional portfolio.
- It must be relevant to the work you are doing and/or plan to do in the near future.
- It must help you to provide the highest possible standards of care for your patients and clients.

*Source*: NMC, 2004a.

the three years prior to renewal of your registration. You will need to demonstrate where, what and how:

- *Where* you were practising when the learning activity took place.
- *What* the learning activity was concerned with.
- *How* the learning influenced or informed your practice, how it related to your practice.

The next section of this chapter discusses the personal professional portfolio (your portfolio) and ways in which you can maintain it.

## PERSONAL PROFESSIONAL PORTFOLIOS

As a student nurse you may have been required to complete and develop a portfolio during your programme of study. The portfolio might have been used for professional development and assessed as part of your overall academic and practical performance. The portfolio may also have been used as a reflective tool. There are several ways in which this may have been undertaken, depending on your educational institution's preference.

Brown (1992) defines a personal portfolio as:

> *A private collection of evidence, which demonstrates the continuing acquisition of skills, knowledge, attitudes, understanding and achievement. It is both retrospective and prospective, as well as reflecting the current stage of development of the individual.*

It is, she continues, a collection of evidence with a particular purpose, for a particular audience. Driscoll and Teh (2001) suggest it is a snapshot in time, outlining where you have come from, where you are now and where you are going, along with the methods you chose to use to get there. Goodfellow (2004) states that the portfolio is a planned and organised collection of artifacts and reflections relating to professional qualities and practices. Compilation of a portfolio can contribute to lifelong learning as part of your continuing professional development. Table 16.4 outlines other ways in which the portfolio can help the nurse.

**Table 16.4** Ways in which a portfolio can help you

- Reflect on clinical, academic experiences and personal growth.
- Make decisions about the quality of your work and performance.
- Encourage reflective thinking.
- Provide empowerment to take on responsibility for your own learning.
- Develop within you a more critical, reflective practitioner.
- Provide documentary evidence of your achievements.
- Enhance self-esteem by demonstration of your ability to accomplish activities you have set out to achieve.

*Source*: Adapted from Pearce, 2003.

Reflection as a tool should feature often in a portfolio. Reflective practice allows the nurse to recognise learning and development that has taken place, either formally or informally, and is a useful tool when developing your portfolio. According to Driscoll and Teh (2001), one of the key skills in compiling a portfolio is the ability to communicate with yourself through critical reflection. This critical ability to reflect can occur by seeing yourself and your practice through different lenses or perspectives. There is more on reflection later in this chapter.

## THE PORTFOLIO: THE PRODUCT

The portfolio as a product (how it looks) can come in many guises. Often it is described as a file. This can be a hard-copy folder (often a looseleaf ring binder) or an electronic file or CD-ROM. There is no definitive requirement for the contents of the folder. The collection of artifacts described by Goodfellow (2004) can be varied and the evidence you choose to include is up to you.

Below are some suggestions on how to document learning activities that you have undertaken. You may be required to provide evidence of your learning activities to the NMC if it requests you to do so as a part of its auditing procedures (NMC, 2004a). The NMC (2004a) suggests the template in Table 16.5 be used, but points out that this is only a suggestion.

In the template suggested, the three key attributes of a professional portfolio can be identified: where, what and how. It may help you if you keep records of learning as described in a professional portfolio.

It is not how you present your collection of artifacts that you will be assessed or judged on. However, you must be able to demonstrate the where, what and how described earlier. A combination of both the process and the finished product is required in order to develop the portfolio. A professional portfolio can help you keep together evidence of your learning and other important facts related to professional development activities.

Portfolios take many forms and there is no set structure. You may wish to use a straightforward version, for example a folder that includes all your achievements, your development activities, work experiences, specific work or personal activities that have informed or influenced your practice. There are many ways in which to structure your portfolio.

## PORTFOLIO OF EVIDENCE

A portfolio of evidence is a collection of important material that you choose to collect to demonstrate some aspects of your professional development, including your evidence of learning. You may already be using a portfolio as a requirement for your programme of study in order to demonstrate your proficiency in relation to nursing practice. However, this varies with different

**Table 16.5** A suggested template for the recording of PREP

*PREP (CPD) PERIOD* – **the three-year registration period to which this learning applies**
From: To:

*WORK PLACE* – **where were you working when the learning activity took place?**
Name of organisation:
Brief description of your work/role:

*NATURE OF THE LEARNING ACTIVITY*
Date:

Briefly describe the learning activity: for example, reading a relevant clinical article, attending a course, observing practice:

State how many hours this took:

*DESCRIPTION OF THE LEARNING ACTIVITY* – **of what did it consist?**
**Describe what the learning activity consisted of** – include for example: why did you decide to do the learning activity or how the opportunity came about; where, when and how you did the learning activity; and what you expected to gain from it.

*OUTCOME OF THE LEARNING ACTIVITY* – **How did the learning relate to your work?**

Give a personal view of how the learning informed and influenced your work – what effect has this learning had on the way in which you work, or intend to work in the future? Do you have any ideas or plans for any follow-up learning?

**The way in which this activity has influenced my work is. . . .**

*Source*: NMC, 2004a.

universities. Some students are introduced to the use of a professional portfolio at the beginning of their studies, others may use a portfolio later on in the programme. If your university requires you to use and compile a portfolio you must follow the guidance provided. The guidelines here are intended to complement that.

The formulation and how you present your portfolio is your responsibility. This approach actively encourages you to take part in your learning as well as emphasising the need for lifelong learning. Regardless of when you begin using a professional portfolio, you will be engaging in a lifelong practice of reflecting, evaluating and recording your professional development.

The portfolio should focus on the process of learning (including evidence of reflective practice), demonstrating, through the collection of evidence, how you have made and can make associations between the theoretical aspects of your programme of study, and what relation this has to the art and science of nursing practice. This can be seen as an ideal method of relating theory to practice and one way of beginning to reduce the practice–theory gap. The portfolio is your own personal record of your achievements.

## ORGANISING YOUR PORTFOLIO

You can purchase ready-made, commercially produced portfolios. Portfolios are highly personalised and unique to the person producing them; because of this ownership belongs to you (Hull et al., 2005). The commercially produced portfolios are convenient to use and can help organise your thoughts; they cannot, however, accomplish your achievements.

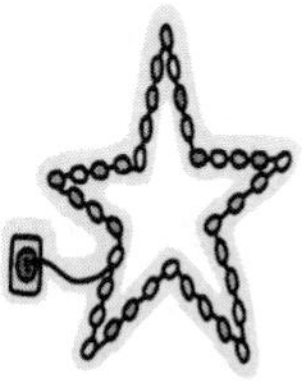

Make a list of things you think you might want to include in your professional portfolio.

The list below is not an exhaustive list of what can be included in a professional portfolio, merely suggestions (beware, however, that you do not unintentionally breach confidentiality with any items you choose to include):

- Items related to reflective practice, e.g. critical incidents.
- Your curriculum vitae.
- Feedback from mentors.
- Feedback from tutors.
- Letters/cards of thanks from patients/families.
- Testimonials.
- Certificates of achievement.
- Study days attended.
- Descriptions of supplementary roles you may have undertaken, for example student ambassador.
- Action plans and learning outcomes constructed in response to feedback.
- Evidence of achievement.
- Learning contracts.
- Elective experiences.
- Self-assessment of your performance.
- Nursing skills/clinical procedures you have performed, observed or assisted with.

- Key documentation produced by organisations such as the NMC, e.g. the code of professional conduct.
- Protocols, policies and procedures.
- Details from/about appraisals.
- Issues concerning and associated with the knowledge and skills framework.
- Details related to AP(E)L (assessment of prior (experiential) learning).
- Details about membership of particular professional fora, for example the RCN's School Nurses Forum.

Ensure that you organise your information thoroughly, for example identify each section of the portfolio clearly. Take some time to ensure you consider the proposed contents carefully. Construct a contents page and cross-tabulate the pages of your portfolio to this. Use dates to help you recall events; a chronological approach may be appropriate for all or just some of the sections. Try to update the contents of your portfolio on a regular basis, updating items and documents that have been superseded by later materials.

Putting together your biographical details may be the first step towards creating your own portfolio. A part of this might be the creation of your curriculum vitae. You must remember that it is the quality of the evidence you include in your portfolio that matters, not the quantity; bigger does not necessarily mean better (Northern Ireland Practice and Education Council for Nursing and Midwifery, 2004). Table 16.6 is an example of a contents list that may be used in a portfolio.

**Table 16.6** A proposed contents list for a professional portfolio

| |
|---|
| Personal details |
| Academic and professional achievements |
| Current role |
| Employment history |
| Personal achievements |
| Learning activities log |
| Evidence log |
| Reflective diary |
| Other information |

*Source*: NIPEC, 2004.

## BIOGRAPHICAL DETAILS

In this section include the following.

### Personal Details

- Name.
- Address.

- E-mail address.
- Phone number (work and home).
- NMC PIN and expiry date.
- Membership details for professional organisations, for example your RCN membership number.

**Introduction**

In this section provide details about who you are and your reasons for wanting to develop your professional portfolio. Include your current role and responsibilities. It is up to you what you put here, but try to give the person looking at your profile a 'flavour' of who you are, what you want (career aspirations) and how you intend to get there (action plan).

**General Education**

In this section and the next two, use a format that is chronological:

- Name(s) of the school(s) you attended and the educational qualifications you gained.
- Name(s) of the university you attended and your educational achievements.

Include any specific roles and responsibilities you held at these educational institutions, for example member of the debating society.

**Professional Education**

List here any qualifications that are recordable with the NMC and the qualifications that led to registration with the NMC (on any part of the register). Include the school/college of nursing or university you attended in order to gain your professional qualification.

Ensure that you include any awards associated with the qualification gained, such as a university prize. Provide details of the classification of your degree (if appropriate).

Include any specific roles and responsibilities you held at these educational institutions, for example member of the curriculum planning group, student ambassador, set rep.

**Work Experience**

A chronological approach must be used. Start with your most recent post and work backwards (as you would on a conventional application form). Include:

- Names of employers.
- Position held.
- A brief account of the duties and responsibilities associated with the post.

**Table 16.7** A profile checklist

| Item | Tick |
|---|---|
| Is the table of contents clear with cross-tabulated page numbers? | |
| Is it well presented and organised? | |
| Is your portfolio user friendly? | |
| Could others easily navigate their way around it – do you need more signposts? | |
| Have you cross-referenced your work? | |
| Have you used a variety of appropriate sources to support your learning? | |
| Have you used the most appropriate media to demonstrate learning? | |
| Can you demonstrate clear reflective action? | |
| Is your evidence genuine? | |
| Does the evidence provided do justice to what you claim to have achieved? | |
| Are the contents true, accurate and your own work? | |
| Have you ensured that the principle of confidentiality has been respected? | |
| Are the contents of your profile up to date? | |

*Source*: NIPCE, 2004.

- Salary paid (if you wish).
- Any voluntary or temporary posts.

In the next section of the portfolio you will need to include details of your continuing professional development as described above (e.g. reflective accounts, learning activities). You should also list any study activity with dates and venues, for example:

- Cardio pulmonary resuscitation updates.
- Moving and handling updates.
- Any other statutory requirements such as fire or health and safety-related activity.
- Project work.
- Clinical supervision activity.

Table 16.7 is a checklist that you may wish to use to ensure that your portfolio is as complete as possible.

There are many skills required of you in an attempt to develop and maintain your professional portfolio. As you become more competent and confident with portfolio development, you will find it easier to maintain.

## REFLECTIVE PRACTICE

Fowler (2003) states that refelection is central to continuing professional practice. The term reflection may be seen by some as a buzzword. Some may feel they do not have enough time for reflection and others may think it helps them provide safe, high-quality care. Reflective practice has the potential to help the nurse become, among other things, a lifelong learner; reflective practice then becomes reflective learning.

## REFLECTIVE LEARNING AND LIFELONG LEARNING

Reflective learning is learning from experience formally or informally, allowing the learner to consider his/her practice honestly and critically (Moon, 2004). The outcome may be the development of a deeper understanding of personal skills, enhanced self-awareness and individual learning needs. The NMC (2001) states that through reflection, nurses can develop further and enhance their understanding of practice.

Continuing professional development is a process of lifelong learning, and as such is an integral aspect of nursing practice. Lifelong learning can be defined as:

> *The continuous development of skills and knowledge to enhance quality of life and employment prospects.*

Pre-registration nurse education provides the foundation for lifelong learning (Department of Health, 2001). Having experienced this foundation, you are expected to continue as a lifelong learner, especially when related to your professional practice.

Reflective practice means that the nurse must engage in an active and conscious process when he/she encounters a problematic aspect of care provision and make an attempt to make sense of it. Reflective practice is a process that can be used for engaging in lifelong learning (Douglas, 2002).

There are several definitions of reflection available in the literature and because of this there may be confusion about what constitutes reflection. Boud et al. (1985) suggest that reflection occurs when individuals engage in activities that aim to explore their experiences in order to lead to new understanding and appreciation of the situation(s). Johns (2000) states that reflection is a window allowing practitioners to view themselves within the context of their own lived experience. By doing this practitioners can confront, understand and work towards resolving issues that arise in practice.

In order to maintain competency, Boud et al. (1985) suggest that you must learn through practice. Johns (1994) is of the opinion that practitioners, through an active and reflective approach, develop and create their own practice.

## REFLECTIVE MODELS

Just as there are many definitions of reflection available, there are also a number of models that you may use to help you consciously reflect. There are several techniques available to help you reflect with purpose. They may offer guidance and structure, but no one technique is better than the others (Platzer

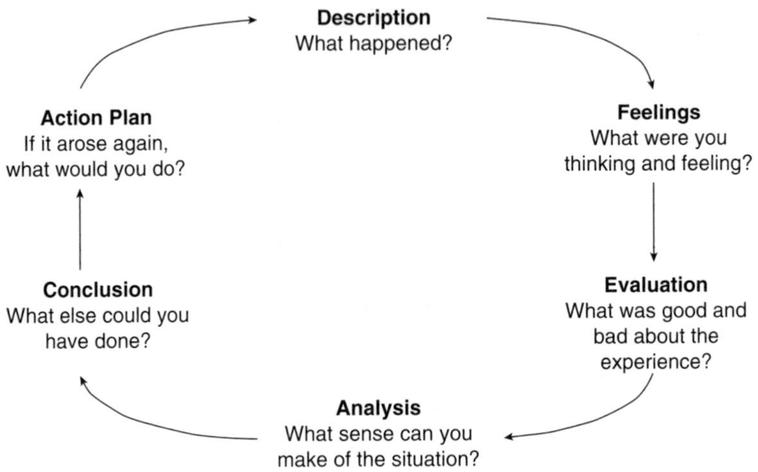


**Figure 16.2** Gibbs' reflective model
*Source*: Gibbs, 1988.

et al., 1997). The choice of model may be individual or it may have been dictated to you, for example your higher education institution may require you to use a particular model.

Driscoll (2000) considers three stages in his approach to reflection:

- *What?* describes the event.
- *So what?* analyses the event.
- *Now what?* proposes actions after the event.

Three models of reflection with a brief explanation of their use are discussed below.

## Gibbs' Model of Reflection

Gibbs (1988) enables those who engage in reflective activity to consider events in a cyclical manner (see Figure 16.2). Gibbs' model is one that promotes a simple approach to refection (Gibbs, 1988). Gibbs (1992) points out that deep learning takes place when reflective practice is used. It goes beyond the memorisation of information, and becomes an active, as opposed to a passive, activity.

## Johns' Model of Reflection

Johns' model of reflection (Johns, 1994) provides a framework that has five components (see Table 16.8).

**Table 16.8** An outline of the components of Johns' reflective model

| Component | Description |
|---|---|
| **Description** | • Describe the experience, document what happened.<br>• What aspects of this experience do I need to pay particular attention to? |
| **Reflection** | • What was it that I was trying to achieve?<br>• What was it that made me act the way I did?<br>• What are the consequences of my actions – for myself, the patient and my colleagues?<br>• How did I feel about the experience as it was happening?<br>• How did the patient feel?<br>• How do I know how the patient felt? |
| **Influencing** | • What internal factors impinged on my decision making and actions?<br>• What external factors impinged on my decision making and actions?<br>• What sources of knowledge did or should have influenced my decision making and actions? |
| **Alternative strategies** | • Could I have dealt better with the situation?<br>• What other choices did I have?<br>• What would be the consequences of these other choices? |
| **Learning** | • How can I make sense of this experience in the light of past experience and future practice?<br>• How do I now feel about this experience?<br>• Have I taken effective action to support myself and others as a result of this experience?<br>• How has this experience changed my way of knowing in practice? |

*Source*: Adapted from Johns, 1994.

### Atkins and Murphy's Model of Reflection

Atkins and Murphey (1994) state that for reflection to make a real difference to nursing practice, the outcome of the activity must include a commitment to action. There are five stages to Atkins and Murphy's model (Atkins and Murphy, 1994); see Figure 16.3.

A summary of the overall benefits of reflection are presented in Table 16.9.

Try to set some time aside to write up your reflective accounts on a regular basis. This way they will be fresh in your mind and they will be truer accounts. Try to remember that you are expected to record how you feel and to be honest about this. Keep the reflective account simple; often it is best to be spontaneous, writing, drawing or making a record in the most appropriate way as it happens or occurs to you.

## CLINICAL SUPERVISION

Associated with reflective practice is clinical supervision (Dooher et al., 2001).

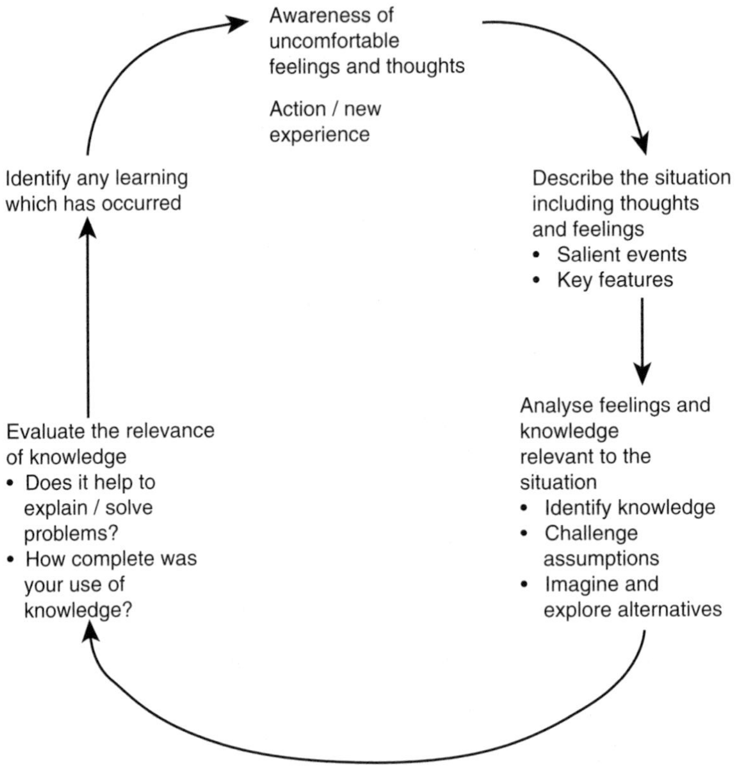


**Figure 16.3** Atkins and Murphy's model of reflection
*Source*: Atkins and Murphy, 1994.

**Table 16.9** The benefits of reflection in summary format

| |
|---|
| • Allows you to consider your practice objectively. |
| • Helps you recognise what you do well. |
| • Improves your professional judgement. |
| • Allows you to learn from your successes and mistakes and as a result enhance your performance. |
| • Helps you to plan for future incidents and respond more positively to change. |
| • It is a critical component of the continuing professional development cycle. |
| • Allows you to resolve uncertainty. |
| • Encourages and fosters independent learning. |

*Source*: Adapted from Institute of Health Care Management, 2004.

Clinical supervision is a term that has been used by nurses and other healthcare professionals to provide a purposeful, practice-focused relationship that enables the nurse to reflect on practice with the support of a skilled supervisor. Clinical supervision has its roots in counselling and psychotherapy.

The RCN (2002) states that clinical supervision in the workplace has been introduced as one method of using reflective practice as part of continuing professional development. However, in some areas where clinical supervision should and could be used by nurses in relation to critical reflection and innovation, this is not always the case (Bishop and Freshwater, 2000). The Foundation of Nursing Studies (2003) points out that the implementation of clinical supervision is patchy.

Midwives have a statutory system of clinical supervision for practice, as dictated by the Midwives Rules and Standards (NMC, 2004b).

The National Health Service Executive (Department of Health, 1993) has produced a strategy for the future, associated with the contribution the nurse, midwife and health visitor should make to the health of the nation. It provided a definition of clinical supervision. Clinical supervision is said to be a formal process of professional support and learning, enabling practitioners to develop knowledge and competence, assuming responsibility for their own practice and, as a result, improving public safety in complex clinical situations. This definition provided, for the first time, a systematic structure for supervision (Fowler, 2003).

As well as providing a relationship between clinical supervision and reflective practice, clinical supervision also has the potential to enable the practitioner to contribute in an effective manner to organisational objectives, such as clinical governance (UKCC, 1996). Chapter 12 of this text discusses the concepts associated with clinical governance. By participating in the clinical supervision process, practitioners are demonstrating commitment to their responsibilities associated with clinical governance. There is a clear symbiotic relationship with the overall framework of clinical governance. Clinical supervision, like clinical governance, is not an activity that is carried out in isolation; successful partnerships are developed and maintained through clinical supervision.

Bond and Holland (1998) suggest that clinical supervision occurs on a regular basis to enable facilitated in-depth reflection on clinical practice through focused support and development. They also emphasise that those focused support sessions should occur as time-protected sessions. The development and establishment of effective clinical supervision, according to the RCN (2002) and the United Kingdom Central Council (1996), allow the practitioner to:

- Reflect on nursing practice.
- Identify room for improvement.
- Develop expertise and promote standards of care.
- Devise new ways of learning.
- Gain professional support.
- Develop a deeper understanding of professional issues.

## WHAT IT IS AND WHAT IT IS NOT

Clinical supervision is suited to a variety of areas of clinical practice, for example with those nurses working in the mental health field, nurses working in the prison service and those nurses who are engaged in activities associated with child protection. Indeed, Barker (1992) suggests that clinical supervision is needed to protect patients from nurses and nurses from themselves. He makes this statement as he notes that the professional relationships nurses have with others may seriously affect how the nurse behaves towards those other people. Nursing, by the nature of the role and the relationship the nurse has with others, has the ability to provoke intimate feelings that, in turn, have the potential to affect the care provided. As a result of this, the nurse must investigate and explore these feelings. One method of doing this in a safe and supportive environment is during clinical supervision.

There are several definitions available that are associated with clinical supervision, but a plethora of definitions can lead to confusion and misunderstanding. It may be more beneficial to state what clinical supervision is *not*, as opposed to what it *is*. It is not, according to Yegdich (1999), psychotherapy or counselling, while Cutcliffe et al. (2001) state that it is distinct from mentoring. Importantly, clinical supervision is not an opportunity for managers to review staff performance; using clinical supervision in this manner may lead to resistance to the concept (Yegdich, 1998; Grant, 2000). See Table 16.10 for a summary of what clinical supervision is and what it is not.

When engaging in clinical supervision, opportunities arise that enable practitioners, in either a one-to-one setting or in a group context, to discuss areas of their practice that may be problematic or challenging. The encounter should aim to be:

**Table 16.10** What clinical supervision is and is not

| | |
|---|---|
| **What clinical supervision is not** | |
| ✗ | A disciplinary channel |
| | A route to make complaints |
| | An opportunity to reprimand poor performance |
| | An opportunity to criticise other team members |
| | Time out to chat about things in general |
| **What clinical supervision is** | |
| ✓ | A chance to openly, safely and honestly examine practice |
| | An opportunity to consider future development need |
| | An opportunity to identify and improve poor practices |
| | An opportunity to improve the delivery of care to patients (wherever they may be, e.g. institutional settings or within the home) |
| | A method to feel professionally supported and to minimise professional isolation |
| | A way of identifying good effective practice |

*Source*: Adapted from Department of Health, HM Prison Service and Welsh Assembly Government, 2004.

- supportive
- encouraging
- explorative
- reflective

## SOME PRACTICAL ISSUES

Prior to commencing clinical supervision an action plan needs to be established. Meetings will be needed to determine the best way forward and, most of all, to determine 'where you are at now'. Decisions need to be made about who will act as clinical supervisor and whether the session will be a one-to-one or group session. These details are important and from the outset they need to be addressed. Local factors will also need to be taken into account. When these issues have been addressed the process can be owned and moved forward. Consider the issues in Table 16.11.

Driscoll (2000) suggests that there are six skills that are essential to the supervisee if effective clinical supervision is to occur. You will become more competent and confident when using the skills listed below as you develop into your role:

- Make the session work for you.
- Identify pertinent issues to disclose in the session.
- Start to be aware of yourself in clinical practice.
- Be open to receiving feedback regarding your performance in the clinical area.
- Write as well as talking about issues that arise during clinical supervision sessions.
- Adopt a more proactive approach to problems that you encounter in clinical practice.

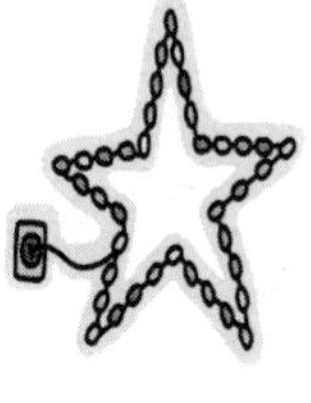

Having read this chapter you should be able to engage in some reflective activity of your own. Think about a recent situation (make it as recent as possible) that you can reflect on. When you have done this, choose one of the three models described in this chapter. Follow the model, addressing all aspects associated with it. When you have completed the activity, consider the following:

- How easy was it?
- How hard was it?

**Table 16.11** Some practicalities for consideration in relation to clinical supervision

| Frequency of interactions | Location | Protecting time | Group vs individual sessions | Professional and ethical issues |
|---|---|---|---|---|
| Determine how often clinical supervision should take place. Often this takes place on a monthly basis. In the initial periods this may be more often and as time progresses this may become less frequent. *Ad hoc* sessions may be required if the need arises. | It is important that the location in which clinical supervision takes place is jointly agreed by both the supervisee and the supervisor. The environment must be comfortable, free from interruption and distractions, as well as the possibility of the conversation being overheard. Careful consideration must be given to conducting clinical supervision in the clinical area as this may be counter-productive. | When the frequency and location have been agreed it is vital that both supervisee and supervisor are committed to the meetings. You should aim to be punctual and only in absolute emergencies should the session be cancelled. | The decision to use group as opposed to one-to-one clinical supervision sessions should be mutually agreed and not prescribed. | The content of the discussion must be confidential and all parties must be reminded of this. Boundaries must be established and respected. Documenting that a session has occurred is necessary and this can be done in the professional portfolio. Details of what was discussed will not be necessary although this can be done privately if desired, but the principles of confidentiality must be respected.<br><br>All nurses must be cognisant of the fact that there may be times when there is a need to disclose records. If this is the case advice must be sought. |

*Source*: Adapted from Faugier and Butterworth, 1994; Freshwater et al., 2002.

- Did you enjoy it?
- Did you feel uncomfortable?
- Did you learn anything?
- Would you do anything differently next time if the same or a similar situation arose?

## CONCLUSIONS

Most nurse education programmes (pre-registration) require student nurses to use a professional portfolio; this may be assessed or used as an opportunity to develop your skills. Using the portfolio and engaging in reflective practice are preparation for when you become a registered nurse. Becoming a registered nurse confers many things on you, and one of those is to engage in lifelong learning.

The Nursing and Midwifery Order 2001 demands that the registered nurse update his/her professional development. These mandatory requirements are part of post-registration education practice requirements – the practice component of PREP and the continuing professional development aspect.

Providing evidence to the NMC when it requests and requires it can be done in a variety of ways. Often nurses use a professional portfolio in order to present and organise their continuing professional development activities. Professional portfolios are varied. You may choose to devise your own or use one that has been commercially produced. The choice is yours, but remember it is not how you arrange and present your portfolio that is important, it is what it contains that will be judged.

Reflective practice is seen as one of the central components of continuing professional development. Three models have been briefly outlined here, but there are many more and you must choose the one that suits you and your situation. Closely related to reflective practice is the notion of clinical supervision. Clinical supervision provides you with an opportunity to engage in professional debate, to enhance care provision and to voice opinion (Allan, 2001). This chapter has pointed out what clinical supervision is and what it is not.

## REFERENCES

Allan, F. (2001) 'Advanced neonatal nursing practice' in Boxwell, G. (ed.) *Neonatal Intensive Care Nursing*. Routledge. London. Ch 1 pp 1–13.

Atkins, S. and Murphy, K. (1994) 'Reflective practice'. *Nursing Standard*. Vol 8, No 39, pp 49–56.

Barker, P. (1992) 'Psychiatric nursing' in Butterworth, T. and Faugier, J. (eds) *Clinical Supervision and Mentorship in Nursing*. Chapman Hall. London. Ch 5 pp 66–80.

Bishop, V. and Freshwater, D. (2000) *Clinical Supervision: Examples and Pointers for Good Practice*. Report for University of Leicester Hospitals Education Consortium. Leicester.

Bond, M. and Holland, S. (1998) *Skills of Clinical Supervision for Nurses*. Open University. Buckingham.

Boud, D., Keogh, R. and Walker, D. (1985) *Reflection: Turning Experience into Learning*. Kogan Page. New York.

Brown, R.A. (1992) *Portfolio Development and Profiling for Nurses*. Quay Books. Lancaster.

Chartered Society of Physiotherapists (2005) *Keeping a CPD Portfolio: Using Your CD ROM*. CSP. London.

Cutcliffe, J.R., Butterworth, T. and Proctor, B. (2001) *Fundamental Themes on Clinical Supervision*. Routledge. London.

Department of Health (1993) *A Vision for the Future: The Nursing, Midwifery and Health Visiting Contribution to Health and Social Care*. HMSO. London.

Department of Health (1998) *A First Class Service: Quality in the New NHS*. Department of Health. London.

Department of Health (2001) *Working Together – Learning Together: A Framework for Lifelong Learning for the NHS*. Department of Health. London.

Department of Health, HM Prison Service and Welsh Assembly Government (2004) *Clinical Supervision in Prison – Getting Started*. Department of Health. London.

Dooher, J., Clark, A. and Fowler, J. (2001) *Case Studies on Practice Development*. Quay Books. Wiltshire.

Douglas, I. (2002) 'Reflective practice' in Hogston, R. and Simpson, P.M. (eds) (2nd edn) *Foundations of Nursing Practice: Making the Difference*. Palgrave. Basingstoke. Ch 18 p 393.

Driscoll, J. (2000) *Practising Clinical Supervision: A Reflective Approach*. Bailliere Tindall. London.

Driscoll, J. and Teh, B. (2001) 'The contribution of portfolios and profiles to continuing professional development'. *Journal of Orthopaedic Nursing*. Vol 5, pp 151–156.

Faugier, J. and Butterworth, T. (1994) *Clinical Supervision: A Position Paper*. Manchester University. Manchester.

Foundation of Nursing Studies (2003) *Establishing Clinical Supervision in Prison and Healthcare Settings*. FONS Dissemination Series. London.

Fowler, J. (2003) 'Supporting practitioners in giving high quality care' in Hinchliff, S., Norman, S. and Schober, J. (eds) (4th edn) *Nursing Practice and Health Care*. Arnold. London. Ch 17 pp 391–413.

Freshwater, D., Walsh, L. and Storey, L. (2002) 'Prison healthcare: Developing leadership through supervision'. *Nursing Management*. Vol 8, No 8, pp 10–14.

Gibbs, G. (1988) *Learning by Doing: A Guide to Learning and Teaching Methods*. Further Education Unit, Oxford Polytechnic. Oxford.

Gibbs, G. (1992) *Improving the Quality of Student Learning*. Technical and Education Services. Plymouth.

Goodfellow, J. (2004) 'Documenting professional practice through the use of a professional portfolio'. *Early Years*. Vol 24, No 1, pp 63–74.

Grant, A. (2000) 'Clinical supervision and organisational power: A qualitative study'. *Mental Health and Learning Disabilities Care*. Vol 3, No 12, pp 398–401.

Health Professions Council (2005) *HPC in Focus*. November, No 1, p 1.

HSC 1999/194 *Continuing Professional Development (Quality in the New NHS)*. Department of Health. London.

Hull, C., Redfern, L. and Shuttleworth, A. (2005) (2nd edn) *Profiles and Portfolios: A Guide for Health and Social Care*. Palgrave. Basingstoke.

Institute of Health Care Management (2004) *Developing Through Partnership: CPFD Portfolio for Health Managers*. IHCM. London.

Johns, C. (1994) 'Guided reflection' in Palmer, A., Burns, S. and Bulman, C. (eds) *Reflective Practice in Nursing*. Blackwell Scientific. Oxford. pp 110–130.

Johns, C. (2000) *Becoming a Reflective Practitioner: A Reflective and Holistic Approach to Clinical Nursing, Practice Development and Clinical Supervision*. Blackwell Scientific. Oxford.

Moon, J. (2004) *A Handbook of Reflective and Experiential Learning*. Routledge. London.

Northern Ireland Practice and Education Council for Nursing and Midwifery (2004) *Your Development Framework: Part 1*. NIPEC. Belfast.

Nursing and Midwifery Council (2001) *Clinical Supervision*. NMC. London.

Nursing and Midwifery Council (2004a) *The PREP Handbook*. NMC. London.

Nursing and Midwifery Council (2004b) *Midwives Rules and Standards*. NMC. London.

Nursing and Midwifery Order 2002, Statutory Instrument 2002, No 253.

Pearce, R. (2003) *Profiles and Portfolios of Evidence*. Nelson Thornes. Cheltenham.

Platzer, H., Blake, D. and Snelling, J. (1997) 'A review of research into the use of groups and discussion to promote reflective practice in nursing'. *Research in Post-Compulsory Education*. Vol 2, No 2, pp 193–204.

Royal College of Nursing (2002) *Clinical Supervision in the Workplace: Guidance for Occupational Health Nurses*. RCN. London.

United Kingdom Central Council (1996) *Position Statement on Clinical Supervision*. UKCC. London.

Yegdich, T. (1998) 'How not to do clinical supervision in nursing'. *Journal of Advanced Nursing*. Vol 28, No 1, pp 193–202.

Yegdich, T. (1999) 'Lost in the crucible of supportive clinical supervision: Supervision is not therapy'. *Journal of Advanced Nursing*. Vol 29, No 5, pp 1265–1275.

# 17 Teaching and Learning in Clinical Practice

Leaders, mentors and teachers are vital for the next generation of practitioners. Nurses are required to enhance the professional development and the safe practice of others (NMC, 2004a). This can be realised through peer support, leadership, supervision and teaching.

As a student of nursing 50 per cent of your learning takes place within the clinical environment. In this chapter information and advice are provided to help you get the best from your clinical placement. It is in this environment that you are expected to apply your knowledge, learn new skills, and achieve the required learning outcomes and proficiencies. Because of this it is important that things go right when you are in your clinical placement.

As a registered nurse you will be expected to teach as well as update your own knowledge, therefore teaching and learning become lifelong activities. You are required to be both teacher and learner. Examples of how to provide environments that are conducive to teaching and learning are offered. This chapter presents practical and contemporary guidance for the development of teachers in many situations. There are several circumstances where the nurse is required to teach, for example when teaching more junior members of staff, or when providing patients with opportunities to learn about their health. The skills and qualities of a successful teacher are outlined in the chapter.

Emphasis is placed on teaching in the clinical area with a particular focus on teaching nurses and other health-care professionals. The principles related to the teaching of nurses and other health-care professionals can be applied (with care) to the teaching of patients.

It is not possible to provide you with authoritative guidelines when it comes to teaching and learning in the clinical area in a chapter of this size, as there are so many situations that may arise providing you with the opportunity to engage in teaching and learning activities. The discussions in this chapter are offered in order to whet your appetite with respect to teaching and learning. You are encouraged to delve deeper and seek out more substantial and definitive resources (both human and material) that address the multifaceted issue of teaching and learning in the clinical environment.

## TEACHING AND LEARNING IN THE CLINICAL ENVIRONMENT: THEORETICAL FRAMEWORKS

Teaching and learning in clinical practice can take place anywhere, as health care has many contexts. The terms 'clinical area' and 'clinical practice' are used in this chapter, but in the broadest context. Teaching and learning may occur in many places and can be associated with many situations, for example a busy acute mental health ward, a hospice, a patient's own home and so forth. There are a range of theories and approaches that you can choose from that most suit the situation; there is no right or wrong way to teach.

### DEFINITIONS

Definitions of teaching and learning are varied and there is no one 'best' definition. The definition chosen may well reflect the situation you find yourself in and it is unlikely that there is a definition of teaching that will satisfy all circumstances. Teaching is described by Curzon (1990) as a system of activities with the intention of inducing learning. It is a deliberate and methodological activity with a controlling element. This definition is often seen as a mechanistic definition of teaching (Dean and Kenworthy, 2000b). Schön (1987) uses a more reflective approach and emphasises the coaching analogy, whereby the learner is encouraged to seek explanations and the teacher provides advice and clarification.

Learning may be defined as a change of behaviour. It is an outcome, an end product. The assumption with this definition is that learning can be recognised or seen. Learning therefore, in this instance, assumes that a person has to perform in order to learn. This definition is associated with behaviouralist theory. Nicklin and Kenworthy (1995) move away from this perspective, suggesting that a description of learning when applied to the clinical setting would result in the measurable effect of the sum total of the intended and unintended encounters on the students, both in qualitative and quantitative terms.

The processes by which learning occurs are complex; over time psychologists have tried to describe them. It may help you to gain some understanding of these processes in order to teach and promote learning. Three theories and the theorists associated with them are briefly described. You are strongly advised to gain further insight and understanding of the theoretical concepts associated with teaching and learning.

### BEHAVIOURAL THEORY

Learning associated with behaviour is linked with the early theorists such as Pavlov. In simple terms these theorists, the behaviourists, demonstrated that if a repeated incentive – for example a negative stimulus such as an electric shock, or as a positive stimulus the provision of food – is used enough times to reward or punish, then eventually the subject learns. McKenna (1998a) suggests that with this approach the learner, when learning, engages in little thinking and that it is the observed change in behaviour that provides evidence that learning has taken place. The crux of the theory is the reinforcement of punishment or reward, rehearsal of a task over time. If there is a positive outcome, this can result in perfection. Behaviourist theory is associated with:

- Activities that aid learning.
- Repetitive activity and continued practice that aid learning.
- Small bite-size steps that aid learning.
- Reinforcement that aids learning.

## COGNITIVE THEORY

This theoretical approach suggests that learning occurs by receiving information, processing it, storing it and retrieving it. McKenna (1998b) suggests that unlike the behaviourists' perspective, cognitivism is associated with engaging in purposeful processes that encourage thinking, perception, organisation and insight. Dean and Kenworthy (2000a) note that cognitivism seeks to build on the insights of the student by stimulating the development of perception, as opposed to the 'stimulus–response' associated with behaviourism.

The psychologist Ausubel uses both educational and psychological theories (Quinn, 2000) when considering teaching and learning strategies. This approach focuses on the importance of experience, meaning, problem solving and the development of insights (Burns, 1995). Burns (1995) suggests that cognitive theory accepts that individuals have different needs and concerns occurring at different times. Those who subscribe to cognitive theory believe that:

- Learning comes from understanding.
- The organisation of teaching and how this is structured will aid learning.
- Cognitive feedback aids learning.
- Individual differences must be considered and taken into account.

## HUMANISM

The individual is the crucial component of this theoretical approach. There are two key theorists associated with the humanist approach to teaching and learning: Rogers (1983) and Knowles et al. (2005). Both these theorists support the notion that adults and children learn differently. Adults have:

- life experiences
- prior knowledge
- personalities

The role of the teacher is to facilitate learning; he/she is not seen as the font of all knowledge. Learning (or growth) takes place when feelings and experiences have been taken into consideration. Learning will only take place, however, if the learner feels comfortable and safe. This is related very closely to Maslow's hierarchy of needs (Maslow, 1954); see Chapter 6 for more detail regarding Maslow's hierarchy.

Rogers (1983) advocated a student-centred approach to learning, believing that the learning that takes place must be significant and meaningful, incorporating both thoughts and feelings. Rogers supports a shift in focus from what the teacher does to what is happening in the student. Knowles et al. (2005) suggest that there are five basic assumptions associated with Roger's thoughts on student-centred learning:

- We cannot teach a person directly, we can only facilitate his/her learning.
- A person will only learn significantly those things that he/she perceives as being involved in the maintenance of, or enhancement of, or the structure of self.
- In order to learn the learner needs to be ready to learn.
- Learning can often threaten an individual, therefore supportive climates that accept the person and enhance student responsibility should be created.
- If the self is not being threatened and supportive environments are in place, then this will promote significant learning.

Much of the theoretical underpinnings associated with humanism can be found in the practice of purposeful reflection. See Chapter 16 for more discussion regarding reflective practice.

To summarise the beliefs of the humanist's perspective:

- Learning is a natural process.
- Motivation, purpose and goals are important.
- The social situation can have an effect on learning.
- Choice, relevance and responsibility aid learning.
- Anxiety, discomfort and emotion affect learning.

When beginning to apply the theories to practice, it may be more appropriate to delve into and out of each one of them, adopting a 'pick-and-mix' approach as the situation dictates. All of the above theoretical approaches can be used and adapted for use in any given clinical setting.

## THE ADULT LEARNER

If you are engaged in teaching fellow health-care professionals, the approach you utilise will need to acknowledge the specific needs of the adult learner. The methods used will be very different from those employed when teaching children. Merriam and Brockett (1996) define adult learning as:

> *Activities intentionally designed for the purpose of bringing about learning among those whose age, social roles, or self perception define them as adults.*

Table 17.1 provides insight into some of the characteristics of adult learning.

Effective teaching in higher education demands that the individual teacher, the organisational culture and the policies and procedures in place meet the needs of the learner. Ramsden (1992) described six key principles associated with teaching in higher education; these beliefs also apply to those who teach in the clinical environment:

- Teachers should have an interest in the subject and be able to explain it to others.
- There should be a concern and respect for students and student learning.
- Appropriate assessment and feedback should be provided.
- There should be clear goals and intellectual challenge.
- Learners should have independence, control and active engagement.
- Teachers should be prepared to learn from students.

By acting as a teacher you also become a role model to other staff (this may include other members of the health-care team, not only nurses) as well as patients. Teaching as a skill, along with all the other skills cited in this text, can be learned and developed. Good teachers are created, not born. Table 17.2 describes the personal attributes of the nurse who also acts as a clinical educator. The skills listed have been adapted to reflect the skills required by the nurse.

**Table 17.1** The main characteristics of adult learning

- The learning is purposeful.
- Participation is voluntary.
- Participation should be active not passive.
- Clear goals and objectives should be set.
- Feedback is required.
- Opportunities for reflection should be provided.

*Source*: Brookfield, 1986.

**Table 17.2** Some of the personal qualities required by the nurse with respect to clinical teaching

- An enthusiasm and commitment to high-quality nursing care.
- A personal commitment to teaching and learning.
- Sensitivity and responsiveness to the educational needs of students.
- The capacity to promote development of the required professional attitudes and values.
- An understanding of the principles of education applied to nursing.
- The command of practical teaching skills and the willingness to enhance these.
- A willingness to develop as a good nurse as well as a teacher.
- A commitment to evaluation and audit of teaching practices.
- The willingness to undertake both summative and formative assessment of student progress.

*Source*: Adapted from General Medical Council, 1999.

The principles above should be taken into account when preparing to teach. The following five steps will be used as a framework to help you with your teaching in the clinical area:

1. Create a positive learning environment.
2. Know who your learners are.
3. Know what it is that you want them to know.
4. Prepare.
5. Ask for feedback.

## CREATE A POSITIVE LEARNING ENVIRONMENT

Creating a positive learning environment is paramount. No matter what you intend to teach, or what the learner wishes to learn, it is vital that the learning environment is a positive one. The humanist approach described earlier suggests that the creation of a safe environment will enhance and aid learning. There are some factors that will be outside of your control in the clinical environment, for example noise and interruptions. Despite these possibilities you should strive to provide an atmosphere that encourages enquiry and is nonthreatening.

If you have any control over the physical environment, always try to ensure that the room or area where you are teaching is warm; open windows if it feels stuffy. Observe the learners and suggest a break if they appear to be tiring. Let people know about taking 'comfort breaks', where the facilities are, and try to provide some idea about how long the session will last. The impact of the room will have implications for learning, therefore consideration should be directed towards seating arrangements. Issues such as seating arrangements are seen as resources. Poor use of resources can have a substantial impact on the learning experience.

Provide the student with evidence that you have their needs at the forefront of your mind. For example, at the beginning of the session determine what the students' needs are and when you conclude the session assess if you have met their needs. Student-centred learning means that the teacher must put the needs of the learner at the centre of teaching activities. Emphasis is needed on encouraging the facilitation of learning as opposed to the delivery of teaching. The facilitator should aim to guide the learner towards resources and sources of knowledge (human and material) just as much as being the source of knowledge him/herself. Bellack (2005) suggests that when a learning-centred approach is used the learner learns as much about how to learn as about the specific content. She adds that the teacher's role is to enable students to discover and experiment.

Learning environments are wide and varied and can be the patient's own home, the operating theatre, the clinic and at the bedside. Nearly every activity that the nurse undertakes is potentially a learning opportunity. The nurse may be required to teach in more formal settings such as in a classroom or a lecture theatre. Other venues may be associated with e-learning, for example a virtual learning environment.

## KNOW WHO YOUR LEARNERS ARE

Research your audience. You must have some insight into who it is you are going to teach, what programme of study they are attending, the academic level and how far they have progressed in the programme so far. How many of them will there be? Find out about previous life experiences (as a professional and as a layperson), determine what the students already know about the topic you are teaching. Avoid making assumptions and stereotyping the learners. Find out what they will be going on to learn next.

## KNOW WHAT IT IS THAT YOU WANT THEM TO KNOW

When using a cognitivist or behaviourist approach you must know what it is you want the learner to know; objectives must be set. Take time considering these carefully: the aims and objectives decided on will result in you applying the correct teaching methods. If you are teaching a rote-based task, for example cardiopulmonary resuscitation, you will need to provide instructions to the learners, and this needs to be broken down into smaller chunks. There will be a need to repeat in order to reinforce learning. If, on the other hand, the points you are trying to convey are concerned with ethics your approach will be different: you may need to seek opinions from the learners, exploring and unravelling these opinions and beliefs, challenging responses in a safe and comfortable manner.

## PREPARE

Just as with any activity that is undertaken, the outcome of teaching will be more beneficial if it has been prepared. The amount of preparation needed to provide a teaching session that is effective and meaningful cannot be overestimated. Even opportunist teaching sessions need to have some degree of planning. Preparation of the patient (if appropriate), the environment and the teaching tools to be used are some examples of issues that need planning consideration. Determine if there will be any pre-reading materials required for the session: if so, how will the learners access them?

## ASK FOR FEEDBACK

Feedback, evaluation and reflection are activities that are synonymous with each other. There are many methods that can be used to provide feedback concerning performance and how the learners felt about the teaching session, as well as you providing the learners with feedback regarding their performance. Reflective activity has been discussed in detail in Chapter 16; the concepts discussed in that chapter can be used by the teacher and the learner.

Formal evaluation in the form of feedback questionnaires can be administered and the results analysed; this has the potential to provide both quantitative and qualitative data depending on how the questionnaire is formulated and structured. Peer review is another alternative. This occurs when a colleague is asked to observe your performance. This can be done in a highly structured manner, for example if a checklist approach is used and you are graded on the outcome, or alternatively an unstructured approach can be used where you are provided with feedback in a more general manner. Feedback given to you can only help you become even better when teaching in the clinical environment.

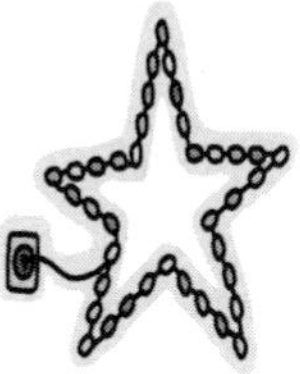

Consider a recent teaching session where you were a learner. Provide evidence and make comments on the how the session addressed the issues described in Table 17.3.

Do you think the session could have been better? If so, how?

## USING RESOURCES TO ENHANCE TEACHING AND LEARNING

The best resource available to you to enhance and encourage teaching and learning in the clinical environment is you once you have become an

**Table 17.3** Evaluating a teaching session

| Aspect of the teaching session | Evidence/comments |
|---|---|
| Did you experience a positive learning environment? | |
| Did you feel that the teacher 'knew' you/the learners? | |
| Was he/she aware of your needs? | |
| Did you know what was expected of you? | |
| Were you aware of the aims and objectives of the session? | |
| Was the session adequately prepared? | |
| Were you able to provide feedback? | |
| How was this done? | |

experienced nurse. You should respect students in acknowledging that you are not the font of all knowledge, simply a conduit to facilitate the activity of learning.

It has already been stated that the poor use of resources can have a considerable effect on learning and teaching; hence the importance of dedicating a section of this chapter entirely to teaching resources. The resources discussed here are resources that can be used in variety of settings. Bear the following points in mind when explaining or facilitating learning (see Table 17.4).

**Table 17.4** Some points to be taken into account when teaching or facilitating learners

| Point | Action |
|---|---|
| Be clear | • If possible teach in a quiet area.<br>• Speak slowly and clearly – enunciate.<br>• Ensure clarity with your teaching resources and materials, e.g. are your transparencies and handouts clear and easy to read?<br>• Use short sentences when speaking.<br>• Do not be tempted to provide too much information. |
| Generate interest | • Use a variety of resources and approaches in order to stimulate.<br>• Be enthusiastic about the topic. |
| Use logical organisation | • Build slowly from one concept to the next.<br>• As with essay writing, ensure that there is an introduction, body and conclusion. |
| Spell out the relevance | • Explain why this topic is important.<br>• Link with the overall assessment strategy.<br>• Explain how patient care can be enhanced by further understanding. |
| Emphasise important points | • Clearly state what the important points are.<br>• Use different emphasis for important points, e.g. different-coloured writing on handouts, use of bold/italics or an increase in font size.<br>• Explain why these points are important. |
| Use examples | • Provide clinical examples, e.g. refer to patients who you are currently caring for.<br>• Use anecdotes – but with caution. |
| Avoid unnecessary jargon | • Speak plainly.<br>• If jargon is used ensure you provide a definition of the terms used. |
| Check out understanding | • Use your skills to determine if learners have understood, be alert to nonverbal communications.<br>• Do not patronise learners.<br>• Listen and respond. |

**Table 17.5** Some dos and don'ts when using an overhead projector

**Do**
- Use permanent marker pens, as water-soluble pens have a tendency to smudge.
- Leave space to add to the transparency as the session progresses.
- Use large fonts; too small a font and the audience may not be able to read it.
- Know how to turn the projector on and what to do if the bulb blows.
- Face the audience.

**Don't**
- Use colours that are difficult to read when projected – red, orange and yellow are particularly difficult to read.
- Use too much text on the transparency; use key words only.
- Use complex diagrams – consider supplementing with hard copies or direct the audience to an electronic source.
- Block the audience's view by standing in front of the projection.
- Rush through the presentation; the audience may wish to be given time to write down what you have projected.

## OVERHEAD PROJECTORS

Projectors can be free standing, fixed, permanent or portable. They require the use of transparencies to project the image onto a suitable screen.

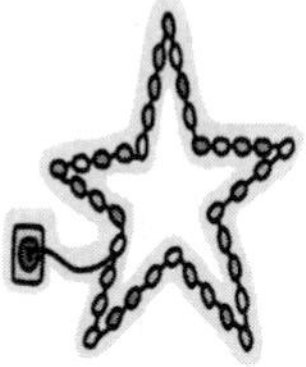

Take some time now to reflect on times when you as a learner have experienced a teacher using the overhead projector. Think about the size of the font used by the teacher: was it too small or too large? Was there too much text on the transparency?

Table 17.5 provides a list of dos and don'ts to be considered when using overhead projectors. Presentation skills are important and can have as much impact as the content that is being provided.

## POWERPOINT PRESENTATIONS

Prior to the arrival of PowerPoint® as software used in presentations, overhead and 35 mm slide projecting were the tools of choice. PowerPoint is a powerful teaching tool enabling the user to prepare a selection of slides to be projected using a data projector. The PowerPoint package enables the user to:

**Table 17.6** Hints and tips for PowerPoint presentations

- Use a sans serif font, for example Arial, for slide presentations in order to prevent blurring of the text during projection.
- Use different font sizes for main titles and text.
- Be judicial with the number of lines used on each slide; seven is a maximum.
- A dark-coloured font should be used against a light background (not white).
- Always have a prepared set of overhead transparencies to hand in case of technological failure.

*Source*: Adapted from Lowe and Jasmine, 1999.

- Use templates.
- Add colours to stimulate the audience.
- Incorporate photographic images.
- Use animation to build up a 'show'.
- Enhance the presentation by using transitions – a function that provides a variety of ways of changing from one slide to another.

As with overhead projection, practice makes perfect. Table 17.6 provides some hints and tips associated with PowerPoint.

## FLIPCHARTS AND WHITEBOARDS

These resources are often used when working with small groups. If used in small groups the participants can be invited to become actively involved in the session. The group could be asked to brainstorm an activity, for example the possible causes of urinary tract infection (Mackway-Jones and Walker, 1999). Excessive use of this approach may not suit all participants, however, and it needs to be employed with care.

After the session has ended, the teacher must treat the used flipchart sheet with respect. It is advocated that the used sheets are folded up (not ripped off the wall and screwed up) and if they are not to be retained then they should be disposed of sensitively.

## HANDOUTS

The mainstay of teaching for many years has been handouts. They are often used by nurses in many situations and settings. Handouts are normally used to supplement or reinforce learning. They are also used as one way of ensuring that all students receive the same information. The creation of handouts should be given much thought if they are to succeed. Thompson and Sheckley (1997) state that students like handouts as they can come away from the lecture with the learning in hand – a record or transcript of learning.

When designing handouts Sakraida and Draus (2005) suggest that the items in Table 17.7 should be considered.

**Table 17.7** Some considerations for the preparation of handouts

| | |
|---|---|
| Type and layout | • Font sizes should be 12 to 14, with bold print to promote ease of reading.<br>• Too long a handout can be a distraction.<br>• Brief handouts can enhance attention as a presentation is being made. |
| Purpose | • The purpose of the handout will determine when it is distributed to the students.<br>• The following are types of handout:<br>  • Complete notes.<br>  • Skeleton notes with blank spaces for students to fill in.<br>  • Notes that emphasise one aspect of the session, for example complex concepts or diagrams. |
| Focus | • A handout should only be concerned with a single topic.<br>• Key points can be used.<br>• Definitions of key terms may be considered. |
| Visual appeal | • Visual appeal can communicate that the teacher has a professional approach.<br>• A creative approach is advocated with the use of various fonts and colours.<br>• Printing on coloured paper is visually appealing.<br>• Spacing of material and design layout must be given some consideration. |

*Source*: Miller, 1999; Heinich et al., 2002; Topps, 2002.

Handouts are still used in various clinical settings for health-care professionals and patients and can be produced as hard copy or electronically. The better the quality of the handout, the more potential there is for learning to take place. The teacher must remember not only to evaluate his/her teaching on a regular basis but also the use of any resources, including handouts.

## LEARNING IN THE PRACTICE PLACEMENT

The NMC (NMC, 2004b) requires that 50 per cent of your time as a student (2300 hours) is to be spent in the practice area. As a result of this, it should be noted that there will be serious implications for the student if things do not go well (RCN, 2005). While undertaking learning experiences in the practice setting you will be able to apply the theory you have learnt to practice, experiencing the various challenges and issues that occur.

### PRACTICE PLACEMENTS

Students have a crucial role to play in ensuring that they get the best from their practice placement. Students have responsibilities as well as other key stakeholders in the practice placement relationship. Practice placements can be defined as opportunities where you can undertake practice under supervision. During your time in a practice placement a mentor assesses learning and facilitates the achievement of required learning outcomes and proficiencies.

The RCN (2002) states that there are several different titles used for nurses who provide support to students in practice, for example:

- mentors
- preceptors
- assessors
- practice educators

With so many titles there is the potential to cause confusion. In order to ensure consistency, the ENB (2001) prefers the term 'mentor' as the title of choice. The quality of a clinical placement (including the mentor) has the potential to impinge on your educational experience. You are encouraged to take personal responsibility for directing your own learning and making the best use of human and material resources in order to achieve the proficiencies required for entry to the professional register.

The RCN (2002) suggests that practice placements that meet the needs of the student can help:

- Meet statutory and regulatory requirements.
- Achieve the required proficiencies as stipulated by the regulator (NMC).
- Provide opportunities to take part in health-care activities in a wide range of rapidly changing health and social-care environments.
- Make available a full range of nursing-care activities to a variety of patients.
- Offer experiences that will enable the student to appreciate the unpredictable and dynamic nature of nursing care in a clinical setting.
- Create the feeling of working as a member of a multidisciplinary team.
- Identify appropriate learning opportunities.

Practice placements must also ensure that the student is provided with opportunities to identify the community focus of care, the continuing nature of care, the need for acute and critical care, as well as a multiprofessional approach to care. These requirements are cited in the European Directive 77/453/EEC. Placements, therefore, should be varied, reflecting care in the independent sector as well the NHS and in both health and social-care settings. They must provide the student with the ability to meet the proficiencies deemed essential by the NMC (NMC, 2004b).

## KEY STAKEHOLDERS ASSOCIATED WITH THE PRACTICE PLACEMENT

The ultimate stakeholder is the patient. There are other stakeholders who will be providing support to help the student gain as much from their clinical learning experience as possible. The United Kingdom Central Council (1999) has stated that all significant stakeholders have a responsibility for ensuring that at the point of registration the nurse is fit for:

- *Purpose* – can function as a competent practitioner in the clinical setting.
- *Practice* – can fulfil the needs of registration.
- *Award* – has attained the breadth and depth of learning that is commensurate with the award, i.e. diploma or degree.

Below is a list of those who could be considered as key stakeholders in the practice placement (the patient has already been mentioned):

- The student.
- The NHS and independent sector.
- The higher education institution (the university).
- Service providers (those in the clinical placement, e.g. mentors, lecturer practitioners) – these are part of the tripartite arrangements.
- The commissioning bodies for education – these are also part of the tripartite arrangements.

Figure 17.1 provides a diagrammatic representation of the stakeholders.

Below are some issues that you may need to consider to get the most out of your clinical placement. Remember that all other members of the tripartite arrangement also have responsibilities to make the experience a valuable and

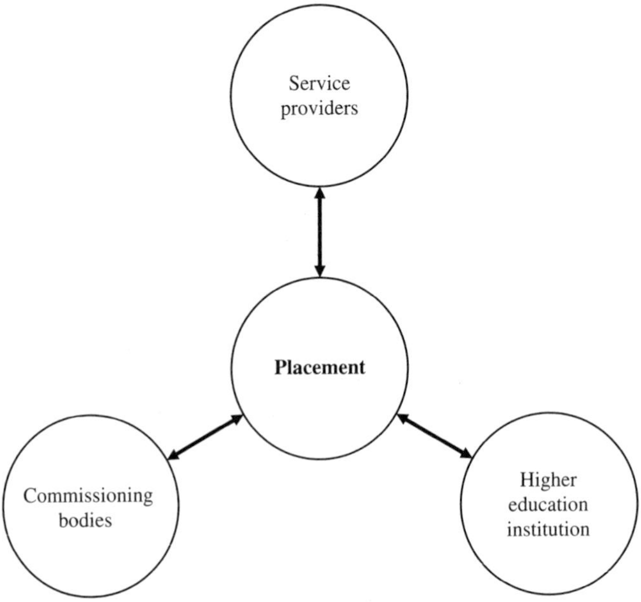


**Figure 17.1** The tripartite approach associated with the practice placement

meaningful one. The prospect of a new placement may seem daunting (Harrison, 2006). Preparation prior to arriving at the placement may help alleviate any anxiety or apprehensions you may have. Prior to your placement:

- Ensure you know about any specific issues related to clinical placements that may be contained in your student handbook. This handbook may include details concerning the assessment of practice and what you are required to achieve while on clinical placement.
- Determine what the purpose of the placement experience is and also what the expectations of the service provider are.
- Contact your link lecturer prior to the placement commencing to find out if there are any specific issues associated with the placement, e.g. whether you have to wear uniform.
- Contact relevant people at the placement.
- Ensure you are cognisant with how you are to be assessed, what are the assessment tools to be used, whether you need to keep a reflective diary, whether there are any learning contracts that need to be drawn up.

While on clinical placement:

- Be punctual, maintain confidentiality, be aware of the image you portray and your attitude and act professionally at all times.
- Be proactive in seeking out learning opportunities with the help of your mentor.
- Take every opportunity available and be willing to work as a member of the team.
- Express your needs.
- Make use of your named mentor and other resources to achieve your learning outcomes.
- Seek help and advice if you feel that the mentor relationship is not working.
- Work under supervision when achieving clinical skills.
- Take every opportunity to work outside the practice placement to work with specialist practitioners.
- Be willing to provide constructive feedback as well as receiving the same.
- Undertake reflective activity to assess your own confidence and competence.
- If you take time off during your placement, for example if you are sick, you may be required to inform the university and the clinical placement with details of your circumstances. You may need to provide self-certification if you are off sick for three consecutive days. If your sickness extends and you are off longer than eight days you may have to produce a doctor's sick certificate. Find out what the requirements are prior to starting your placement.
- If during placement you are of the opinion that you have witnessed bad practice, you must first inform your mentor or the nurse in charge. You may feel your concerns have not been adequately addressed; if this is the case contact your link lecturer.

- During your placement you will be supernumerary to the placement staffing levels. This means that students are additional to staffing establishment figures. However, you must make a contribution to the work of the practice placement area to enable you to learn how to care for patients.

After the placement experience:

- Evaluate your achievements – what you have enjoyed and how you have benefited from the placement.
- Evaluate the placement against requirements, e.g. by completing an online evaluation form.
- Participate in classroom discussion regarding the placement if this is required.
- Ensure you submit on time any placement documentation required as a part of your assessment.
- Reflect on your experiences.

## TEACHING IN THE PRACTICE PLACEMENT

Once you are qualified you may be required to act as a resource for teaching junior members of the multidisciplinary team and this may mean teaching student nurses. In time you can choose to become a mentor who holds the relevant mentor qualifications. If you do become a mentor you will be required to have your name placed on an up-to-date mentors' register and undertake a programme of study that prepares you for teaching and assessing in the clinical area.

## MENTORSHIP

Mentors and teachers are central to the preparation of the next generation of practitioners. It is vital that student nurses are taught by those with practical and recent experience of their profession (English National Board and Department of Health, 2001). During your pre-registration programme of study you will have been allocated a mentor. The allocation of a mentor is one way in which the NMC can ensure that the proficiencies required for registration have been achieved. The mentor, having been prepared to teach and assess in clinical practice, is a key person in ensuring that the student receives clinical education opportunities that are commensurate with achieving learning outcomes associated with the proficiencies (ENB and Department of Health, 2001; NMC, 2004b).

The NMC (2002) states that in order to record a teaching qualification on the NMC register the nurse will need to undertake additional preparation and education that reflects the standards set by the NMC. Originally there were eight advisory standards published by the NMC (2002) for mentors and mentorship (see Table 17.8). This was altered in 2003 (NMC, 2003) from 'advisory' to 'required'.

The NMC (2002) stipulates that mentors must have a current registration with the NMC. They must also have a minimum of 12 months' full-time

**Table 17.8** The standards and expectations required of a mentor

| Required standard | Expectations |
|---|---|
| **Communication and working relationships** | • Development of effective relationships based on mutual trust and respect.<br>• An understanding of how students integrate into practice settings and assisting with this process.<br>• Provision of ongoing and constructive support for students. |
| **Facilitation of learning** | • Demonstration of sufficient knowledge of the student's programme to identify current learning needs.<br>• Demonstration of strategies that will assist with the integration of learning from practice and education settings.<br>• Creation and development of opportunities for students to identify and undertake experiences to meet their learning needs. |
| **Conducting assessment** | • Demonstration of a good understanding associated with assessment and ability to assess.<br>• Implementation of approved assessment procedures. |
| **Role model** | • Demonstration of effective relationships with patients and clients.<br>• Contribution to the development of an environment in which effective practice is fostered, implemented, evaluated and disseminated.<br>• Assessment and management of clinical developments to ensure safe and effective care. |
| **Creating an environment for learning** | • Ensuring effective learning experiences and opportunities to achieve learning outcomes for students by contribution to the development and maintenance of a learning environment.<br>• Implementation of strategies for quality assurance and quality audit. |
| **Improving practice** | • Contribution to the creation of an environment in which change can be initiated and supported. |
| **Knowledge base** | • Identification, application and dissemination of research findings within the area of practice. |
| **Course development** | • Contribution to the development and/or review of courses. |

*Source*: Adapted from NMC, 2002; NMC, 2003.

experience (or a part-time equivalent) before becoming a mentor. The ENB and Department of Health (2001) describe a mentor as a registered nurse, midwife or health visitor who facilitates learning and supervises and assesses students in the practice setting.

There are several approaches to supporting students in clinical practice and each NHS Trust and higher education institution will have its own approved methods of doing this. The use of an appropriately qualified and approved mentor has already been outlined. The terms 'associate mentor', 'co-mentor' and 'secondary mentor' may also be used to identify health-care professionals (not necessarily nurses) who are relevant to the practice experience in which the student is placed. These individuals may be registered nurses who have not completed a recognised programme of study leading to a qualification as a mentor; they may be social workers or teachers. The latter professionals play a significant part in teaching and learning in the practice placement.

Assessment of the student can only be undertaken by a person who is entered on a live register of mentors. The following is a list of those who can carry out the assessment of student performance; however, the titles of the programmes of study may vary from institution to institution. A registered nurse who has undertaken any of the following programmes of study or their equivalent:

- ENB 998 approved assessor.
- Mentorship and Support for Professional Practice Module.
- Preparation for Mentorship and Proceptorship in Professional Education.
- Postgraduate Certificate in Education.
- A1/2 D32/33. These qualifications are associated with those who undertake work-based assessments, such as vocational courses and City and Guilds programmes. They are verifiers' qualifications.

You should seek advice from your university if you are unsure about who will be able to assess your performance while on clinical placement.

The growth in the number of terms and the roles associated with mentors in relation to teaching and learning may be seen as evidence that practice-based teaching and learning are generally achieving a higher profile in nurse education. This growth in interest will continue, particularly in relation to the expansion of interprofessional education, as well as government initiatives such as the knowledge and skills framework and Agenda for Change. Agenda for Change aims to determine new frameworks for the employment of health-care staff (apart from doctors) and recognises the contribution nurses are making to the effective delivery of health care. It might also be suggested that recognition is forthcoming regarding the important role nurses play in teaching and assessing in the clinical area (Department of Health, 2004).

## CONCLUSIONS

Half of your time as a student nurse is associated with work-based learning and the remaining 50 per cent is related to theory, for example by attending your programme of study at the university. This theory and practice split means you will be assessed from both a theoretical and a practical perspective. University staff (lecturers) generally assesses theory and a recognised and registered practice assessor or your mentor assesses practice. A variety of terms are used to describe those who undertake teaching and assessing roles and much confusion can occur as a result of this. Some of the terms used have been discussed.

This chapter had addressed several key concepts associated with teaching and learning in the clinical environment. Although the bulk of the chapter is focused on the teaching and learning needs of student nurses and other health-care professionals, the principles outlined can (with care) be applied to the patient in a variety of settings.

The processes associated with learning are complex and much of the theory used to explain and enhance teaching arises in psychology. Three theoretical approaches have been briefly outlined. It is important to gain a fundamental understanding of the theoretical approaches if the teaching of nurses and other health-care professionals in the health-care environment is to be effective. All the approaches discussed can be used and applied simultaneously; the reader is encouraged to pick and mix approaches to suit the situation.

Practical tips and hints have been provided with the aim of helping the student to get the most out of the clinical experience from a teaching and learning perspective, either as a learner and/or a teacher. A framework is used relating to five areas in order to provide advice and each aspect of the framework offers the reader pointers to enhance teaching and learning. The use of various resources such as overhead projection and handouts in order to enhance teaching and learning opportunities is outlined.

Practice placements have the potential to provide students with opportunities to achieve their learning outcomes as well as the proficiencies required by the regulator (NMC). The mentor is seen as one member of a tripartite arrangement who can help students achieve the statutory requirements. The role and function of the mentor are described.

## REFERENCES

Bellack, J.P. (2005) 'Teaching for learning and improvement'. *Journal of Nursing Education.* Vol 44, No 7, pp 295–296.

Brookfield, S.D. (1986) *Understanding and Facilitating Adult Learning: A Comprehensive Analysis of Principles and Effective Practice.* Open University Press. Milton Keynes.

Burns, J. (1995) *The Adult Learner at Work.* Business and Professional Publishing. Sydney

Curzon, L.B. (1990) *Teaching in Further Education.* Cassell. London.

Dean, J. and Kenworthy, N. (2000a) 'The principles of learning' in Nicklin, P.J. and Kenworthy, N. (eds) (3rd edn) *Teaching and Assessing in Nursing Practice.* Bailliere Tindall. London. Ch 4 pp 45–67.

Dean, J. and Kenworthy, N. (2000b) 'The principles of teaching' in Nicklin, P.J. and Kenworthy, N. (eds) (3rd edn) *Teaching and Assessing in Nursing Practice.* Bailliere Tindall. London. Ch 5 pp 69–100.

Department of Health (2004) *Agenda for Change: Final Agreement.* Department of Health. London.

English National Board for Nursing, Midwifery and Health Visiting and Department of Health (2001) *Preparation of Mentors and Teachers: A New Framework for Guidance.* ENB. London.

General Medical Council (1999) *The Doctor as Teacher.* GMC. London.

Harrison, P. (2006) 'Perspectives on adult nursing' in Schrober, J. and Ash, C. (eds) *Student Nurses' Guide to Professional Practice and Development.* Arnold. London. Ch 4 pp 35–45.

Heinich, R., Molenda, M., Russell, J.D. and Smaldino, S.E. (2002) (7th edn) *Instructional Media and Technologies for Learning.* Merill-Prentice Hall. New Jersey.

Knowles, M., Holton, E.F. and Swanson, R.A. (2005) (6th edn) *The Adult Learner: The Definitive Classic in Adult Education and Human Resource Development.* Elsevier. Burlington.

Lowe, D. and Jasmine, G. (1999) *PowerPoint for Dummies.* Hungry Minds. Indianapolis.

Mackway-Jones, K. and Walker, M. (1999) *Pocket Guide to Teaching for Medical Instructors.* BMJ Books. London.

Maslow, A. (1954) *Motivation and Personality.* New York. Harper and Row.

McKenna, G. (1998a) 'Learning theories made easy: Behaviourism' in Downie, C.M. and Basford, P. (eds) (2nd edn) *Teaching and Assessing in Clinical Practice: A Reader.* Greenwich University Press. Greenwich. Ch 9 pp 95–100.

McKenna, G. (1998b) 'Learning theories made easy: Congitivism' in Downie, C.M. and Basford, P. (eds) (2nd edn) *Teaching and Assessing in Clinical Practice: A Reader.* Greenwich University Press. Greenwich. Ch 10 pp 100–107.

Merriam, S.B. and Brockett, R.G. (1996) *The Process and Practice of Adult Education.* Jossey-Bass. San Francisco.

Miller, C.A. (1999) (3rd edn) *Nursing Care of Older Adults: Theory and Practice.* Lippincott. Philadelphia.

Nicklin, P.J. and Kenworthy, N. (1995) (2nd edn) *Teaching and Assessing in Nursing Practice.* Scutari Press. London.

Nursing and Midwifery Council (2002) *Standards for the Preparation of Teachers of Nursing and Midwifery.* NMC. London.

Nursing and Midwifery Council (2003) *QA Fact Sheet O/2003: NMC Requirements for Mentors and Mentorship.* NMC. London.

Nursing and Midwifery Council (2004a) *The NMC Code of Professional Conduct: Standards for Conduct, Performance and Ethics.* NMC. London.

Nursing and Midwifery Council (2004b) *Standards of Proficiency for Pre-registration Nursing Education.* NMC. London.

Quinn, F. (2000) (4th edn) *Principles and Practice of Nurse Education.* Nelson Thornes. Cheltenham.

Ramsden, P. (1992) *Learning to Teach in Higher Education.* Routledge. London.

Rogers, C.R. (1983) *Freedom to Learn.* Merril. Ohio.

Royal College of Nursing (2002) *Helping Students Get the Best from Their Practice Placements.* RCN. London.

Royal College of Nursing (2005) *The Practice Placement Experience A Survey of RCN Student Members: Executive Summary.* RCN. London.

Sakraida, T.J. and Draus, P.J. (2005) 'Quality handout development and use'. *Journal of Nursing Education.* Vol 44, No 7, pp 326–329.

Schön, D. (1987) *Educating the Reflective Practitioner.* Jossey Bass. San Francisco.

Thompson, C. and Sheckley, B.G. (1997) 'Differences in classroom teaching preferences between traditional and adult BSN students'. *Journal of Nursing Education.* Vol 36, pp 163–170.

Topps, D. (2002) 'Visual handouts for hand held computers'. *Medical Education.* Vol 36, p 1101.

United Kingdom Central Council (1999) *Fitness to Practice, Nursing and Midwifery Education. Report of the UKCC's Commission for Nursing and Midwifery Education.* UKCC. London.

# Review Responses

1. What date was the current Code of Conduct published?
   a. 1994
   b. 2001
   **c. 2004**
   d. 2005

2. How many sections are there in the Code of Conduct?
   a. 10
   **b. 9**
   c. 14
   d. 16

3. The Code of Conduct is:
   a. A legal document
   b. A document produced to protect the nurse
   **c. An advisory document**
   d. A document used for disciplinary purposes for the student

4. Who does the document concern?
   a. Children and families
   b. Children's Nurses
   **c. All nurses, midwives and community public health nurses**
   d. All health-care professionals

5. Where can copies be obtained?
   a. The university learning resource centre
   b. The NMC Web site
   c. The NMC
   **d. All of the above**

6. Which of the following are documents that the NMC does not produce?
   a. Administration of medicines
   b. Records and record keeping
   **c. National service frameworks**
   **d. Manual removal of faeces**

7. The key aim of the NMC is to:
   **a. Protect and serve the public**
   b. Protect the best interests of the nurse
   c. Provide an annual report to the ombudsman
   d. Generate income

8. How many parts are there to the professional register?
   a. 1
   b. 14
   **c. 3**
   d. 16

9. Which of the following statements is true?
   a. The NMC is a commercial enterprise
   b. All doctors must have live registration with NMC in order to practise
   **c. The NMC is an organisation set up by Parliament to ensure nurses and midwives provide high standards of care to their patients and clients**
   d. Membership to the NMC is open to all health-care professionals

10. When was the NMC created?
   a. December 2002
   b. April 2003
   **c. April 2002**
   d. December 2003

# Glossary of Terms

| Word/Phrase | Meaning |
|---|---|
| Accountability | Process that mandates that individuals are answerable for their actions and have an obligation (or duty) to act. |
| Active listening | Listening that focuses on the feelings of the individual who is speaking. |
| Acute care | Short-term hospital care provided to patients with conditions of short duration requiring stays of, on average, fewer than 30 days. |
| Acute illness | Disruption (usually reversible) in functional ability characterised by a rapid onset, intense manifestations and a relatively short duration of illness. |
| Acute pain | Discomfort identified by sudden onset and relatively short duration, mild to severe intensity, and a steady decrease in intensity of pain over several days or weeks. |
| Addiction | The physical and psychological dependence on using a substance, e.g. tobacco or alcohol. |
| Adverse drug event | Harm resulting from medical intervention related to a drug. |
| Adverse health-care event | An event or omission arising during clinical care and causing physical or psychological injury to a patient. |
| Advocate | A person who pleads the cause of another. |
| Aeitiology | The cause or contributing factors of a health problem. |
| Analysis | A mental process that enables a person to gain a better understanding of something. |
| Antidiscriminatory practice | Acknowledging the sources of oppression in a person's life and actively seeking to reduce them. |

| Word/Phrase | Meaning |
|---|---|
| Anxiety | A vague, uneasy feeling of discomfort or dread accompanied by an autonomic response. |
| Assumption | Something that is taken for granted without any proof. |
| Attitude | Mental stance that is composed of several beliefs. Often involves a negative or positive judgement towards a person, object or idea. |
| Autonomy | The state of being independent, self-governing, with no outside control, the ability to make one's own decisions. |
| Bar graph | A chart that displays data by comparing the height or length of bars of equal width. |
| Behaviour | Observable response of an individual to external stimuli. |
| Beliefs | Interpretations or conclusions that are accepted as accurate. |
| Beneficence | Ethical principle regarding the duty to promote good and prevent harm. |
| Bereavement | Period of grieving following the death of a loved one. |
| Blame culture | An organisational culture that inhibits openness regarding reporting incidents as staff are fearful of being personally penalised for making errors. |
| Body image | Individual's perception of physical self, including appearance, function and ability. |
| Caring | The intentional action that suggests physical and emotional support and security. A genuine connectedness with another person or a group of people. |
| Categorical imperative | Concept that states that one should act only if the action is based on a principle that is universal. |
| Chronic acute pain | Discomfort that occurs almost daily over a long period (months or years) and that has a high probability of ending; also known as progressive pain. |
| Chronic illness | Disruption in functional ability usually characterised by a gradual, insidious onset of illness with lifelong changes that are usually irreversible. |

| Word/Phrase | Meaning |
|---|---|
| Chronic pain | Discomfort that is persistent, nearly constant and long-lasting (six months or longer); or recurrent pain that produces significant negative changes in a person's life. |
| Client/patient advocate | Person who speaks up or acts on behalf of the client/patient. |
| Clinical decision making | An organised, sequential reasoning process that includes assessment, analysis, planning, implementation and evaluation. |
| Clinical governance | A framework whereby NHS organisations are accountable for continuously improving the quality of services and safeguarding high standards of care. |
| Clinical supervision | A formal process of professional support and learning that enables individual practitioners to develop knowledge and competence. |
| Closed question | A communication technique that consists of questions that can be answered briefly with yes–no or one-word responses. |
| Cognition | The mental process of faculty by which knowledge is acquired. |
| Cognitive skills | Intellectual skills that can include problem solving, critical thinking and decision making. |
| Communication | The complex, active process of relating to individuals and groups, which may include health team members, by written, verbal and nonverbal means. The goal is to understand and be understood and involves the transmission of ideas, messages, emotions and information by various means, between individuals and groups. Therapeutic communication promotes caring relationships between nurses and patients. |
| Competency | Ability, qualities and capacity to function in a particular way. |
| Compliance | The degree to which the patient follows the recommendations made by nurses and other health-care professionals (this is also sometimes called adherence). |
| Concept(s) | Vehicle of thought. Abstract ideas or mental images of reality. |
| Conceptual framework (model) | Structure that links global concepts together to form a unified whole. |

| Word/Phrase | Meaning |
|---|---|
| Conceptualisation | Process of developing and refining abstract ideas. |
| Consent | Voluntary act by which a person agrees to allow someone else to do something. |
| Construct | Abstraction or mental representation inferred from situations, events or behaviours. |
| Context | The circumstances in which a particular event or events occur. |
| Coping | A complex of behavioural, cognitive and physiological responses that aim to prevent or minimise unpleasant or harmful experiences that challenge one's personal resources. |
| Counselling | The process of helping an individual to recognise and cope with problems that may cause stress. An attempt to develop interpersonal growth with the aim of promoting personal growth. |
| Criteria | Standards that are used to evaluate whether the behaviour demonstrated indicates accomplishment of the goal. |
| Critical thinking | A purposeful, deliberate method of thinking used in search for meaning. |
| Cultural competence | Process through which the nurse provides care that is appropriate to the patient's cultural context. |
| Cultural diversity | Individual differences among people that result from racial, ethnic and cultural variables. |
| Culture | Dynamic and integrated structures of knowledge, beliefs, behaviours, ideas, attitudes, values, habits, customs, language, symbols, rituals, ceremonies and practices that are unique to a particular group of people; growing micro-organisms to identify a pathogen. |
| Data | Pieces of information about health, for example the patient's vital signs (also known as cues). |
| Decision making | The consideration and selection of interventions that facilitate the achievement of a desired outcome. |
| Delegation | Process of transferring a selected nursing task in a situation to an individual who is competent to perform that task. |

| **Word/Phrase** | **Meaning** |
|---|---|
| Democratic leadership style | Style of leadership (also called participative leadership) that is based on the belief that every group member should have input into the development of goals and problem solving. |
| Demography | The study of populations. Statistics related to distribution by age and place of residence, mortality and morbidity. |
| Deontology | Ethical theory that considers the intrinsic moral significance of an act itself as the criterion for determination of good. |
| Diagnosis | Classification of a disease, condition or human response that is determined by scientific evaluation of signs and symptoms, patient history and diagnostic studies. |
| Disability | A lack of ability to perform an activity a normal person can perform. |
| Disease | An alteration in body function resulting in a reduction of capabilities in the ability to perform the activities of living, or contributing to the shortening of the normal life span. |
| Distress | Experienced when stressors evoke an ineffective response. |
| Duty | Obligation created either by law or contract, or by any voluntary action. |
| Efficacy | The extent to which nursing and/or medical interventions achieve health improvements under ideal conditions. |
| Empathy | Understanding another person's perception of a situation. The ability to discriminate what the other person's world may be like. |
| Emotion | Any strong feeling for example, joy, hate, sorrow, love. |
| Empowerment | Process of enabling others to do things for themselves. |
| Epidemic | The situation in which the occurrence of a health problem has increased quickly. |
| Equity | Fair distribution of resources or benefits. |
| Ethical dilemma | Situation that occurs when there is a conflict between two or more ethical principles. |
| Ethical principles | Tenets that direct or govern actions. |

| Word/Phrase | Meaning |
|---|---|
| Ethical reasoning | Process of thinking through what one ought to do in an orderly, systematic manner in order to provide justification of actions based on principles. |
| Ethics | Branch of philosophy concerned with determining right from wrong on the basis of a body of knowledge. |
| Ethnicity | Culture group's perception of themselves (group identity) and others' perception of them. |
| Ethnocentrism | Assumption of cultural superiority and an inability to accept other cultures' ways of organising reality. |
| Ethnography | A type of qualitative research whose approach involves anthropology, in which a person's culture is examined by studying the meanings of the actions and events of the culture's members. |
| Ethnomethodology | A type of qualitative methodology in which interpretations of ethnography are made in a particular social world. |
| Eustress | Type of stress that results in positive outcomes. |
| Euthanasia | Intentional action or lack of action causing the merciful death of someone suffering from a terminal illness or incurable condition; derived from the Greed work *euthanatos*, which literally means 'good or gentle death'. |
| Evaluation | Fifth step in the nursing process; involves determining whether patient goals have been met, partially met or not met. |
| Express | To manifest or communicate, to make known. |
| Extended family | Family members from previous generations, such as grandparents, uncles and aunts. |
| Fear | Anxiety caused by consciously recognised and realistic danger. It can be a perceived threat, real or imagined. |
| Fidelity | Ethical concept that means faithfulness and keeping promises. |
| Gender (biology, sex) | Biological structure of a person's genitals that designates them as male, female or intersexed. |
| Gender identity | View of one's self as male or female in relationship to others. |

| **Word/Phrase** | **Meaning** |
|---|---|
| Gender role | Masculine or feminine role adopted by a person; often culturally and socially determined. |
| Goal | Aim, intent or end. |
| Grief | The emotional suffering often caused by bereavement. |
| Group communication | A complex level of communication that occurs when three or more people meet in face-to-face encounters or through another communication medium, such as a conference call. |
| Group dynamics | Study of the events that take place during small-group interaction and the development of sub-groups. |
| Hazard | Anything that can cause harm. |
| Healing | Process of recovery from illness, accident or disability. |
| Healing touch | Energy-based therapeutic modality that alters the energy fields through the use of touch, thereby affecting physical, mental, emotional and spiritual health. |
| Health | Process through which a person seeks to maintain an equilibrium that promotes stability and comfort; includes physiological, psychological, sociocultural, intellectual and spiritual wellbeing. |
| Health and Safety Executive | A statutory body that reports to the Health and Safety Commission, with day-to-day responsibility for making arrangements for the enforcement of safety legislation to ensure that risks to health and safety due to work activities are properly controlled. |
| Health Care Commission | Promotes improvement in quality of the NHS and independent health care. Assess performance of health-care organisations, awarding annual ratings. |
| Health promotion | Process undertaken to increase levels of wellness in individuals, families and communities. |
| Health Protection Agency | An independent body that protects the health and wellbeing of the population of the UK, particularly with regards to infectious diseases, chemical hazards, poisons and radiation. |

| Word/Phrase | Meaning |
|---|---|
| Health-seeking behaviours | Activities that are directed towards attaining and maintaining a state of wellbeing. |
| Heterosexism | Perspective or assumption that people are heterosexual. |
| Heterosexual | Describes sexual activity between a man and a woman. |
| Holism | The belief that individuals function as complete units that cannot be reduced to the sum of their parts. |
| Holistic nursing | Nursing practice that has as its aim the healing of the whole person. |
| Homosexuality | Sexual activity between two members of the same sex. |
| Hopelessness | A subjective state in which an individual sees limited or no alternatives or personal choices available and is unable to mobilise energy on his/her own behalf. |
| Hospice | Type of care for the terminally ill founded on the concept of allowing individuals to die with dignity and surrounded by those who love them. |
| Hypothesis | Statement of an asserted relationship between dependent variables. |
| Iatriogenic disease | A condition or disease that is caused by medical or surgical intervention, for example the side effects of some drugs. |
| Identity | What sets one person apart as a unique individual; it may include a person's name, gender, ethnic identity, family status, occupation and various roles. |
| Illness | Inability of an individual's adaptive responses to maintain physical and emotional balance that subsequently results in an impairment in functional abilities. |
| Illness stage | Time interval when patient is presenting or manifesting specific signs and symptoms of an infectious agent. |
| Implementation | Fourth step in the nursing process; involving the execution of the nursing plan of care formulated during the planning phase of the nursing process. |
| Implied contract | Contract that recognises a relationship between parties for services. |

| **Word/Phrase** | **Meaning** |
|---|---|
| Incidence | Refers to the prevalence of a disease in a population or community. The predictive value of the same test can be different when applied to people of differing ages. |
| Individualism | A predominant cultural type that focuses on an independent lifestyle that flourishes in urban settings. |
| Informed consent | The patient understands the reason for the proposed intervention, its benefits and risks, and agrees to the treatment by signing a consent form. |
| Interpersonal communication | Process that occurs between two people in face-to-face encounters over the telephone, or through other communication media. |
| Intersexed | Person born with both sets of or ambiguous genitalia. |
| Interview | Therapeutic interaction that has a specific purpose. |
| Intrapersonal communication | Messages one sends to oneself, including 'self-talk' or communication with oneself. |
| Intuition | Knowing something without evidence, the learning of things without the conscious use of reasoning. |
| Justice | Ethical principle based on the concept of fairness that is extended to each individual. |
| Knowledge and skills framework | Describes the knowledge and skills required by NHS staff to deliver quality services in their work. It also supports personal development and career progression. |
| Leadership | Interpersonal process that involves motivating and guiding others to achieve goals. |
| Leadership theory | Conceptual support framework for leadership. |
| Leading question | A question that influences the patient to give a specific answer. |
| Learning | Process of assimilating information with a resultant change in behaviour. |
| Learning plateau | A temporary slowdown in learning. |
| Lesbian | Female who has affectional and sexual tendencies towards females. |
| Liability | Obligation one has incurred or might incur through any act or failure to act. |

| **Word/Phrase** | **Meaning** |
|---|---|
| Life events | Major occurrences that occur in a person's life that require some element of psychological adjustment. |
| Lifestyle | The values and behaviours that have been taken on by a person in daily life. |
| Line graph | A graph that compares two variables through a line. |
| Living will | Document prepared by a competent adult that provides direction regarding medical care should the person become incapacitated or otherwise unable to make decisions personally. |
| Locus control | A person's perception of the sources of control over events and situations affecting the person's life. |
| Measurable | Able to be quantified. |
| Medication error | Any preventable harm that may cause or lead to inappropriate medication use or patient harm while the medication is in the control of the health-care professional, patient or customer. |
| Mentor | A knowledgeable person, someone with insight, someone to trust and confide in, helps a person to clarify thinking. |
| Minority group | Group of people who constitute less than a numerical majority of the population and who, because of their cultural or physical characteristics, are labelled and treated differently from others in society. |
| Morality | Behaviour in accordance with custom or tradition that usually reflects personal or religious beliefs. |
| Morbidity | The condition, illness, injury or disability in the population. |
| Mortality | Refers to death, often associated with a large population. |
| Motivation | The internal drive or externally arising stimulus to action or thought. |
| Mourning | Period of time during which grief is expressed and resolution and integration of the loss occur. |
| National Institute for Health and Clinical Excellence | An independent organisation responsible for providing national guidance on the promotion of good health and the prevention and treatment of ill health. |

| **Word/Phrase** | **Meaning** |
| --- | --- |
| National Service Frameworks | One of a range of measures to raise quality and decrease variations in service, containing long-term strategies. |
| Need | Anything that is absolutely essential for existence. |
| Negligence | Failure of an individual to provide the care in a situation that a reasonable person would ordinarily provide in a similar circumstance. |
| Negotiation | A method of conflict management whereby the parties decide what they must retain and what they are willing to give up in order to reach a compromise position. |
| Nonmaleficence | Ethical principle that means the duty to cause no harm to others. |
| Nursing | An art and a science that assists individuals to learn to care for themselves whenever possible; it also involves caring for others when they are unable to meet their own needs. |
| Nursing leadership | Interpersonal process in nursing that involves motivating and guiding others to achieve goals. |
| Nursing process | Systematic method of providing care to patients; consists of four or five steps:<br>1. Assessment.<br>2. Diagnosis.<br>3. Outcome identification and planning.<br>4. Implementation.<br>5. Evaluation. |
| Nursing research | Systematic application of formalised methods for generating valid and dependable information about the phenomena of concern to the discipline of nursing. |
| Objective data | Observable and measurable data that are obtained through both standard assessment techniques performed during the physical examination, and laboratory and diagnostic tests. |
| Observation | The skill of watching with thought, using all the senses. |
| Open-ended questions | Interview technique that encourages the patient to elaborate about a particular concern or problem. |

| Word/Phrase | Meaning |
|---|---|
| Open family system | A family system that interacts with the environment and in doing so maintains growth and balance. |
| Pain | State in which an individual experiences and reports the presence of physical discomfort; may range in intensity from uncomfortable sensation to severe discomfort. Pain is what the patient says it is, existing whenever he/she says it does. |
| Paradigm | A pattern of collective understandings and assumptions about reality and the world. |
| Paraverbal communication | The way in which a person speaks, including voice tone, pitch and inflection. |
| Paraverbal cue | Verbal message accompanied by cues, such as tone and pitch of voice, speed, inflection, volume and other nonlanguage vocalisations. |
| Participative leadership style | Leadership style where every person's viewpoints are considered as valuable and have equal voice in making decisions. |
| Passive euthanasia | Process of cooperating with the patient's dying process. |
| Paternalism | Practice by which health-care providers decide what is 'best' for patients and then attempt to coerce patients to act against their own choices. |
| Perception | Person's sense and understanding of the world. |
| Personality | The cognitive, affective or behavioural predispositions of people in different situations, over a period of time. |
| Phenomenon | Observable fact or event that can be perceived through the senses and is susceptible to description and explanation. |
| Philosophy | Statement of beliefs that is the foundation for one's thoughts and actions. |
| Pictograph | Pictorial (usually symbols) representation of statistical data on a graph. |
| Pie chart | A graph that is made up of a circle that is divided into sectors; each sector represents a proportion of the whole. |
| Planning | Third step of the nursing process; includes the formulation of guidelines that establish the proposed course of nursing action in the |

| Word/Phrase | Meaning |
|---|---|
| | resolution of nursing diagnoses and the development of the patient's plan of care. |
| Portfolio | A collection of personal evidence selected for a particular purpose. |
| Posology | The science of quantity, the science of dosage. |
| Power | Ability to do or act, resulting in the achievement of desired results. |
| Prejudice | A negative belief that is generalised about a group and this leads to prejudgement. |
| Prevalence | The total number of cases existing at a given period of time. |
| Profession | Group (vocational or occupational) that requires specialised education and intellectual knowledge. |
| Professional organisation | Members engaged in the same professional pursuit, often with similar goals and concerns. |
| Professional regulation | Process by which nursing ensures that its members act in the public interest by providing a unique service that society has entrusted to them. |
| Professional standards | Authoritative statements developed by the profession by which quality of practice, service and/or education can be judged. |
| Qualitative research | Systematic collection and analysis of subjective narrative materials, using procedures for which there tends to be a minimum of research-imposed control. |
| Quality assurance framework | Traditional approach to quality management in which monitoring and evaluation focus on individual performance, deviation from standards and problem solving. |
| Quality improvement | A process for change using a multidisciplinary approach to problem identification and resolution. |
| Quantitative research | Systematic collection of numerical information, often under conditions of considerable control. |
| Racism | Discrimination directed towards individuals who are misperceived to be inferior because of biological factors. |
| Radiation | Loss of heat in the form of infrared rays. |
| Rapport | Mutual trust and understanding in a relationship. |

| Word/Phrase | Meaning |
|---|---|
| Rationale | Explanation based on the theories and scientific principles of natural and behavioural sciences and the humanities. |
| Reflective diary | A personal aid to reflection, a document used to structure and document reflective accounts. |
| Relationship | An interaction of individuals over a period of time. |
| Religion | A system of beliefs and practices that usually involves a community of like-minded people. |
| Research | Systematic method of exploring, describing, explaining, relating or establishing the existence of a phenomenon, the factors that cause changes in the phenomenon, and how the phenomenon influences other phenomena. |
| Risk | The chance of something happening that will have an impact on individuals and/or organisations. Risk is measured in terms of likelihood and consequence. |
| Risk management | A method of reducing risks of adverse events occurring in organisations by systematically assessing, reviewing and seeking ways to prevent the occurrence of risks. |
| Role | Set of expected behaviours associated with a person's status or position. |
| Role ambiguity | Role expectations that are unclear. People do not know what or how to do what is expected of them. |
| Role conflict | When the expectations of one role compete with the expectations of other roles. |
| Scattergram | A graph that plots data, however the points are not joined into lines (sometimes called scatter plot or scatter diagram). |
| Scope of practice | Legal boundaries of practice for health-care providers as defined in statute. |
| Self-concept | The collection of ideas, feelings and beliefs one has about oneself. |
| Self-esteem | A sense of pride in oneself; self-love. |
| Sexual dysfunction | Physical inability to perform sexually, but can also be a psychological inability to perform sexually. |

| Word/Phrase | Meaning |
|---|---|
| Sexual health | Ability to form mutually consensual, developmental-appropriate sexual relationships that are safe and respectful of self and others; includes emotional, physical and psychological components. |
| Sexuality | Human characteristic that refers not just to gender but to all the aspects of being male or female, including feelings, attitudes, beliefs and behaviour. |
| Sexual orientation | Individual's preference for ways of expressing sexual feelings. |
| Sick role | A set of social expectations met by an ill person, such as being exempt from the usual social role responsibilities and being obligated to get well and to seek competent help. |
| Socialisation | The ways in which people learn about the ways of a group or society in an attempt to become a functioning partner. |
| Sociocultural | Involving social and cultural features or processes. |
| Spirituality | Relationship with one's self, a sense of connection with others, and a relationship with a higher power or divine source. |
| Standard of care | Delineates the extent and character of the nurse's duty to the patient; defined by organisational policy or professional standards of practice. |
| Stress | Body's reaction to any stimulus. |
| Stressors | Circumstances or events that a person perceives as threatening or harmful. |
| Subjective data | Data from the patient's point of view, including feelings, perceptions and concerns. |
| Teaching | Active process in which one individual shares information with another as a means to facilitate behavioural changes. |
| Teaching–learning process | Planned interaction promoting a behavioural change that is not a result of maturation or coincidence. |
| Teaching strategies | Techniques employed by the teacher to promote learning. |
| Team | Group of individuals who work together to achieve a common goal. |

| **Word/Phrase** | **Meaning** |
|---|---|
| Theory | Set of concepts and propositions that provide an orderly way to view phenomena. |
| Therapeutic | Describes actions that are beneficial to the patient. |
| Therapeutic communication | Use of communication for the purpose of creating a beneficial outcome for the patient. |
| Therapeutic range | Achievement of constant therapeutic blood level of a medication within a safe range. |
| Therapeutic touch | Holistic technique that consists of assessing alterations in a person's energy fields and using the hands to direct energy to achieve a balanced state. |
| Therapeutic use of self | Process in which nurses deliberately plan their actions and approach the relationship with a specific goal in mind before interacting with the patient. |
| Transcultural nursing | Formal area of study and practice focused on comparative analysis of different cultures and sub-cultures with respect to cultural care, health and illness beliefs, and values and practices, with the goal of providing health care within the context of the patient's culture. |
| Transgender | Person who dresses and engages in roles of the person of the opposite gender. |
| Utility | Ethical principle that states that an act must result in the greatest amount of good for the greatest number of people involved in a situation. |
| Values | Principles that influence the development of beliefs and attitudes. |
| Variable | A characteristic that is measurable on people, objects or events that may change in quantity or quality. |
| Veracity | Ethical principle that means that one should be truthful, neither lying nor deceiving others. |
| Verbal message | Message communicated through words or language, both spoken and written. |
| Whistle-blowing | Calling attention to the unethical, illegal or incompetent actions of others. |

# Abbreviations Commonly Used in Health Care

| | |
|---|---|
| AAA | Abdominal aortic aneurysm |
| ABC | Airway breathing and circulation |
| ABG | Arterial blood gases |
| ACE | Angiotensin converting enzyme |
| A&E | Accident and emergency |
| AF | Atrial fibrillation |
| AFB | Acid-fast bacilli |
| AFP | Alpha-fetoprotein |
| AHP | Allied health professional |
| AIDS | Acquired immune deficiency syndrome |
| ALOS | Average length of stay |
| AP(E)L | Assessment of prior (experience/experiential) learning |
| APL | Assessment of prior learning |
| ARD | Adult respiratory disease |
| ARF | Acute renal failure |
| ASW | Approved social worker |
| AXR | Abdominal Xray |
| BMI | Body Mass Index |
| BUPA | British United Provident Association |
| CABG | Coronary artery bypass graft |
| CAMHS | Child and adolescent health services |
| CAT | Computerised axial tomography |
| CATS | Credit Accumulation and Transfer Scheme |
| CCF | Congestive cardiac failure |
| CCU | Coronary care unit |
| CDSC | Communicable Disease Surveillance Centre |
| CHD | Coronary heart disease |
| CNM | Clinical nurse manager |
| CNO | Chief nursing officer |
| CNS | Central nervous system |
| COSHH | Control of Substances Hazardous to Health |
| CPAP | Continuous positive airway pressure |
| CPD | Continuing professional development |

| | |
|---|---|
| CPN | Community psychiatric nurse |
| CPR | Cardiac pulmonary resuscitation |
| CRF | Chronic renal failure |
| CSF | Cerebro spinal fluid |
| CSSD | Central sterile services/supplies department |
| CT | Computerised tomography |
| CVA | Cerebrovascular accident |
| CVP | Central venous pressure |
| CXR | Chest Xray |
| DIC | Disseminated intravascular coagulation |
| DNA | Did not attend |
| DSU | Day surgery unit |
| DVT | Deep vein thrombosis |
| EBM | Evidence-based medicine |
| EBP | Evidence-based practice |
| ECDL | European Computer Driving License |
| ECG | Electro cardiograph |
| ECT | Electro convulsive therapy |
| EEG | Electro encephalograph |
| EMG | Electro myograph |
| EMI | Elderly mentally infirm |
| ENP | Emergency nurse practitioner |
| ENT | Ear, nose and throat |
| ERCP | Endoscopic retrograde cholangiopancreatography |
| ET | Endotracheal tube |
| FE | Further education |
| FPA | Family Planning Association |
| GFR | Glomerular filtration rate |
| GI | Gastro intestinal |
| GMS | General medical services |
| GP | General practitioner |
| HAI | Hospital acquired infection |
| HCA | Health care assistant |
| HEI | Higher education institution |
| HFEA | Human Fertilisation and Embryology Authority |
| HIV | Human immuno deficiency virus |
| HPA | Health Protection Agency |
| HRT | Hormone replacement therapy |
| HSE | Health and Safety Executive |
| HV | Health visitor |
| IBD | Inflammatory bowel disease |
| ICN | Infection control nurse |
| ICP | Intracranial pressure |

| | |
|---|---|
| ICPU | Intensive care psychiatric unit |
| ICU | Intensive care unit |
| IHD | Ischaemic heart disease |
| IM | Intramuscular |
| IM&T | Information management and technology |
| IPCU | Intensive psychiatric care unit |
| IT | Information technology |
| ITU | Intensive therapy/treatment unit |
| IUD | Intrauterine device |
| IV | Intra venous |
| IVF | In vitro fertilisation |
| IVI | Intra venous infusion |
| JVP | Jugular venous pressure |
| LFT | Liver function test |
| LVF | Left ventricular failure |
| LP | Lumbar puncture |
| MC+S | Microscopy, culture and sensitivity |
| MI | Myocardial infarction |
| MIU | Minor injuries unit |
| MRI | Magnetic resonance imaging |
| MRSA | Methicillin resistant staphylococcus aureus |
| MS | Multiple sclerosis |
| NAO | National Audit Office |
| NATN | National Association of Theatre Nurses |
| NBM | Nil by mouth |
| NFA | No fixed address/abode |
| NGT | Naso gastric tube |
| NHS | National Health Service |
| NHS(S) | National Health Service in Scotland |
| NICE | National Institute for Health and Clinical Excellence |
| NMAS | Nursing and Midwifery Admissions Service |
| NMC | Nursing and Midwifery Council |
| NSAID | Nonsteroidal anti-inflammatory drug |
| NSFs | National Service Frameworks |
| NTD | Neural tube deficit |
| OA | Osteo arthritis |
| ODP | Operating department practitioner |
| OP | Outpatient |
| OPA | Outpatient attendances (appointments) |
| OPD | Outpatient department |
| OT | Occupational therapist/therapy |
| PAM | Professions allied to medicine |
| PAS | Patient administration system |

| | |
|---|---|
| PBL | Practice-based learning |
| PCA | Patient controlled analgesia |
| PCT | Primary Care Trust |
| PD | Peritoneal dialysis |
| PE | Pulmonary embolism |
| PEG | Percutaneous endoscopic gastrostomy |
| PEJ | Percutaneous endoscopic jejunostomy |
| PHCT | Primary health care team |
| PHLS | Public Health Laboratory Service |
| PID | Pelvic inflammatory disease |
| POM | Prescription only medicine |
| PR | Per rectum |
| PREP | Post registration education and practice |
| PSA | Prostate specific antigen |
| PV | Per vagina |
| PVD | Peripheral vascular disease |
| QA | Quality asurance |
| RA | Rheumatoid arthritis |
| RBC | Red blood cell |
| RCN | Royal College of Nursing |
| ROM | Range of movement |
| RTA | Road traffic accident |
| SAH | Sub arachnoid haemorrhage |
| SC | Subcutaneous |
| SCBU | Special care baby unit |
| SHAs | Strategic Health Authorities |
| SL | Sublingual |
| SLE | Systemic lupus erythematosus |
| SOB | Short of breath |
| SODoH | Scottish Department of Health |
| STI | Sexually transmitted infection |
| TB | Tuberculosis |
| TENS | Transcutaneous electrical nerve stimulation |
| TOD | Took own discharge |
| TOP | Termination of pregnancy |
| TPN | Total parenteral nutrition |
| TQM | Total quality management |
| TSO | The Stationery Office |
| TSSU | Theatre sterile supplies unit |
| TURP | Trans-urethral resections of the prostate |
| U+Es | Urea and electrolytes |
| UCAS | Universities and Colleges Admissions Service |
| URTI | Upper respiratory tract infection |
| US | Ultra sound |

| | |
|---|---|
| UTI | Urinary tract infection |
| VF | Ventricular fibrillation |
| VT | Ventricular tachycardia |
| WBC | White blood cell |
| WHO | World Health Organisation |

# Index